Hormones
and the Brain

Hormones and the Brain

Papers presented at a workshop organized and sponsored by the International Health Foundation on the theme 'The brain as an endocrine target organ in health and disease'. The workshop was held in Bordeaux, France, under the auspices of the Université de Bordeaux II and the Unité d'Enseignement et de Recherche de Médecine I

Edited by

David de Wied and Pieter A. van Keep

The editors were assisted by Pamela Freebody

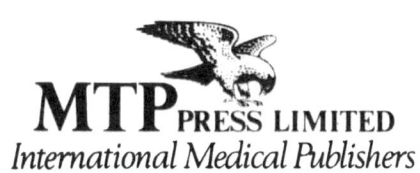

MTP PRESS LIMITED
International Medical Publishers

Published by
MTP Press Limited
Falcon House
Lancaster, England

Copyright © 1980 MTP Press Limited
Softcover reprint of the hardcover 1st edition 1980

First published 1980

British Library Cataloguing in Publication Data

Hormones and the brain.
  1. Brain chemistry – Congress
  2. Hormones – Congresses
  I. Wied, David de   II. Keep, Pieter A van
  612',822   QP376
  ISBN-13:978-94-009-8711-1   e-ISBN-13:978-94-009-8709-8
  DOI: 10.1007/978-94-009-8709-8

Filmset and printed by Mather Bros (Printers) Ltd, Preston, England

Contents

CONTENTS

Contributors

H. Akil
Assistant Professor,
Mental Health Research Institute,
University of Michigan,
205 Washtenaw Place,
Ann Arbor, MI 48109, USA

J. C. Ballenger
Biological Psychiatry Branch,
National Institute of Mental Health,
9000 Rockville Pike,
Building 10, Room 3S239,
Bethesda, MD 20205, USA

J. D. Barchas
Nancy Friend Pritzker Professor,
Department of Psychiatry and Behavioral
 Sciences,
Stanford University School of Medicine,
Stanford, CA 94305, USA

B. Bohus
Associate Professor,
Rudolf Magnus Instituut voor Farmacologie.
Medische Faculteit,
Rijksuniversiteit Utrecht,
Vondellaan 6,
3521 GD Utrecht. The Netherlands

F. Brambilla
Director of the Psychoendocrine Service,
Ospedale Psichiatrico Paolo Pini,
Via Ippocrate 45,
Milano Affori, Italy

E. van Cauter
Institut de Recherches Interdisciplinaires,
Université Libre de Bruxelles,
Rue Evers 2,
1000 Bruxelles, Belgium

P. Chiodera
Département de Clinique et de Pathologie
 Médicales,
C.H.U., local 4/12,
Université de Liège,
Sart Tilman par Liège 1, Belgium

G. Copinschi
Head of the Department of Endocrinology,
Clinique Médicale et Laboratoire de
 Médecine Expérimentale,
Université Libre de Bruxelles,
Rue Evers 2,
1000 Bruxelles, Belgium

J. C. Crabbe
Research Service,
Veterans Administration Medical Center,
Portland, OR 97201, USA

D. Désir
Laboratoire de Médecine Expérimentale,
Université Libre de Bruxelles,
Rue Evers 2,
1000 Bruxelles, Belgium

B. Dufy
Maître de Recherche CNRS,
Institut National de la Santé et de la
 Recherche Médicale,
Unité de Recherches de Neurobiologie des
 Comportements, U176,
Rue Camille Saint-Saëns,
33077 Bordeaux-Cedex, France

R. H. Ehrensing
Chairman, Department of Psychiatry,
Ochsner Clinic,
1514 Jefferson Highway,
New Orleans, LA 70121, USA

CONTRIBUTORS

G. Elliott
Visiting Fellow,
Institute of Medicine,
National Academy of Sciences,
2101 Constitution Avenue, NW,
Washington, DC 20418, USA

V. S. Fang
Endocrinology Laboratory,
Department of Medicine,
University of Chicago,
950 East 59th Street,
Chicago, IL 60637, USA

M. Fink
Professor of Psychiatry,
Department of Psychiatry and Behavioral
  Science,
Health Sciences Center—School of Medicine,
State University of New York at Stony Brook,
Stony Brook, NY 11794, USA

R. Fog
Sct Hans Hospital,
Department E,
DK-4000 Roskilde, Denmark

P. Franchimont
Laboratoire de Radioimmunologie,
Institut de Médecine,
Université de Liège,
Tour de Pathologie,
CHU, Bâtiment B23,
Sart Tilman par Liège 1, Belgium

A. Galatzer
Chief Clinical Psychologist,
Beilinson Medical Center,
Petah-Tiqva, Israel

P. W. Gold
Chief, Unit on Neuroendocrine Studies,
Clinical Psychobiology Branch,
National Institute of Mental Health,
9000 Rockville Pike,
Building 10, Room 4S239,
Bethesda, MD 20205, USA

J. Golstein
Institut de Recherches Interdisciplinaires,
Université Libre de Bruxelles,
Rue Evers 2,
1000 Bruxelles, Belgium

F. K. Goodwin
Chief, Clinical Psychobiology Branch,
National Institute of Mental Health,
9000 Rockville Pike,
Building 10, Room 4S239,
Bethesda, MD 20205, USA

H. M. Greven
Organon International BV,
Scientific Development Group,
Research Laboratory for Peptide Chemistry,
PO Box 20,
5340 BH Oss, The Netherlands

K. Hall
Department of Endocrinology,
Karolinska Hospital,
S-104 01 Stockholm 60, Sweden

R. B. Innis
Department of Pharmacology and
  Experimental Therapeutics,
The Johns Hopkins University School of
  Medicine,
725 North Wolfe Street,
Baltimore, MD 21205, USA

C. Jadot
Service de Psychiatrie,
Université Libre de Bruxelles.
Hôpital Erasme.
Route de Lennick 808.
1070 Bruxelles. Belgium

A. J. Kastin
Professor, Department of Medicine,
Tulane University School of Medicine,
New Orleans,
and
Chief, Endocrinology Section of the
  Medical Service,
Veterans Administration Medical Center.
1601 Perdido Street.
New Orleans. LA 70146. USA

H. Kopera
Clinical Pharmacology Unit.
Department of Experimental and Clinical
  Pharmacology,
Universität Graz,
Universitätsplatz 4,
A-8010 Graz, Austria

G. Langer
Psychiatrische Universitätsklinik,
Lazarettgasse 14,
A-1097 Wien, Austria

CONTRIBUTORS

Z. Laron
Professor of Pediatric Endocrinology,
Sackler School of Medicine,
Tel Aviv University, Israel
and
Director, Institute of Pediatric and
  Adolescent Endocrinology,
Beilinson Medical Center,
Petah-Tiqva, Israel

J. J. Legros
Secteur de Neuroendocrinologie,
Laboratoire de Radioimmunologie,
Département de Clinique et de Pathologie
  Médicales,
Université de Liège,
CHU, local 4/12,
Sart Tilman par Liège 1, Belgium

E. Martino
Thyroid Study Unit,
Department of Medicine,
University of Chicago,
950 East 59th Street,
Chicago, IL 60637, USA

B. S. McEwen
Associate Professor,
The Rockefeller University,
1230 York Avenue,
New York, NY 10021, USA

J. Mendlewicz
Professor of Psychiatry,
Université Libre de Bruxelles,
Hôpital Erasme,
Route de Lennick 808,
1070 Bruxelles, Belgium

D. J. Micco
Assistant Professor,
The Rockefeller University,
1230 York Avenue,
New York, NY 10021, USA

C. Mormont
Département de Psychiatrie,
Université de Liège,
Rue St Laurent,
Liège, Belgium

I. Munkvad
Sct Hans Hospital,
Department E,
DK-4000 Roskilde, Denmark

R. M. Post
Biological Psychiatry Branch,
National Institute of Mental Health,
9000 Rockville Pike,
Building 10, Room 3S239,
Bethesda, MD 20205, USA

H. M. van Praag
Professor of Psychiatry,
Psychiatric University Clinic,
Academic Hospital Utrecht,
Catharijnesingel 101,
3500 CG Utrecht, The Netherlands

A. Randrup
Sct Hans Hospital,
Department E,
DK-4000 Roskilde, Denmark

J. M. van Ree
Rudolf Magnus Instituut voor Farmacologie,
Medische Faculteit,
Rijksuniversiteit Utrecht,
Vondellaan 6,
3521 GD Utrecht, The Netherlands

S. Refetoff
Thyroid Study Unit,
Department of Medicine,
University of Chicago,
950 East 59th Street,
Chicago, IL 60637, USA

H. Rigter
Organon International BV,
Scientific Development Group,
CNS Pharmacology Department,
PO Box 20,
5340 BH Oss, The Netherlands

G. L. Robertson
Department of Medicine,
University of Chicago School of Medicine,
Billings Hospital,
Chicago, IL, USA

R. M. Rose
Professor *and* Chairman,
Department of Psychiatry and Behavioral
  Sciences,
University of Texas Medical Branch,
Galveston, TX 77550, USA

V. R. Sara
Karolinska Institute,
Department of Psychiatry,
St Göran's Hospital,
Box 12500,
S-112 81 Stockholm, Sweden

CONTRIBUTORS

J. Servais
Département de Psychiatrie,
Université de Liège,
Boulevard de la Constitution.
Liège, Belgium

S. H. Snyder
Distinguished Service Professor of
  Pharmacology and Psychiatry,
Department of Pharmacology and
  Experimental Therapeutics,
The Johns Hopkins University School of
  Medicine,
725 North Wolfe Street,
Baltimore, MD 21205, USA

D. F. Swaab
Director, Nederlands Instituut voor Hersen-
  onderzoek (Netherlands Institute for Brain
  Research),
Ijdijk 28,
1095 KJ Amsterdam, The Netherlands

L. Terenius
Department of Pharmacology.
Uppsala Universitets,
Biomedicinska Centrum,
Box 573,
S-751 23 Uppsala, Sweden

W. M. A. Verhoeven
Psychiatric University Clinic.
Academic Hospital Utrecht,
Catharijnesingel 101,
3500 CG Utrecht, The Netherlands

J. D. Vincent
Scientific Director.
INSERM, U.176.
Rue Camille Saint Saëns.
33077 Bordeaux-Cedex. France

S. J. Watson
Assistant Professor,
Mental Health Research Institute,
University of Michigan,
205 Washtenaw Place,
Ann Arbor, MI 48109, USA

H. Weingartner
Laboratory of Psychology and
  Psychopathology,
National Institute of Mental Health,
9000 Rockville Pike,
Building 31, Room 4C35B,
Bethesda, MD 20205, USA

L. Wetterberg
Karolinska Institute,
Department of Psychiatry,
St Göran's Hospital,
Box 12500,
S-112 81 Stockholm, Sweden

R. E. Whalen
Scientific Director,
Long Island Research Institute,
Health Sciences Center 10T,
State University of New York at Stony Brook,
Stony Brook, NY 11794, USA

D. de Wied
Professor of Pharmacology,
Rudolf Magnus Instituut voor Farmacologie.
Medische Faculteit,
Rijksuniversiteit Utrecht,
Vondellaan 6,
3521 GD Utrecht, The Netherlands

CONTRIBUTORS

The following people. although not contributing papers to the present volume, attended the workshop and took part in the discussions:

A. A. Haspels
Head, Universiteitskliniek voor Obstetrie en
  Gynaecologie,
Academisch Ziekenhuis Utrecht,
Catharijnesingel 101,
3500 CG Utrecht, The Netherlands

P. A. van Keep
Director General,
International Health Foundation,
Rue de Rhône 40,
1204 Genève, Switzerland

F. Lembeck
Head, Department of Experimental and
  Clinical Pharmacology,
Universität Graz,
Universitätsplatz 4,
A-8010 Graz, Austria

M. Le Moal
Laboratoire de Psychophysiologie,
Faculté des Sciences,
Université de Bordeaux,
Domaine Universitaire,
351 cour de la Libération,
33401 Bordeaux-Talence, France

N. Matussek
Psychiatrische Klinik und Poliklinik,
Nervenklinik der Universität München,
Nussbaumstrasse 7,
8000 München 2, West Germany

L. Rauramo
Professor, Department of Obstetrics and
  Gynecology,
The University Central Hospital of Turku,
20520 Turku 52, Finland

L. H. Rees
Professor, Department of Chemical
  Endocrinology,
St Bartholomew's Hospital,
West Smithfield,
London EC1A 7BE, United Kingdom

W. H. Utian
Associate Professor,
Department of Reproductive Biology,
MacDonald House,
University Hospitals of Cleveland,
University Circle,
Cleveland, OH 44106, USA

Preface

During the last decade it has become evident that the brain is an important target for hormones. Although it has been discovered only recently that the brain contains numerous peptide hormones, the role of pituitary and hypo-thalamic hormones in brain activity has been the subject of basic studies for quite some time. Peptide hormones are involved in mental performance, pain perception, food and water metabolism, sleep, sexual behaviour and nursing behaviour, and disturbances in the hormonal climate of the brain may be associated with psychopathology, cognitive disturbances and, possibly, addiction. The clinical influence of neurohypophysial hormones and their fragments is studied today on learning and memory, on inadequate behaviour and addiction, in Parkinson's disease, Lesch–Nyhan syndrome, depression and schizophrenia. Fragments of adrenocorticotrophin have been shown to affect motivation, concentration and attention, and neuropeptides derived from β-lipotrophin are probably involved in psychopathology. Thyrotrophin-releasing hormone has been implicated in depression, and lutein-releasing hormone in sexual disturbances.

In spite of the impressive experimental data, clinical results to date have been controversial and, to some extent, anecdotal. In some cases they have been exciting, and in others disappointing.

It was against this background that the International Health Foundation decided to organize and sponsor their workshop on 'The brain as an endocrine target organ in health and disease' at which the papers appearing in this book were presented. This workshop was held in Bordeaux under the auspices of the Université de Bordeaux II and the Unité d'Enseignement et de Recherche de Médecine I.

The first part of the programme centred upon basic information. It dealt with hormone receptors in the brain, hormone–receptor interactions, and peptidergic pathways. In the second part attention was given to animal experiments on the effects of peptide hormones on various brain functions. These laboratory studies have laid the foundation for clinical research, and this was the next area of discussion, the main topics being psychopathology as a consequence of hormone dysfunction and, conversely, hormonal changes in psychopathology.

When presenting their reports on their current work and opinions, the authors were asked to look also to the future, and hints as to the direction of future research are clearly discernible in the papers published here.

The Bordeaux meeting was an exciting and an encouraging one at which to be present. It is hoped that in the papers published in this book the reader will similarly find much of interest, and will come to share the optimism of those of us working in this field, that this work on hormones, and, in particular, neuropeptides, will soon lead to the development of new psychopharmacological agents, agents which are more specific and less toxic than those used at the present time.

DAVID DE WIED
Rudolf Magnus Instituut voor Farmacologie,
Medische Faculteit,
Rijksuniversiteit Utrecht,
The Netherlands

PIETER A. VAN KEEP
International Health Foundation,
Geneva,
Switzerland

Section 1
Receptors and peptidergic pathways in the brain

1.1
Hormone receptors in the brain

R. E. WHALEN

ABSTRACT

Reproductive behaviours are regulated by gonadal steroids. In most mammalian species sexual activities decline or disappear following gonadectomy and can be reinstated by administering exogenous steroids systemically or by direct application to the brain. It is generally believed that the gonadal hormones act in the brain as they do in peripheral target tissues by binding selectively to cytoplasmic protein 'receptors' with subsequent translocation of the hormone-receptor complex to the nuclear chromatin material. Chromatin binding is thought to induce genomic activation, RNA and protein synthesis and, thereby, the regulation of cell function.

Evidence is presented here that indicates that chromatin binding of oestradiol in hypothalamic cells is correlated with the potential to display sexual behaviour. For example, female rats which display receptive behaviour when given oestradiol bind more oestradiol in hypothalamic chromatin than do male rats which are relatively insensitive to oestradiol.

The role of cytoplasmic oestradiol receptors in hormone action is also discussed. The hypothesis is advanced that oestradiol regulates the molecular configuration of the receptor in a dose-dependent fashion and that receptor configuration determines chromatin acceptor site binding and functional activity. Kinetic data are presented which indicate that hypothalamic receptors change their characteristics as a function of hormone dose.

INTRODUCTION

The reproductive behaviours of the two sexes usually differ dramatically. In mammalian species the male typically displays mounting responses followed by penile insertion, thrusting and ejaculation. Sexually receptive females often show two types of behaviours which Beach (1976) has termed *proceptive* and *receptive*. Proceptive behaviours are those by which the female seeks the male and/or stimulates him to initiate mounting; receptive behaviours are those 'reflexive' responses and postural adjustments which permit the male to mount. In rats, the model species for the present discussion, proceptive behaviours include a distinctive hopping and darting response and a rapid head vibration usually described as ear-wiggling. Receptivity in the rat is characterized by the lordosis response, a deep concave arching of the back which exposes the perineum.

The reproductive behaviours of both male and female rats are under hormone control. When the gonads are removed, these behaviours cease; they can be reinstated by the administration of exogenous hormones. Moreover, these effects are mediated by the action of the hormones upon the central nervous system. The local application of testosterone, oestradiol or progesterone to limited regions of the brain can restore sexual activity in animals which have ceased copulating following gonadectomy. For this reason we, and several other laboratories, have been studying hormone receptor systems in the brain.

The first question is: what is a receptor? By current usage a steroid hormone receptor is a specific, high affinity, low capacity binding site located on or within a cell. Studies of the uterus, the cell system most used in the development of the receptor concept, indicate that gonadal hormone binding sites are of two types, cytoplasmic and nuclear. Cytoplasmic receptors are thought to be soluble proteins which bind their ligand specifically and then undergo a transformation or activation process. The activated hormone-receptor complex is translocated to the cell nucleus where it binds to the nuclear chromatin material at an 'acceptor' site. Nuclear binding is followed by genomic activation, RNA synthesis and ultimately protein synthesis and alterations in cell function. When known targets of a gonadal steroid such as the uterus are stimulated by their specific hormone, such as oestradiol, cytoplasmic receptors are depleted coincident with an increase in nuclear binding. The cytoplasmic receptors are subsequently replenished either by recycling of receptors or by de novo receptor synthesis, or possibly by both processes. The details of these processes are ably reviewed by several authors in recent reviews edited by O'Malley and Birnbaumer (1978).

BRAIN RECEPTORS

While the receptor concept and the currently accepted model of steroid hormone action were developed using peripheral hormone target tissues, the basic ideas were rapidly applied to the brain. For example, as early as 1965 Eisenfeld and Axelrod reported the selective concentration of oestradiol by the hypothalamus of rats and Kato and Villee (1967) noted a declining gradient of oestradiol concentration from anterior to posterior hypothalamus. The cerebral cortex did not concentrate oestradiol relative to blood. Subsequent biochemical analyses have demonstrated cytoplasmic binding (Eisenfeld, 1970), nuclear binding (Zigmond and McEwen, 1970) and chromatin binding (Whalen and Olsen, 1978) of oestradiol within the hypothalamus of rats. Similarly, androgen (Naess et al., 1975) and progesterone receptors (Lee et al., 1979) have been detected in the brain biochemically, and autoradiographic studies have confirmed that gonadal hormone binding within the brain is regionally located.

Clearly, gonadal steroids are bound selectively to cytoplasmic proteins and cell nuclei within the brain. The major question is whether the binding is to *receptors* in the traditional sense of that term, i.e. transducers of information. That question is difficult to answer for any hormone system and is particularly difficult to resolve for neuroendocrine systems. Consider, for example, the neural binding of oestradiol. It is widely distributed throughout basal diencephalon and amygdala (Pfaff and Keiner, 1973) and presumably subserves a variety of functions: the regulation, both positive and negative, of gonadotropin secretion, the regulation of sexual behaviour, and the regulation of body weight to name a few. Since these functions are not clearly segregated anatomically within the brain, it is not possible to assign the oestrogen binding observed in any particular site to a specific function. Moreover, for each given functional system, difficult problems are faced. Receptive behaviour, for example, cannot be detected until more than 15 hours have passed after the intravenous administration of oestradiol (Green et al., 1970). The initial dynamic events of cytoplasmic receptor binding, translocation and nuclear binding begin within minutes of hormone administration. The relationship between binding and behaviour indeed becomes difficult to assess.

SEX DIFFERENCES IN BINDING

One strategy we have adopted in an attempt to distinguish between oestradiol binding which is related to sexual behaviour from that serving other functions is to compare receptor binding in animals which do and do not readily display lordosis when given oestradiol. The sexes differ in this regard. Female rats gonadectomized in adulthood respond to oestradiol treatment, whereas males castrated at the same time rarely display a full lordosis response when oestrogen treated, even though oestrogen can inhibit gonadotrophin secretion and cause weight loss in both sexes.

There is some controversy about the hormonal basis for this sex difference which is relevant to our strategy. It has been suggested that males differ from females primarily in their response to progesterone rather than to oestrogen (Clemens *et al.*, 1969). Progesterone facilitates receptivity in oestrogen-primed females. We, however, found that males do not show lordosis even when administered large doses of oestradiol over long periods of time. Males castrated at birth respond to oestrogen treatment like females, while females given a large dose of testosterone at birth, like males, fail to respond to oestradiol (Whalen *et al.*, 1971). Thus, although the sexes may indeed differ in their responsiveness to progesterone, they differ also in their responsiveness to oestradiol. We have, therefore, attempted to relate this sex difference in behavioural response to oestradiol to possible sex differences in the nuclear binding of the hormone.

In our first study we found a sex difference in the kinetics of [³H]oestradiol binding by hypothalamic nuclei. The hypothalamic nuclei of both sexes accumulated oestradiol, but higher levels were attained in the female and the hormone was retained for a longer period of time (Whalen and Massicci, 1975). In more recent work, we detected sex differences in hypothalamic chromatin binding as well (Whalen and Olsen, 1978).

Most recently, Olsen and I (1980) have compared the chromatin binding in rats which do or do not display receptivity in adulthood as a result of hormonal manipulation at birth. These rats were gonadectomized and/or hormone treated at birth and examined for both behavioural potential and chromatin binding in adulthood. To ensure that we were observing maximum behavioural potential the animals were tested for sexual receptivity following combined oestrogen and progesterone treatment. These high levels of hormone were allowed to dissipate before the animals were given tracer levels of radio-labelled oestradiol.

Again we found that neonatal hormonal stimulation does not eliminate hypothalamic chromatin binding. However, the magnitude of binding did vary with behavioural potential, being highest in females, slightly lower in neonatally castrated males and in females made anovulatory by a low dose of testosterone given at birth, still lower in females given a large dose of testosterone at birth, and lowest in males castrated 10 days after birth. Thus, there is a relationship between behaviour and chromatin binding suggesting that such binding may be critical for the behavioural action of the hormone.

There are several questions which findings such as these raise. For example:

(1) Are there quantitative relationships between binding and behavioural action?

(2) How is the information represented by chromatin binding translated into behaviour? That is, what are the critical molecular events (RNA synthesis? protein synthesis? protein phosphorylation?) which lead to changes in behaviour?

(3) What is the nature of the sex difference in chromatin binding? Does it

reflect quantitative or qualitative differences in cytoplasmic receptors? Does it reflect differences in the non-histone proteins which are associated with the nuclear DNA?

I expect that these questions will be answered within the next decade. The most difficult question, both experimentally and conceptually, is: What is the precise nature of the translation between hormone binding and the neurophysiology of hormone action? I would not dare to speculate as to when this problem will be solved. The problems associated with detecting relevant electrical events which follow the initial biochemical events by over 18 hours are indeed enormous.

CYTOPLASMIC RECEPTORS

It is generally thought that neural cell membranes pose no barrier to the lipid soluble gonadal steroids and that the interaction of the steroid with a specific cytoplasmic protein is the first critical step in hormone action. Although specific cytoplasmic binding in the hypothalamus was first noted in 1970, little is yet known about the oestradiol receptors. In sucrose gradients they appear to behave like uterine receptors sedimenting as 8S aggregates under low salt conditions and 4S monomers (?) in high salt. They are thermolabile and react to sulfhydryl reagents. Their binding of [^{3}H]oestradiol is blocked by oestradiol, oestrone, diethylstilbestiol and by various anti-oestrogens, but minimally, if at all, by testosterone or progesterone.

Lately we have been using anti-oestrogens as probes to detect some of the characteristics of these cytoplasmic binding elements in hypothalamic tissue. The functional activity of three anti-oestrogens, CI-628, nafoxidine and tamoxifen* was studied first (Etgen, 1979). All three inhibited oestrogen-induced sexual receptivity in a dose- and time-dependent manner.

The nature of the anti-oestrogen inhibitory process is usually thought to be one of simple competition by the anti-oestrogen molecule for the oestradiol binding site on the receptor protein. Hahnel et al. (1973), however, found evidence that in uterine cells the inhibition might be allosteric rather than competitive. In such an interaction the anti-oestrogen would prevent oestradiol binding by altering the conformation of the receptor protein rather than by occupying the oestradiol binding site.

It is possible to distinguish competitive from other forms of inhibition using an enzyme kinetic model. In this model competitive inhibition is reflected by

---

*CI-628 (Parke-Davis Co.): 1-(2-(p-(α(p-methoxy)-β-nitrostyryl)phenoxy)ethyl)pyrrolidine.
Nafoxidine (Upjohn Co.): 1,2-(p-(3,4-dihydro-6-methoxy-2-phenyl-1-naphthyl)phenoxy)pyrrolidine hydrochloride.
Tamoxifen (Stuart Pharmaceuticals): trans-(1-(p-α-dimethylaminoethoxyphenyl)-1,2-diphenylbut-1-ene)citrate.

an increase in the apparent value of K_d, a parallel reduction in B_{max}/K_d with no change in B_{max}. We therefore determined the kinetic parameters of [³H]oestradiol binding using unlabelled oestradiol, presumably a competitive inhibitor, nafoxidine and tamoxifen as antagonists. All three inhibited [³H]oestradiol binding in a dose-dependent manner. However, neither oestradiol nor the anti-oestrogens behaved as simple competitive inhibitors. The kinetic patterns of the anti-oestrogens are not easily classified, but must represent some complex form of mixed inhibition.

The pattern of changes found using oestradiol as an antagonist, although unexpected, is simpler. As the dose of unlabelled oestradiol was increased from 10^{-12} mol to 10^{-10} mol, K_d rose, B_{max}/K_d declined and B_{max} remained stable as expected for a competitive inhibitor. At doses higher than 10^{-10} mol oestradiol behaved as a non-competitive inhibitor of [³H]E2 binding.

These findings suggest that oestradiol is capable of binding to more than a single site on the receptor. At low doses the receptor remains stable and unlabelled oestradiol acts as a competitive inhibitor. At high doses, possibly after all 'preferred' high affinity/low capacity sites are occupied, oestradiol also binds to secondary sites with such binding altering the conformation of the receptor. It would be interesting to know whether such a process occurs *in vivo* and whether changes in the conformation in the receptor alter its physiological activity. One could speculate that, at low doses, when the oestradiol-receptor complex is in 'configuration A', chromatin binding is to a set of 'configuration A' acceptor sites, while at higher doses 'configuration B' is induced, thereby activating a different set of acceptor sites on the genome. For example, low doses of oestradiol will induce sexual receptivity only when combined with progesterone. At high oestradiol doses progesterone is not necessary. Possibly the progesterone-independent induction of receptivity reflects the action of the 'B configuration' of the hormone-receptor complex.

One can extend this speculation to make predictions about the kinetic behaviour of oestradiol in other neurobehavioural test systems. For example, the sexually receptive behaviour of the golden hamster is as dependent upon oestradiol as is that of the rat. Relative to the rat, however, the hamster is considered to be insensitive to the behavioural effects of oestradiol. Moreover, relative to the rat, the brain accumulates relatively little oestradiol when examined either biochemically (Feder et al., 1974) or autoradiographically (Krieger et al., 1976). One might expect the opposite to be the case: if the hamster has limited binding sites for oestradiol it should be possible to saturate these sites with a low dose of oestradiol and readily induce behaviour. This does not occur. High doses may be required because, in this species, the behaviour is controlled by the activation of the 'B configuration' acceptor sites on the neural cell chromatin. A kinetic analysis of hamster receptors, using the 'double-dose-response' competition procedure we have used with rat receptors, might reveal that the point of change from simple competitive inhibition to non-competitive inhibition occurs at a higher antagonist dose than we found in the rat. This would indicate that in the hamster a higher dose of oestradiol is needed to induce 'configuration B'. Such a finding would be consistent with the hypothesis that steroid regulated receptor configuration determines the function of the hormone-receptor complex.

Speculations about the relationship between receptor configuration and function are no more than speculations at this time. However, the model is not inherently weak. We already accept the notion that to become functional, that is, to bind to nuclear chromatin, the 4S receptor must be 'activated' to a 5S form and there is some evidence that the nuclear-bound receptor has two forms, a salt-extractable form and a salt-resistant form (Ruh and Baudendistel, 1977). We may well find that receptor configuration determines behavioural function as well.

Acknowledgement

This research was supported by grant HD-00893 from the National Institute of Child Health and Human Development.

References

Beach, F. A. (1976). Sexual attractivity, proceptivity and receptivity in female mammals. *Horm. Behav.*, **7**, 105

Clemens, L. G., Hiroi, M. and Gorski, R. A. (1969). Induction and facilitation of female mating behavior in rats treated neonatally with low doses of testosterone propionate. *Endocrinology*, **84**, 1430

Eisenfeld, A. J. (1970). [³H]Estradiol: *in vitro* binding to macromolecules from the rat hypothalamus, anterior pituitary and uterus. *Endocrinology*, **86**, 1313

Eisenfeld, A. J. and Axelrod, J. (1965). Selectivity of estrogen distribution in tissues. *J. Pharmacol. Exp. Ther.*, **150**, 469

Etgen, A. M. (1979). Anti-estrogens: effects of tamoxifen, nafoxidine and CI-628 on sexual behavior, cytoplasmic receptors and nuclear binding of estrogen. *Horm. Behav.*, **13**, 97

Feder, H. H., Siegel, H. and Wade, G. N. (1974). Uptake of 6,7[³H]estradiol-17β in ovariectomized rats, guinea pigs and hamsters: correlations with species differences in behavioral responsiveness to estradiol. *Brain Res.*, **71**, 93

Green, R., Luttge, W. G. and Whalen, R. E. (1970). Induction of receptivity in ovariectomized female rats by a single intravenous injection of estradiol-17β. *Physiol. Behav.*, **5**, 137

Hahnel, R., Twaddle, E. and Ratajczak, T. (1973). The influence of synthetic anti-estrogen on the binding of tritiated estradiol-17β by cytosols of human uterus and human breast carcinoma. *J. Steroid Biochem.*, **4**, 687

Kato, J. and Villee, C. A. (1967). Preferential uptake of estradiol by the anterior hypothalamus of the rat. *Endocrinology*, **80**, 567

Krieger, M. S., Morrell, J. I. and Pfaff, D. W. (1976). Autoradiographic localization of estradiol-concentrating cells in the female hamster brain. *Neuroendocrinol.*, **22**, 193

Lee, H., Davies, I. J. and Ryan, K. J. (1979). Progesterone receptor in the hypothalamic cytosol of female rats. *Endocrinology*, **104**, 791

Naess, O., Attramadal, A. and Aakvaag, A. (1975). Androgen binding proteins in the anterior pituitary, hypothalamus, preoptic area and brain cortex of the rat. *Endocrinology*, **96**, 1

Olsen, K. L. and Whalen, R. E. (1980). Sexual differentiation of the brain: effects on mating behavior and [³H]-estradiol binding by hypothalamic chromatin in rats. *Biol. Reprod.*, **22**, 1086

O'Malley, B. W. and Birnbaumer, L. (1978). *Receptors and Hormone Action II*. (New York: Academic Press)

Pfaff, D. W. and Keiner, M. (1973). Atlas of estradiol concentrating cells in the central nervous system of the female rat. *J. Comp. Neurol.*, **151**, 121

Ruh, T. H. and Baudendistel, L. J. (1977). Different nuclear binding sites for anti-estrogen and estrogen receptor complexes. *Endocrinology*, **100**, 420

Whalen, R. E., Luttge, W. G. and Gorzalka, B. B. (1971). Neonatal androgenization and the development of estrogen responsivity in male and female rats. *Horm. Behav.*, **2**, 83

Whalen, R. E. and Massicci, J. (1975). Subcellular analysis of the accumulation of estrogen by the brain of male and female rats. *Brain Res.*, **89**, 255

Whalen, R. E. and Olsen, K. L. (1978). Chromatin binding of estradiol in the hypothalamus and cortex of male and female rats. *Brain Res.*, **152**, 121

Zigmond, R. E. and McEwen, B. S. (1970). Selective retention of oestradiol in specific brain regions of the ovariectomized rat. *J. Neurochem.*, **17**, 889

Address for correspondence

Dr R. E. Whalen, Scientific Director, Long Island Research Institute, State University of New York at Stony Brook, Health Sciences Center 10T, Stony Brook, NY 11794, USA

1.2
Toward an understanding of the multiplicity of glucocorticoid actions on brain function and behaviour

B. S. McEWEN and D. J. MICCO

ABSTRACT

Glucocorticoids have a multiplicity of effects on brain biochemistry, neural excitability and behaviour. This article attempts to relate certain of the biochemical and neurological effects of glucocorticoids to some of the behavioural actions related to extinction of learned behaviour and retrograde amnesia, as well as to behaviours related to function of the hippocampus. It is suggested from this analysis that there is no unitary biochemical mechanism for these various glucocorticoid effects.

We summarize in greater detail progress in one of the more fruitful lines of biochemical investigation of glucocorticoid action in the nervous system, namely, the study of the neural receptor sites for this class of hormones. These studies have focused on the limbic system, and especially the hippocampus, as the major neuronal glucocorticoid target sites of the central nervous system. We attempt to relate findings regarding receptors to recent studies which implicate a role for adrenocortical secretion in behaviours which are dependent upon hippocampal function.

INTRODUCTION

It has long been recognized that mood and affective state are influenced by adrenocortical secretions (Brown, 1975; Sachar, 1975; Quarton et al., 1955). This and the fact that the most important factors causing glucocorticoid output are psychological (Selye, 1973; Bush, 1962; Mason, 1958) has made the nervous system an obvious site in which to investigate glucocorticoid action. Yet, as will be indicated in this article, the effects of glucocorticoids on behaviour and neural activity are subtle and subject to many problems of interpretation, and the sites and types of hormone effects are rather more numerous than might have been anticipated.

One of the more fruitful lines of investigation has been the study of the neural receptor sites for glucocorticoids, and these studies have focused on the limbic system, and especially the hippocampus, as the major neuronal glucocorticoid target sites of the central nervous system. This article summarizes the major features of the CNS glucocorticoid receptor system as well as the biochemical actions of glucocorticoids in neural tissue and then summarizes some of the major glucocorticoid effects on neuroendocrine function and behaviour. An attempt is made to apply the biochemical information regarding sites and mechanisms of glucocorticoid action to some of the various neuroendocrine and behavioural effects.

GLUCOCORTICOID RECEPTORS

Based upon the model emerging in the mid-1960s concerning steroid action via intracellular receptors (Jensen and Jacobson, 1962), we began to look at the uptake and binding of [^{3}H]corticosterone (CORT) in brains of adrenal-ectomized (ADX) rats. Much to our surprise, the highest uptake sites were in hippocampus, septum and amygdala and not in hypothalamus or pituitary (McEwen et al., 1972b and 1968) (Figure 1). These observations were subsequently extended to the primate brain (Gerlach et al., 1976), thus suggesting that there may be a common plan of the limbic glucocorticoid target sites across mammalian species. Studies of the receptors themselves revealed that there are both soluble (Grosser et al., 1973 and 1971; McEwen et al., 1972a) and cell nuclear (McEwen et al., 1972b and 1970; McEwen and Plapinger, 1970) binding sites which can be distinguished from the serum binding protein, transcortin. Of particular importance to subsequent behavioural studies is the observation that the potent adrenocorticotrophin hormone-(ACTH)-suppressing synthetic glucocorticoid, dexamethasone (DEX), has a different pattern of uptake from that of CORT, with higher concentration in pituitary and hypothalamus than in hippocampus (McEwen et al., 1976; de Kloet et al., 1975) (Figure 1). This finding may explain the more potent ACTH-suppressing effects of DEX compared to CORT at the level of the pituitary (McEwen, 1977), while the lesser uptake of DEX compared to

CORT in hippocampus predicts that this steroid might be less potent in eliciting behavioural effects mediated by the hippocampus. Indeed, recent work in our laboratory (Micco and McEwen, unpublished observations) and in Utrecht (Bohus and deKloet, personal communication) supports this prediction.

Autoradiographic studies with [³H]CORT reveal that neurons are labelled (McEwen et al., 1975; Warembourg, 1975a; Gerlach and McEwen, 1972). Neuronal labelling is especially heavy in the pyramidal neurons of CA1 and CA2 of Ammon's horn and in the granule neurons of the dentate gyrus. Precommisural hippocampus and induseum griseum are also labelled. Neurons of the anterior, dorsal and lateral (but not medial) septum are labelled by [³H]CORT, as are neurons in the basomedial and cortical regions of the amygdala. Scattered neurons of the neocortex are also labelled and there appears to be a somewhat higher density of labelled neurons in piriform and entorhinal cortex than in neocortex.

Autoradiographic studies with [³H]DEX confirm the lesser labelling of hippocampus and septum observed after *in vivo* administration of this steroid compared to results with [³H]CORT. and support the heavier labelling reported for [³H]DEX in anterior pituitary (Rhees et al.. 1975; Warembourg, 1975b).

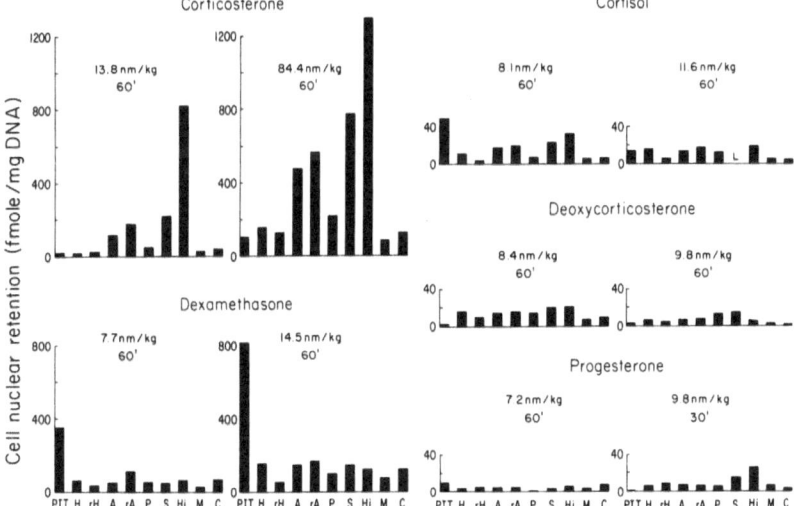

Figure 1   Cell nuclear retention of [³H]steroids by various brain regions after their infusion via tail vein in ADX–OVX rats. Time between injection and sacrifice and dose of [³H]steroid (nmol/kg body weight) is indicated for each experiment. Tissue from three/four identically treated rats, obtained by a dissection procedure described elsewhere (McEwen et al., 1976), was pooled for cell nuclear isolation. Abbreviations: L, lost sample; PIT, pituitary; H, basomedial hypothalamus; rH, rest of hypothalamus; A, corticomedial amygdala; rA, rest of amygdala; P, medial preoptic area; S, septum; Hi, hippocampus; M, midbrain; C, cerebral cortex
(McEwen et al.. 1976; reproduced with permission)

In none of the autoradiographic studies has there been clearcut evidence for glial cell labelling. Yet biochemical evidence on glial tumour cells in culture (de Vellis *et al.*, 1974 and 1971) and on the optic nerve after removal of the eyes (Meyer *et al.*, 1978) points very clearly to the existence of glucocorticoid receptors in oligodendroglial cells which contain a glucocorticoid inducible enzyme, glycerol phosphate dehydrogenase (Leveille *et al.*, 1977).

The explanation for the lack of clearcut evidence for glucocorticoid uptake in glial cells may be that the concentration of receptors is too low to concentrate [^{3}H]glucocorticoid to the degree required for successful auto-radiographic visualization. The logic of this explanation does, however, leave open the possibility that many neurons not presently recognized to have glucocorticoid receptors (based on autoradiography) may in fact contain some receptors. It would therefore be premature to exclude any brain region as a glucocorticoid target on the basis of negative evidence from auto-radiography. Indeed, brain regions such as hypothalamus and cerebellum, which are not heavily labelled by [^{3}H]CORT *in vivo*, do contain glucocorticoid receptors when assayed *in vitro* by biochemical techniques (Olpe and McEwen, 1976; McEwen and Wallach, 1973). The relative contributions of oligo-dendroglial and neuronal cell types to this pool of receptors remain to be determined. Initially promising attempts to subdivide glucocorticoid recep-tors into two subtypes (McEwen, 1979; MacLusky *et al.*, 1977) have not so far been applied to resolution of this question.

GLUCOCORTICOID EFFECTS ON BRAIN CHEMISTRY

Hippocampus

Attempts to find neurochemical correlates of glucocorticoid action in hippo-campus have produced more negative than positive evidence. Of 17 enzymes of carbohydrate and neurotransmitter metabolism assayed in hippocampus from ADX and CORT-treated ADX rats, the only one found to change was the oligodendroglial enzyme, glycerol phosphate dehydrogenase (Meyer *et al.*, 1979a). On the other hand, the high affinity uptake of [^{3}H]gamma-amino-butyric acid (GABA) by synaptosomes from hippocampus increases over several days following bilateral ADX and returns to normal after 4–7 days of CORT replacement therapy (Table 1). This effect is not observed in synapt-osomes from cortex and cerebellum. The hippocampus also is the site of a rapid (≈ 1 h) stimulation of amino acid incorporation into at least one protein band on polyacrylamide gels (Table 1).

Other neural sites

Glucocorticoid effects on other neural structures besides hippocampus (Table 1) include very rapid effects such as the inhibition of corticotrophin releasing

Table 1 Glucocorticoid effects in adult brain‡

Effect	Tissue	Steroid dose		Time	Reference
1. Inhibits CRF release	Hypothalamic fragments, in vitro*	B	$10-10-10^{-7}$ mol	10'	Jones et al., 1977
2. Increases brain tyrosine level	Whole brain, in vivo*	F	20 mg/kg	15'	Diez et al., 1977
3. Increases P/O ratio	Whole brain, in vivo*	F	3–5 mg/kg	60'	Roosevelt et al., 1973
4. Decreases single unit activity	Hippocampus, in vivo*	B	5 mg/kg	30–60'	Pfaff et al. 1971
5. Increases labelling of proteins	Hippocampus, in vitro, slices*	B	10^{-10} mol	60'	Etgen et al., 1979
6. Decreases high affinity GABA transport	Hippocampus, in vivo*	B	solid implant	4–7 days	Miller et al., 1978
7. Increases GPDH activity	Whole brain, nerve, in vivo*	B / B	endogenous / solid implant	7–14 days	Meyer et al., 1979b and 1978; de Vellis and Inglish, 1968
8. Increases DBH activity	Hypothalamus, in vivo*	B	100 mg/kg	4 hr	Shen and Ganong, 1976
9. Increases NA. DA turnover	Whole brain, in vivo†	B	5–15 mg/kg	60'	Iuvone et al., 1977
10. Decreases NA turnover	Whole brain, in vivo*	B / F	endogenous / 25 mg/kg	2 days	Javoy et al., 1968; Fuxe et al., 1970
11. Increases TH activity	Superior cervical ganglion, in vivo*		Dex 3 mg/kg	48 hr	Hanbauer et al., 1975a
12. Potentiates reserpine induction of TH	Superior cervical ganglion, in vivo*	B	endogenous		Hanbauer et al., 1975b
13. Potentiates NGF effect on TH activity	Superior cervical ganglion, culture*	B	5×10^{-6} mol	24–48 hr	Otten and Thoenen, 1977 and 1976
14. Increases TH activity	Median eminence, in vivo*		Dex 0.3 mg/kg/day	7 days	Kizer et al. 1974
15. Induces PNMT	Hypothalamus, medulla, in vivo*		Dex 1 mg kg day	7–13 days	Moore and Phillipson. 1975;
16. Increases NA, DA levels and size of large and small vesicles	Adrenal medulla, in vivo*		Dex 3–5 mg/kg/day	3 days	Pohorecky and Wurtman, 1971
	Carotid body. in vivo*		Dex 1 mg/kg/day	10 days	Hellstrom and Koslow. 1976

* Rat
† Mouse
‡ Abbreviations: CRF. corticotropin releasing factor; P/O ratio. ratio of ATP generated to oxygen used; GABA. gamma aminobutyric acid; NA. noradrenaline; DA. dopamine; DBH. dopamine hydroxylase; GPDH. glycrol phosphate dehydrogenase; TH. tyrosine hydroxylase; NGF. nerve growth factor; PNMT. phenylethanolamine N methyl transferase; B. corticosterone; F. cortisol; Dex. dexamethasone. (McEwen et al. 1979; reproduced with permission)

factor (CRF) release from hypothalamic fragments *in vitro* (Jones *et al.*, 1977) and the acute elevation of brain tyrosine (Diez *et al.*, 1977) and tryptophan (Sze, 1976; Hillier *et al.*, 1975) levels. There are also effects of glucocorticoid treatment over hours and days (Table 1) and many of these effects are concerned with catecholamine metabolism. The metabolism of serotonin (5HT) is also regulated by glucocorticoids (Table 2). This control is exerted

Table 2　Effects of glucocorticoid on the serotonergic system

Effect	Reference
Elevates 5HT synthesis	Millard *et al.*, 1972; Azmitia *et al.*, 1970a; Gal *et al.*, 1968
Acute elevation of 5HT levels	Telegdy and Vermes, 1975
Depression of 5HT levels	Curzon and Green, 1971
Enhances uptake of Tp by synaptosomes; by brain	Neckers and Sze, 1975; Hillier *et al.*, 1975
Enhances uptake and release of 5HT by synaptosomes	Vermes *et al.*, 1976
Inhibition of MAO activity	Petrovic and Janic, 1974; Parvez and Parvez, 1973
Required for elevation of tryptophan hydroxylase activity by	Sze, 1976
Ethanol intoxication	Kuriyama *et al.*, 1971
Morphine	Azmitia *et al.*, 1970b
Reserpine	Sze *et al.*, 1976
Foot shock, cold, ether stress	Azmitia and McEwen, 1974
Required for appearance of:	
Ethanol withdrawal seizures	Sze *et al.*, 1974
Acoustic reduction of susceptibility to audiogenic seizures	Sze and Maxon, 1975

Abbreviations: 5HT, serotonin; Tp, tryptophan; MAO, monoamine oxidase
(McEwen *et al.*, 1979; reproduced with permission)

rapidly, e.g. the elevation of 5HT synthesis seen in intact (but not in ADX) rats exposed to cold stress parallels very closely the elevation and fall of plasma CORT (Table 3). The changes in 5HT formation as a result of CORT are widespread, occurring in forebrain as well as in midbrain (Azmitia and McEwen, 1976).

Table 3　Changes in midbrain tryptophan hydroxylase activity and plasma cortico-sterone level following exposure to cold (4°C)

Treatment group	Tryptophan hydroxylase activity (pmoles/g/h)	Plasma corticosterone (µg/100 ml)
Control	1306 ± 69 (20)	12.0 ± 2.2 (13)
5 h cold	2154 ± 216 (7)*	27.5 ± 5.1 (4)*
8 h cold	1838 ± 101 (7)*	21.3 ± 4.2 (3)*
48 h cold	1319 ± 58 (9)	12.1 ± 3.4 (5)

*$p < 0.001$. Student's t-test compared to control group
Numbers in parentheses refer to number of animals in group
(Azmitia and McEwen, 1974; reproduced with permission)

Comments on mechanism

Rapid glucocorticoid effects such as those on 5HT formation (Tables 2 and 3), CRF release, tyrosine levels, and noradrenaline (NA) and dopamine (DA) turnover (Table 1) may be mediated by receptors other than those described in the previous section (McEwen, 1980; McEwen *et al.*, 1978). The site of action of the hormone may well be the synaptic membrane. On the other hand, changes in enzyme activities brought about by prolonged glucocorticoid treatment (e.g. glycerol phosphate dehydrogenase, tyrosine hydroxylase and phenylethanolamine *N*-methyl transferase) (Table 1) may involve the genomic action of the intracellular receptors described above. By reason of their occurrence in the receptor-rich hippocampus, the glucocorticoid effect on GABA transport (Miller *et al.*, 1978) and the change in labelling of a specific protein band (Etgen *et al.*, 1979) may also be receptor-mediated genomic events. We shall return below to a consideration of mechanism in the discussion of the neuroendocrine and behavioural consequences of glucocorticoid action.

GLUCOCORTICOIDS AND ACTH SECRETION

Glucocorticoids exert a negative feedback control over ACTH secretion and appear to do so both rapidly and after a delay of some hours (McEwen, 1979 and 1977). Although the pituitary is a primary site for this control, especially for the action of DEX (McEwen, 1979), neural structures also show some feedback sensitivity when glucocorticoids are implanted directly into the brain (McEwen, 1977; Bohus, 1975). Neural effects of DEX on CRF release and/or synthesis are likely, since alterations in feedback effectiveness of DEX are reported to result from lesions of afferents to hypothalamus in rodents (Feldman and Conforti, 1976) and from therapy with a serotonin-blocking drug, cyproheptadine, in Cushing's disease patients (Krieger *et al.*, 1975).

The hypothalamus displays both rapid and delayed glucocorticoid feedback when CRF release is studied *in vitro* (Jones *et al.*, 1977). The pituitary responds to suppressive actions of glucocorticoids by two mechanisms: one which is blocked by the RNA synthesis inhibitor, Actinomycin D, and one which is not (McEwen, 1979). Thus the pituitary may also show rapid as well as delayed feedback control.

GLUCOCORTICOIDS AND BEHAVIOURS WHICH ARE LINKED TO HIPPOCAMPAL FUNCTION

Behaviours affected by hippocampal lesions

One approach to the elucidation of the role of glucocorticoid receptors in the limbic system, and especially in hippocampus, is to study adrenal steroid effects on behaviours which depend in some way on hippocampal function. Such behaviours have been recognized in recent years because hippocampal lesions alter them (Kimble, 1968; Douglas, 1967). Using this approach, Micco et al. (1979) established a CORT effect on the extinction, but not on the acquisition, of an appetitively motivated runway task. The CORT effect is to retard extinction and is opposite to the effect of ADX, which facilitates extinction, but is in the same direction as the effect of hippocampal lesions. This suggests that CORT may be suppressing the function of the hippo-campus, which in this particular task may be to attenuate performance in the absence of reward. (See Kimble, 1968, for a discussion of the hippocampus and internal inhibition.) The postulated inhibition by CORT of hippocampal function is apparently selective, since in a subsequent study two other tasks also affected by hippocampal lesions (spontaneous alternation and explora-tory behaviour) showed no response to adrenal steroid manipulations (Micco and McEwen, unpublished observations). As a possible explanation of the differences in hormonal sensitivity of these behaviours, it was suggested that the hormone-sensitive component of the appetitive runway task may be either the level of activation (i.e. motivation and stress) and/or the kind or degree of learning (and therefore extinction) which may be involved. While these notions are not at this point supported by data concerning the differential nature of hippocampal activity in these tasks, it is possible to put this hormone-sensitive extinction behaviour into a broader biological context. As a result of withholding reward, adrenocortical secretion is increased (Coover et al., 1971). According to the results of Micco et al. (1979), this 'stress response' would have the effect of subsequently suppressing the action of the hippocampus to extinguish the behaviour. The resulting 'persistence' of the animal in the absence of reward might be useful in the event that food reward should reappear, thus maintaining foraging in the feral animal.

Support for involvement of the hippocampus as a primary site of CORT action on this behaviour derives not only from the sensitivity of the behaviour to hippocampal lesions but also from the finding that DEX doses known to suppress stress-induced ACTH release are unable to mimic the actions of CORT (Micco and McEwen, unpublished observation*). This is consistent with the uptake pattern of DEX and CORT discussed above and with hippocampal involvement, and it also implies that ACTH suppression is not necessarily a major factor in glucocorticoid action on this behaviour. How-ever, more extensive dose response information is needed for both DEX and CORT before this aspect of the study is complete.

Even then the most definitive evidence for hippocampal involvement in the glucocorticoid effect on extinction may have to come from brain hormone implantation studies. Previous work by Bohus (1975 and 1973) utilized the

---

*See Micco and McEwen, 1980

implant technique to establish a glucocorticoid effect on extinction of avoidance behaviour and to argue for a dissociation of this action from the suppression of ACTH release.

An important question which remains to be investigated concerns cellular mechanism of CORT effects. In both the Micco *et al.* (1979) and Bohus and deKloet (personal communication) studies, the time interval between CORT injection and behavioural testing is in the order of an hour. It is too rapid an effect to be explained by the change in [^{3}H]GABA uptake found after chronic CORT administration (Miller *et al.*, 1978). This is also rather rapid for a genomically mediated effect of a steroid but not too rapid still to be explained by this mechanism. For example, genomic action of glucocorticoids on thymus lymphocytes have been detected within 15–20 min (Makman *et al.*, 1971; Mosher *et al.*, 1971) and a recent study of protein synthesis in hippocampal slices indicates that CORT may increase labelling of one or two protein bands within 1 hour (Etgen *et al.*, 1979). On the other hand, another mechanism which may operate in hippocampus as well as in other brain regions is related to the apparently direct action of CORT to increase serotonin (5HT) formation from tryptophan (Tables 2 and 3). This mechanism has been invoked by Kovács *et al.* (1976) to explain glucocorticoid facilitation of the extinction of avoidance behaviour. These authors reported that inhibition of 5HT formation by *para*-chlorophenylalanine attenuates the facilitatory effects of glucocorticoids on extinction. It is questionable, however, whether extinction of aversively and appetitively motivated tasks are mediated by the same neurological and cellular mechanisms (see below).

Another index of glucocorticoid action in hippocampus is the inhibition of unit electrical activity by CORT (Pfaff *et al.*, 1971) which occurs in pyramidal neurons of dorsal hippocampus within the time frame of the behavioural effects described above. All of the mechanistic considerations described in the preceding paragraph apply to this effect. The inhibition of hippocampal unit activity by CORT fits well with the notion that this hormone inhibits a normally inhibitory output of the hippocampus. However, the selectivity of the behavioural effect noted by Micco *et al.* (1979) suggests that the electrical effect reported by Pfaff *et al.* (1971) may not be widespread throughout Ammon's horn.

Another interaction between hippocampal lesions and the adrenal glands was described by Iuvone and van Hartesveldt (1977). These investigators showed that while ADX had no effect in non-brain damaged rats on the diurnal pattern or the absolute level of locomotor activity in an open field, it did reduce both morning and evening locomotor activity of hippocampal lesioned animals. CORT replacement in these ADX lesioned rats was apparently able to reverse the deficit (Iuvone and van Hartesvelt, 1977). This experiment suggests that glucocorticoid sensitive elements other than those in hippocampus play a role in modulating some behaviours. One interpretation of the lesion effect is that hippocampus normally has a counterbalancing effect on the CNS response to glucocorticoids. Other interactions between brain lesions and ADX will be considered again below.

Behaviours affected by 6-hydroxydopamine lesions

Injection of 6-hydroxydopamine (6-OHDA) into the dorsal adrenergic bundle produces profound depletion of NA in cortex, hippocampus and amygdala and lesser depletions in hypothalamus, septum and thalamus (Mason and Iversen, 1979). DA and 5HT levels are not affected, nor are the activities of two key neurotransmitter enzymes, choline acetyltransferase and glutamic acid decarboxylase, changed. The behavioural deficit resulting from these lesions consists of a general resistance to extinction of various learned behaviours with very little effect on appetitive task acquisition (Mason and Iversen, 1979). The syndrome has been called the dorsal bundle extinction effect (DBEE), and there are many similarities between this syndrome and the effects of hippocampal lesions (Mason and Iversen, 1977), and indeed the hippocampus is one of the major neural sites where neurochemical depletion is observed following dorsal bundle 6-OHDA lesions (Mason and Iversen, 1979).

Of particular interest for the present discussion is the observation that ADX blocks the DBEE (Mason and Iversen, 1979). These authors have proposed that the DBEE may be due to a failure of the lesioned animal to suppress attention to irrelevant cues in the environment: i.e. the dorsal bundle normally inhibits attention to these irrelevant cues. As a result, the lesioned animal associates many cues, both relevant and irrelevant, with the reward or punishment and, like a partially reinforced animal, is slower to extinguish. From the fact that ADX blocks the DBEE, one is tempted to infer that adrenal secretions act in opposition to the normal function of the dorsal bundle: i.e. adrenal secretion normally makes the animal more susceptible to irrelevant cues in opposition to the dorsal bundle input. This view predicts that glucocorticoids would retard extinction, and this is in fact what Micco et al. (1979) found for the extinction of the hippocampally dependent runway task (see above). Such an explanation is somewhat different from the notion of internal inhibition, which Micco et al. (1979) have suggested as an explanation for the CORT effect in their experiments. It should be noted that Mason and Iversen (1979) have considered and rejected the internal inhibition hypothesis as an adequate explanation for the DBEE.

Another effect of ADX on rats with 6-OHDA lesions of the dorsal bundle is to impair acquisition and retention of both passive and active avoidance behaviour, a deficit which is reversed by glucocorticoid replacement therapy (Mason et al., 1979; Ogren and Fuxe, 1977; Roberts and Fibiger, 1977). In contrast to the DBEE, this interaction of adrenal steroids and 6-OHDA lesions may be related more to fear motivation than to a more general deficit related to attention (Mason et al., 1979).

Glucocorticoids, hippocampus and avoidance behaviour

Glucocorticoids facilitate the extinction of aversively-motivated behaviours (Coover *et al.*, 1978; Bohus, 1975 and 1973; de Wied, 1966). Progesterone, as well as a number of other pregnene-steroids which are not glucocorticoids, produces similar effects (van Wimersma Greidanus, 1977; van Wimersma Greidanus *et al.*, 1973).

Local application of glucocorticoids in hippocampus as well as other cerebral sites mimics the actions of systemically administered hormones on extinction of certain avoidance tasks (Bohus, 1975 and 1973). However, these implantation studies give no indication that the hippocampus is an exclusive or even primary site of action.

The facilitation of avoidance extinction by glucocorticoids is opposite to the inhibition of extinction reported by Micco *et al.* (1979) for an appetitive task which appears to involve the hippocampus. There is no single theoretical framework for explaining these opposite effects, and, in fact, extinction of appetitively and aversively motivated behaviours may involve different neural mechanisms. It has been evident for some time that elevated ACTH levels are perhaps the most important hormonal signals relevant to fear-motivated behaviour, and suppression of ACTH secretion by glucocorticoids may thus play a role in determining the level of fear (van Wimersma Greidanus *et al.*, 1977; DiGiusto *et al.*, 1971; Weiss *et al.*, 1969; de Wied, 1966). Since the hippocampus does not appear to play a major role in the feedback control of ACTH secretion (McEwen, 1977; Bohus, 1975), it appears that glucocorticoid actions on other brain structures and possibly on the pituitary may be of greater importance for the avoidance extinction effects. In addition, the enhancement of forebrain (not merely hippocampal) 5HT formation (Tables 2 and 3) has been invoked as a possible mechanism for avoidance extinction effects (Kovács *et al.*, 1976).

The study of retrograde amnesia in rats for conditioned avoidance behaviours provides another example of glucocorticoid effects in which some involvement of hippocampus has been suggested. In particular, the amnesia produced by pre-training administration of protein synthesis inhibitors or post-training electroconvulsive shock is attenuated by glucocorticoid administration (Flood *et al.*, 1978; Nakajima, 1978 and 1975; Barondes and Cohen, 1968). Local injection of glucocorticoids into hippocampus was equally effective to systemic hormone treatment; septal and hypothalamic injection sites were ineffective (Cottrell and Nakajima, 1977). Two explanatory hypotheses were considered and rejected: (1) state dependence of the effects of inhibitor and glucocorticoid (Nakajima, 1978; Cottrell and Nakajima, 1977); (2) deficiency of adrenal steroid formation produced by protein synthesis inhibition (Dunn and Leibmann, 1977; Squire *et al.*, 1976). Perhaps the most viable explanation for these glucocorticoid actions involves the notion of 'arousal' (Flood *et al.*, 1978; Barondes and Cohen, 1968). As noted by these authors, the anti-amnesic effect of glucocorticoid administration is a property shared by a number of CNS excitants, including amphetamine, strychnine and caffeine. This explanation brings to mind two possibly interrelated neuro-chemical correlates of this glucocorticoid effect, namely, the elevation of brain tyrosine and tryptophan levels and NA, DA and 5HT formation produced by acute glucocorticoid administration (Tables 1–3). With respect to the involvement of the hippocampus in the anti-amnesic effect as noted by Cottrell and Nakajima (1977), it should be pointed out that the hippocampus is one of the most sensitive cerebral sites for evoking retrograde amnesia by electrical stimulation (Vardaris and Schwartz, 1971) or by the protein synthesis inhibitors puromycin and cycloheximide (Eichenbaum *et al.*, 1976; Flexner *et al.*, 1967).

CONCLUSIONS

The discovery of putative receptor sites for glucocorticoids in neurons of the hippocampal formation has provided a neuroanatomical focal point for studies of glucocorticoid action on behaviour, effects which are so numerous and subtle as to be elusive. We are by no means in a position to offer a unifying explanation as to how glucocorticoids affect behaviour and how the hippocampus functions as a glucocorticoid target, but there appear to be a number of promising leads, notably the study of behaviours in which hippocampal function is implicated and the dorsal bundle extinction effect (DBEE). We are also, perhaps, in a position to distinguish between glucocorticoid effects which may be mediated by intracellular receptors interacting with the genome (Figure 1) and hormone effects which involve a direct action upon neuronal membranes (e.g. the effects on 5HT, NA and DA formation referenced in Tables 1–3). We have suggested that these latter effects may be able to explain glucocorticoid actions on the extinction of conditioned avoidance behaviour and on retrograde amnesia. It remains to be demonstrated that the intra-cellular receptor sites of hippocampus actually mediate some of the other behavioural effects of glucocorticoids described in this article. A promising step in that direction is provided by the striking difference in hippocampal uptake of corticosterone and dexamethasone and by the initial studies which support a preferential behavioural effect of corticosterone *vs* dexamethasone. Eventually, it will be desirable to demonstrate the involvement of protein synthesis in these actions by means of protein synthesis inhibitors. In this connection, the rapid increase in labelling of a protein component produced by corticosterone in hippocampal slices (Etgen *et al.*, 1979) is very encouraging.

Acknowledgements

The research in our laboratory was supported by NIH Grant NS07080 and NSF Grant GB43558. D.J.M. has received salary support from the Alfred P. Sloan Foundation. We wish to thank Mrs Oksana Wengerchuk for editorial assistance.

References

Azmitia, E. C., Jr, Algeri, S. and Costa, E. (1970a). Turnover rate of *in vivo* conversion of tryptophan into serotonin in brain areas of adrenalectomized rats. *Science*, **169**, 201

Azmitia, E. C., Hess, P. and Reis, D. (1970b). Tryptophan hydroxylase changes in midbrain of the rat after chronic morphine administration. *Life Sci.*, **9**, 633

Azmitia, E. C., Jr and McEwen, B. S. (1976). Early response of rat brain tryptophan hydroxylase activity to cycloheximide, puromycin and corticosterone. *J. Neurochem.*, **27**, 773

Azmitia, E. C. and McEwen, B. S. (1974). Adrenalcortical influence on rat brain tryptophan hydroxylase. *Brain Res.*, **78**, 291

Barondes, S. H. and Cohen, H. D. (1968). Arousal and the conversion of 'short-term' to 'long-term' memory. *Proc. Natl. Acad. Sci. USA*, **61**, 923

Bohus, B. (1975). The hippocampus and the pituitary–adrenal system hormones. In R. L. Isaacson and K. H. Pribram (eds.), *The Hippocampus*. Vol. 1: Structure and development, pp. 323–353. (New York: Plenum Press)

Bohus, B. (1973). Pituitary adrenal influences on avoidance and approach behavior of the rat. *Prog. Brain Res.*, **39**, 407

Brown, G. M. (1975). Psychiatric and neurologic aspects of endocrine disease. *Hospital Practice*, **10**, 71

Bush, I. E. (1962). Chemical and biological factors in the activity of adrenocortical steroids. *Pharmacol. Rev.*, **14**, 317

Coover, G. D., Goldman, L. and Levine, S. (1971). Plasma corticosterone increases produced by extinction of operant behavior in rats. *Physiol. Behav.*, **6**, 261

Coover, G. D., Sutton, B. R., Welle, S. L. and Hart, R. P. (1978). Corticosterone responses, hurdle-jump acquisition, and the effects of dexamethasone using classical conditioning of fear. *Horm. Behav.*, **11**, 294

Cottrell, G. A. and Nakajima, S. (1977). Effect of corticosteroids in the hippocampus on passive avoidance behavior in the rat. *Pharm. Biochem. Behav.*, **7**, 277

Curzon, G. and Green, A. R. (1971). Regional and subcellular changes in the concentration of 5-hydroxytryptamine and 5-hydroxyindoleacetic acid in the rat brain caused by hydrocortisone, DL-α-methyl-tryptophan, L-kynurenine and immobilization. *J. Pharm. Pharmacol.*, **43**, 39

Diez, J. A., Sze, P. Y. and Ginsburg, B. E. (1977). Effects of hydrocortisone and electric footshock on mouse brain tyrosine hydroxylase activity and tyrosine levels. *Neurochem. Res.*, **2**, 161

DiGiusto, E. L., Cairncross, K. and King, M. G. (1971). Hormonal influences on fear-motivated responses. *Psychol. Bull.*, **75**, 432

Douglas, R. J. (1967). The hippocampus and behavior. *Psychol. Bull.*, **67**, 416

Dunn, A. J. and Leibmann, S. (1977). The amnestic effect of protein synthesis inhibitors is not due to the inhibition of adrenal corticosteroidogenesis. *Behav. Biol.*, **19**, 411

Eichenbaum, H., Quenon, B. A., Heacock, A. and Agranoff, B. S. (1976). Differential behavioral and biochemical effects of regional injection of cycloheximide into mouse brain. *Brain Res.*, **101**, 171

Etgen, A. E., Lee, K. S. and Lynch, G. (1979). Glucocorticoid modulation of specific protein metabolism in hippocampal slices maintained *in vitro*. *Brain Res.*, **165**, 37

Feldman, S. and Conforti, N. (1976). Inhibition and facilitation of feedback influences of dexamethasone on adrenocortical responses to ether stress in rats with hypothalamic deafferentations and brain lesions. *Acta Endocrinol. (Kbh.)*, **82**, 785

Flexner, L. B., Flexner, J. B. and Roberts, R. B. (1967). Memory in mice analyzed with antibiotics. *Science*, **155**, 1377

Flood, J. F., Vidal, D., Bennett, D. L., Orme, A. E., Vlasquez, S. and Jarvik, M. E. (1978). Memory facilitating and anti-amnesic effects of corticosteroids. *Pharm. Biochem. Behav.*, **8**, 81

Fuxe, K., Corrodi, H., Hökfeldt, T. and Jonsson, G. (1970). Central monoamine neurons and pituitary adrenal activity. *Prog. Brain Res.*, **32**, 42

Gal, E. M., Heater, R. D. and Millard, S. A. (1968). Studies on the metabolism of 5-hydroxy-tryptamine (serotonin). VI. Hydroxylation and amines in cold-stressed reserpinized rats. *Proc. Soc. Exp. Biol. Med.*, **128**, 412

Gerlach, J. L. and McEwen, B. S. (1972). Rat brain binds adrenal steroid hormone: radio-autography of hippocampus with corticosterone. *Science*, **175**, 1133

Gerlach, J. L., McEwen, B. S., Pfaff, D. W., Moskovitz, S., Ferin, M., Carmel, P. W. and Zimmerman, E. A. (1976). Cells in regions of rhesus monkey brain and pituitary retain radioactive estradiol, corticosterone and cortisol differentially. *Brain Res.*, **103**, 603

Grosser, B. I., Stevens, W., Bruenger, F. W. and Reed, D. J. (1971). Corticosterone binding in rat brain cytosol. *J. Neurochem.*, **18**, 1825

Grosser, B. I., Stevens, W. and Reed, D. J. (1973). Properties of corticosterone-binding macro-molecules from rat brain cytosol. *Brain Res.*, **57**, 387

Hanbauer, I., Guidotti, A. and Costa, E. (1975a). Dexamethasone induces tyrosine hydroxylase in sympathetic ganglia but not in adrenal medulla. *Brain Res.*, **85**, 527

Hanbauer, I., Lovenberg, W., Guidotti, A. and Costa, E. (1975b). Role of cholinergic and glucocorticosteroid receptors in the tyrosine hydroxylase induction elicited by reserpine in superior cervical ganglion. *Brain Res.*, **96**, 197

Hellstrom, S. and Koslow, S. H. (1976). Effects of glucocorticoid treatment on catecholamine content and ultrastructure of adult rat carotid body. *Brain Res.*, **102**, 245

Hillier, J., Hillier, J. G. and Redfern, P. H. (1975). Liver tryptophan pyrrolase activity and metabolism of brain 5HT in rat. *Nature*, **253**, 566

Iuvone, P. M. and van Hartesvelt, C. (1977). Diurnal locomotor activity in rats: effects of hippocampal ablation and adrenalectomy. *Behav. Biol.*, **19**, 228

Iuvone, P. M., Morasco, J. and Dunn, A. J. (1977). Effect of corticosterone on the synthesis of [³H]catecholamines in the brains of CD-1 mice. *Brain Res.*, **120**, 571

Javoy, F., Glowinski, J. and Kordon, C. (1968). Effects of adrenalectomy on the turnover of norepinephrine in the rat brain. *Europ. J. Pharmacol.*, **4**, 103

Jensen, E. V. and Jacobson, H. E. (1962). Basic guides to the mechanism of estrogen action. *Rec. Prog. Horm. Res.*, **18**, 387

Jones, M. T., Hillhouse, E. W. and Burden, J. L. (1977). Dynamics and mechanics of cortico-steroid feedback at the hypothalamus and anterior pituitary gland. *J. Endocrinol.*, **73**, 405

Kimble, D. P. (1968). Hippocampus and internal inhibition. *Psychol. Bull.*, **70**, 285

Kizer, J. S., Palkovits, M., Zivin, J., Brownstein, M., Saavedra, J. M. and Kopin, I. J. (1974). The effect of endocrinological manipulations on tyrosine hydroxylase and dopamine β hydroxylase activity in individual hypothalamic nuclei of the adult male rat. *Endocrinology*, **95**, 799

deKloet, R., Wallach, G. and McEwen, B. S. (1975). Differences in corticosterone and dexa-methasone binding to rat brain and pituitary. *Endocrinology*, **96**, 598

Kovács, G. L., Telegdy, G. and Lissak, K. (1976). 5-Hydroxytryptamine and the mediation of pituitary adrenocortical hormones in the extinction of active avoidance behavior. *Psychoneuroendocrinology*, **1**, 219

Krieger, D. T., Amorosa, L. and Linick, F. (1975). Cyproheptadine-induced remission of Cushing's disease. *New Engl. J. Med.*, **293**, 893

Kuriyama, K., Rauscher, G. E. and Sze, P. Y. (1971). Effect of acute and chronic administration of ethanol on the 5-hydroxytryptamine turnover and tryptophan hydroxylase activity of the mouse brain. *Brain Res.*, **26**, 450

Leveille, P. J., deVellis, J. and Maxwell, D. W. (1977). Immunocytochemical localization of glycerol-3-phosphate dehydrogenase in rat brain: are oligodendrocytes target cells for glucocorticoids? *Abstract No. 1066.* Presented at the *Annual Meeting of Society for Neuroscience,* 1977, Anaheim

MacLusky. N. J.. Turner. B. B. and McEwen. B. S. (1977). Corticosteroid binding in rat brain and pituitary cytosols: resolution of multiple binding components by polyacrylamide gel based isoelectric focusing. *Brain Res.*, **130**, 564

Makman, M. H., Dvorkin, D. and White, A. (1971). Evidence for induction by cortisol *in vitro* of a protein inhibitor of transport and phosphorylation processes in rat thymocytes. *Proc. Natl. Acad. Sci., USA*, **68**, 1269

Mason, J. W. (1958). The central nervous system regulation of ACTH secretion. In H. H. Jasper *et al.* (eds.), *Reticular Formation of the Brain*, pp. 645–662. (Boston: Little. Brown)

Mason, S. T. and Iversen, S. D. (1979). Theories of the dorsal bundle extinction effect. *Brain Res. Rev.*, **1**, 107

Mason, S. T. and Iversen, S. D. (1977). Effects of selective forebrain noradrenaline loss on behavioral inhibition in the rat. *J. Comp. Physiol. Psychol.*, **91**, 165

Mason, S. T., Roberts, D. C. S. and Fibiger, H. C. (1979). Interaction of brain noradrenaline and the pituitary–adrenal axis in learning and extinction. *Pharm. Biochem. Behav.*, **10**, 11

McEwen, B. S. (1980). Steroid hormones and the brain: cellular mechanisms underlying neural and behavioral plasticity. *Psychoneuroendocrinology* (In press)

McEwen, B. S. (1979). Influences of adrenocortical hormones on pituitary and brain function. In G. Rousseau and J. Baxter (eds.), *Mechanisms of Glucocorticoid Action*, pp. 467–492. (Berlin: Springer)

McEwen, B. S. (1977). Adrenal steroid feedback on neuroendocrine tissues. *Ann. N.Y. Acad. Sci.*, **297**, 568

McEwen, B. S., Davis, P. G., Parsons, B. and Pfaff, D. W. (1979). The brain as a target for steroid hormone action. In M. Cowan (ed.), *Annual Review of Neuroscience*, vol. 2, p. 65

McEwen, B. S., Gerlach, J. L. and Micco, D. J., Jr (1975). Putative glucocorticoid receptors in hippocampus and other regions of the rat brain. In R. Isaacson and K. Pribram (eds.), *The Hippocampus: A Comprehensive Treatise*, pp. 285–322. (New York: Plenum Press)

McEwen, B. S., deKloet, R. and Wallach, G. (1976). Interactions *in vivo* and *in vitro* of corticoids and progesterone with cell nuclei and soluble macromolecules from rat brain regions and pituitary. *Brain Res.*, **105**, 129

McEwen, B. S., Krey, L. C. and Luine, V. N. (1978). Steroid hormone action in the neuroendocrine system: when is the genome involved? In S. Reichlin, R. J. Baldessarini and J. B. Martin (eds.), *The Hypothalamus*, pp. 255–268. (New York: Raven Press)

McEwen, B. S., Magnus, C. and Wallach, G. (1972a). Soluble corticosterone-binding macromolecules extracted from rat brain. *Endocrinology*, **90**, 217

McEwen, B. S. and Plapinger, L. (1970). Association of corticosterone-1,2-H^3 with macromolecules extracted from brain cell nuclei. *Nature*, **226**, 263

McEwen, B. S. and Wallach, G. (1973). Corticosterone binding to hippocampus: nuclear and cytosol binding *in vitro*. *Brain Res.*, **57**, 373

McEwen, B. S., Weiss, J. M. and Schwartz, L. S. (1970). Retention of corticosterone by cell nuclei from brain regions of adrenalectomized rats. *Brain Res.*, **17**, 471

McEwen, B. S., Weiss, J. M. and Schwartz, L. (1968). Selective retention of corticosterone by limbic structures in rat brain. *Nature*, **220**, 911

McEwen, B. S., Zigmond, R. E. and Gerlach, J. L. (1972b). Sites of steroid binding and action in the brain. In G. H. Bourne (ed.), *Structure and Function of Nervous Tissue*, vol. v, pp. 205–291. (New York: Academic Press)

Meyer, J. S., Leveille, P. J., McEwen, B. S. and deVellis, J. (1978). Corticoids and glial cells: glycerolphosphate dehydrogenase induction and cytosol binding in normal and degenerated rat optic nerve. Presented at the *Annual Meeting of the Endocrine Society*, 1978, Miami

Meyer, J. S., Luine, V. N., Khylchevskaya, R. I. and McEwen, B. S. (1979a). Glucocorticoids and hippocampal enzyme activity. *Brain Res.*, **166**, 172

Meyer, J. S., Micco, D. J., Stephenson, B. S., Krey, L. C. and McEwen, B. S. (1979b). Subcutaneous implantation method for chronic glucocorticoid replacement therapy. *Physiol. Behav.*, **22**, 867

Micco, D. J. and McEwen, B. S. (1980). Glucocorticoids, the hippocampus, and behaviour: interactive relation between task activation and steroid hormone binding specificity. *J. Comp. Physiol. Psychol.*, **94**, 624

Micco, D. J., McEwen, B. S. and Shein, W. (1979). Modulation of behavioral inhibition in appetitive extinction following manipulation of adrenal steroids in rats: implications for involvement of the hippocampus. *J. Comp. Physiol. Psychol.*, **93**, 323

Miller, A. L., Chaptal, C., McEwen, B. S. and Peck, E. J., Jr (1978). Modulation of high affinity GABA uptake into hippocampal synaptosomes by glucocorticoids. *Psychoneuroendocrinology*, **3**, 155

Millard, S. A., Costa, E. and Gal, E. M. (1972). On the control of brain serotonin turnover rate by end product inhibition. *Brain Res.*, **40**, 545

Moore, K. E. and Phillipson, O. T. (1975). Effects of dexamethasone on phenylethanolamine N-methyl-transferase and adrenaline in the brains and superior cervical ganglia of adult and neonatal rats. *J. Neurochem.*, **25**, 289

Mosher, K. M., Young, D. A. and Munck, A. (1971). Evidence for irreversible, actinomycin D-sensitive, and temperature-sensitive steps following the binding of cortisol to glucocorticoid receptors and preceding effects on glucose metabolism in rat thymus cells. *J. Biol. Chem.*, **246**, 654

Nakajima, S. (1978). Attenuation of amnesia by hydrocortisone in the mouse. *Physiol. Behav.*, **20**, 607

Nakajima, S. (1975). Amnesic effect of cycloheximide in the mouse mediated by adrenocortical hormones. *J. Comp. Physiol. Psychol.*, **88**, 378

Neckers, L. and Sze, P. Y. (1975). Regulation of 5-hydroxytryptamine metabolism in mouse brain by adrenal glucocorticoids. *Brain Res.*, **93**, 123

Ogren, S-O. and Fuxe, K. (1977). On the role of brain noradrenaline and the pituitary–adrenal axis in avoidance learning. I. Studies with corticosterone. *Neurosci. Lett.*, **5**, 219

Olpe, H-R. and McEwen, B. S. (1976). Glucocorticoid binding to receptor-like proteins in rat brain and pituitary: ontogenetic and experimentally induced changes. *Brain Res.*, **105**, 121

Otten, U. and Thoenen, H. (1977). Effect of glucocorticoids on nerve growth factor mediated enzyme induction in organ cultures of rat sympathetic ganglia: enhanced response and reduced time requirement to initiate enzyme induction. *J. Neurochem.*, **29**, 69

Otten, U. and Thoenen, H. (1976). Modulatory role of glucocorticoids on NGF-mediated enzyme induction in organ cultures of sympathetic ganglia. *Brain Res.*, **111**, 438

Parvez, H. and Parvez, S. (1973). The effects of metopirone and adrenalectomy on the regulation of the enzymes monoamine oxidase and catechol-*o*-methyl transferase in different brain regions. *J. Neurochem.*, **20**, 1011

Petrovic, V. M. and Janic, V. (1974). Adrenocortical control of monoamine oxidase activity in the ground squirrel (*Citellus citellus*) during the winter. *J. Endocrinol.*, **62**, 407

Pfaff, D. W., Silva, M. T. A. and Weiss, J. M. (1971). Telemetered recording of hormone effects on hippocampal neurons. *Science*, **172**, 394

Pohorecky, L. A. and Wurtman, R. J. (1971). Adrenocortical control of epinephrine synthesis. *Pharm. Rev.*, **23**, 1

Quarton, G. C., Clark, L. D., Cobb, S. and Bauer, W. (1955). Mental disturbances associated with ACTH and cortisone: a review of explanatory hypotheses. *Medicin*. **34**, 13

Rhees, R. W., Grosser, B. I. and Stevens, W. (1975). The autoradiographic localization of [³H]dexamethasone in the brain and pituitary of the rat. *Brain Res.*, **100**, 151

Roberts, D. C. S. and Fibiger, H. C. (1977). Evidence for interactions between central noradrenergic neurons and adrenal hormones in learning and memory. *Pharm. Biochem. Behav.*, **7**, 191

Roosevelt, T. S., Ruhmann-Wennhold, A. and Nelson, D. H. (1973). Adrenal corticosteroid effects upon rat brain mitochondrial metabolism. *Endocrinology*, **53**, 619

Sachar, E. J. (1975). Hormonal changes in stress and mental illness. *Hospital Practice*, **10**, 49

Selye, H. (1973). The evolution of the stress concept. *Am. Sci.*, **61**, 692

Shen, J-T. and Ganong, W. F. (1976). Effect of variations in pituitary–adrenal activity on dopamine-β-hydroxylase activity in various regions of rat brain. *Neuroendocrinology*, **20**, 311

Squire, L. R., St John, S. and Davis, H. P. (1976). Inhibitors of protein synthesis and memory: dissociation and amnesic effects and effects of adrenal steroidogenesis. *Brain Res.*, **112**, 200

Sze, P. Y. (1976). Glucocorticoid regulation of the serotonergic system of the brain. *Advances in Biochemical Psychopharmacology*, vol. 15, p. 251. (New York: Raven Press)

Sze, P. Y. and Maxon, S. C. (1975). Involvement of corticosteroids in acoustic induction of audiogenic seizure susceptibility in mice. *Psychopharmacologia* (Berl.), **45**, 79

Sze, P. Y., Neckers, L. and Towle, A. C. (1976). Glucocorticoids as a regulatory factor for brain tryptophan hydroxylase. *J. Neurochem.*, **26**, 169

Sze, P. Y., Yanai, J. and Ginsburg, B. E. (1974). Adrenal glucocorticoids as a required factor in the development of ethanol withdrawal seizures in mice. *Brain Res.*, **80**, 155

Telegdy, G. and Vermes, I. (1975). Effect of adrenocortical hormones on activity of the serotoninergic system in limbic structures in rats. *Neuroendocrinology*, **18**, 16

Vardaris, R. M. and Schwartz, K. E. (1971). Retrograde amnesia for passive avoidance produced by stimulation of dorsal hippocampus. *Physiol. Behav.*, **6**, 131

deVellis, J. and Inglish, D. (1968). Hormonal control of glycerol phosphate dehydrogenase in the rat brain. *J. Neurochem.*, **15**, 1061

deVellis, J., Inglish, D., Cole, R. and Molson, J. (1971). Effects of hormones on the differentiation of cloned lines of neurons and glial cells. In D. Ford (ed.), *Influence of Hormones on the Nervous System*, pp. 25–39. (Basel: Karger)

deVellis, J., McEwen, B. S., Cole, R. and Inglish, D. (1974). Relations between glucocorticoid nuclear binding, cytosol receptor activity and enzyme induction in a rat glial cell line. *J. Ster. Biochem.*, **5**, 392

Vermes, I., Smelik, P. G. and Mulder, A. H. (1976). Effects of hypophysectomy, adrenalectomy and corticosterone treatment on uptake and release of putative central neurotransmitters by rat hypothalamic tissue *in vitro*. *Life Sci.*, **19**, 1719

Warembourg, M. (1975a). Radioautographic study of the rat brain after injection of (1,2,³H) corticosterone. *Brain Res.*, **89**, 61

Warembourg, M. (1975b). Radioautographic study of the rat brain and pituitary after injection of [³H]dexamethasone. *Cell Tiss. Res.*, **161**, 183

Weiss, J. M., McEwen, B. S., Silva, M. T. and Kalkut, M. F. (1969). Pituitary–adrenal influences on fear responding. *Science*, **163**, 197

de Wied, D. (1966). Antagonistic effect of ACTH and glucocorticoids on avoidance behavior of rats. Presented at the *Second International Congress on Hormonal Steroids, Milan*. (Amsterdam: Excerpta Medica Int. Congress Series, nr. 11)

van Wimersma Greidanus, T. B. (1977). Pregnene-type steroids and impairment of passive avoidance behavior in rats. *Horm. Behav.*, **9**, 49

van Wimersma Greidanus, T. B., Rees, L. H., Scott, A. P., Lowry, P. J. and de Wied, D. (1977). ACTH release during passive avoidance behavior. *Brain Res. Bull.*, **2**, 101

van Wimersma Greidanus, T. B., Weijnen, H., Deurloo, J. and de Wied, D. (1973). Analysis of the effect of progesterone on avoidance behavior. *Horm. Behav.*, **4**, 19

Address for correspondence

Dr B. S. McEwen, The Rockefeller University, 1230 York Avenue, New York, NY 10021, USA

1.3
Effects of sex steroids on cell membrane excitability: a new concept for the action of steroids on the brain

B. DUFY and J. D. VINCENT

ABSTRACT

The functions of the brain depend largely upon the complex inter-actions of nervous and hormonal factors. Indeed, it is gradually emerging that the only way to account for brain mechanisms which have a physiological relevance is to assume that they depend on the simultaneous action of multiple influences. Steroid hormones have long been considered as a separate entity even though it has been demonstrated that they act at the brain level. They have been thought to act, both at the brain and at the uterus, through the genetic synthesizing system. In this rather rigid scheme, the primary action of a sex steroid, oestrogen for example, is the formation of a cytoplasmic receptor complex which is translocated into the nucleus as the first step leading to the genetic machinery for the synthesis of a protein. The purpose of the present paper is to put forward evidence from several investigators of the action of sex steroids on membrane excitability of brain and pituitary cells. In addition we examine the possibility of interaction between sex steroids and neurotransmitters. These observations open a new field in the understanding of brain mechanisms concerning a regulatory role for steroid hormones in conventional neurotransmission.

INTRODUCTION

Classically we are accustomed to differentiate between nervous elements which are supposed to communicate using neurotransmitters in specific and localized pathways, and endocrine cells which use hormones for a widespread mode of communication. However, such a rigid dichotomy must be revised in the light of recent experiments. We do not intend to discuss here the classic neuroendocrine concept; this was first queried when signs of secretory activity of the type encountered in endocrine cells were found in neurons of basal brain areas (Scharrer and Scharrer, 1940). Rather, we wish to consider more recent observations, findings which will, no doubt, lead to a more generalized but also a more complex concept of neurohormonal communication.

Firstly, recent work has shown definite neuronal characteristics in endocrine cells of various origin (Pearse and Takor, 1976; Pearse, 1968), which is in contrast to the concept developed by the Scharrers. These endocrine cells belong to the APUD system, APUD being an acronym for amine precursor uptake and decarboxylase (Pearse, 1968). As well as the cytochemical and ultrastructural features which they share with neurons, most of these endocrine cells are excitable and are able to display action potentials (Taraskevich and Douglas, 1977; Tischler et al., 1976; Kidokoro, 1975). Secondly, it has been suggested that a number of peptides and various hormones, including posterior and anterior pituitary hormones, play a role in the despatching of information within the brain (Krieger and Liotta, 1979; Barker, 1977). However, such a transfer of information differs from the classical neurotransmission; the neuromodulators, as they have been named, display effects of longer duration and on wider targets (Barker, 1977). Thirdly, evidence has recently been presented giving a true hormonal modality of action to the neurotransmitter dopamine (DA). DA is released from the median eminence, as are other hypothalamic hormones, and has been shown to act on the pituitary cells which secrete prolactin (PRL) (MacLeod and Lehmeyer, 1974). There is also evidence that DA acts on the gonadotrophin-producing cells (Dailey et al., 1978).

In the classic neuroendocrine scheme sex steroids remain a separate entity. A conceptual polarization between the mechanisms of action of sex steroids and those of peptide hormones has been strongly defended. Peptide hormones were known to activate membrane receptor sites as a first step, whereas steroid hormones were thought to passively cross the lipid bilayer of the cell membrane to bind to a cytosolic receptor as the first step in a number of processes leading to the genetic machinery of protein synthesis. Several pieces of evidence were provided to support such a mechanism at the level of the brain (McEwen, 1978; Warembourg, 1978). However, it is now known that sex steroids control or modulate a number of functions in the central nervous system (CNS). A fundamental argument against the concept of there being a single mechanism of action for sex steroids is the wide range of delays which appear to occur before the various physiological effects for which they are responsible become apparent. Some of these effects take place within seconds or minutes, whereas others occur after a delay of hours or even days. The effects of sex steroids are generally biphasic, i.e. there is an early inhibitory effect which is followed by a stimulatory effect some hours later, or vice versa. To date insufficient studies have been done to prove that short-term biological effects of steroids are possible within the classical scheme of genetic protein synthesis, and no alternative possibilities have been provided.

Finally, observation of the early interactions which occur between sex steroids, peptides and neurotransmitters strongly suggests that convergence of influences may occur at specific points (Szego, 1978).

The purpose of the present essay is to put forward evidence of a membrane involvement of steroid hormone effects in the brain and to examine the possibility of interactions at the membrane level of substances involved in neurohormonal communication.

DO SEX STEROIDS AFFECT ELECTRICAL EXCITABILITY OF CENTRAL NEURONS?

The studies of Barraclough and Cross (1963) constituted one of the earliest attempts to answer the important question: do steroid hormones directly influence brain electrical activity? These authors succeeded in recording single unit activity in the hypothalamus of the cyclic female rat. They observed that some stimuli accelerated the firing rate of the majority of neurons tested, and that progesterone was able to induce a selective depression of the response of lateral hypothalamic neurons to cervical probing. This technique has since been used to demonstrate responses of single units in specific brain regions to the administration of oestrogen (Lincoln and Cross, 1967). The spontaneous electrical activity in the anterior hypothalamic areas was noted to be lower in oestrous rats than in ovariectomized animals, and the administration of oestradiol benzoate to ovariectomized rats was noted to reduce the levels of neuronal activity to those observed in oestrous animals. It has been suspected that these modifications could be due to a physiological action of oestrogen in relation to gonadotrophin regulation (Lincoln and Cross, 1967).

Early changes in the electrical activity of hypothalamic neurons have been reported following oestrogen injections (Dufy et al., 1976; Yagi, 1973) (Figure 1). The latencies (in terms of minutes) observed between the systemic administration of the oestrogen and the changes in the electrical activity of the recorded neurons hardly agree with the classical model of a nuclear mode of action and synthesis of a new protein. However, such studies do not provide any information as to the site and mechanism of action of the steroid.

In recent experiments, Kelly et al. (1977) administered 17β-oestradiol hemi-succinate by micro-electrophoresis directly onto the membrane of individual hypothalamic neurons and observed changes in the electrical activity of some hypothalamic neurons within seconds. They suggested, therefore, that a specific membrane and/or cytosol receptor could be responsible for these rapid changes in excitability. Thus, besides a nuclear mode of action revealed by autoradiography and other techniques (McEwen, 1978; Warembourg, 1978), it seems possible that some oestrogen effects may be mediated by membrane phenomena.

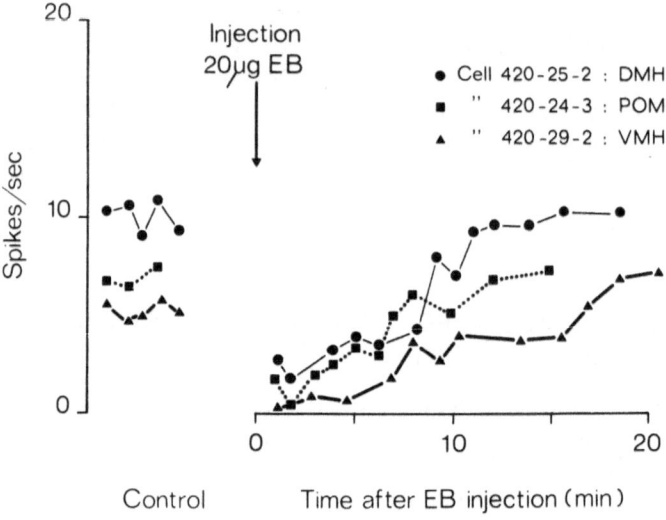

Figure 1   Effect of the injection of 20 µg oestradiol benzoate (EB) on the mean firing rate of three hypothalamic neurons (DMH dorso medial hypothalamus, POM medial preoptic area, VMH ventro medial hypothalamus). These experiments were performed on ovariectomized female rabbits (Dufy *et al.*, 1976). A chronic recording device was stereotaxically implanted under general anaesthesia. This system allowed the introduction of microelectrodes in various hypothalamic areas. The recordings were obtained in unanaesthetized animals accustomed to a restraining box during the recording session. Each point represents the mean firing rate obtained during similar states of arousal as judged by the EEG recording

PITUITARY CELLS IN CULTURE: A WORKING MODEL FOR THE STUDY OF THE EFFECTS OF SEX STEROIDS ON CELL MEMBRANE EXCITABILITY

Though of primary interest from the physiological point of view, the *in vivo* experiments described above involve too many unknown parameters to be of practical use in the understanding of the mechanism of hormone action. Such studies are, indeed, greatly impeded because the responsive elements are embedded within a maze of non-responsive ones. Therefore, studies using cultured cells appear more suitable at the present time. The *in vitro* systems have led to major achievements despite inherent limitations which are beyond the scope of this essay. Cells in culture have been studied morphologically and biochemically as well as electrophysiologically using organotypic cultures, primary cultures of fetal or neonatal materials, and clonal strains of dissociated cells of tumoural origin. Hypothalamic organotypic cultures which are responsive to sex steroids have been developed (Toran-Allerand, 1978). However, to our knowledge, no study of the putative effect of sex steroids on the membrane electrical properties of such cultures has been reported. This apparent lack of interest among investigators has to be attributed to the fact that the possibility of a sex steroid effect at the level of the cell membrane has never been very seriously concerned. Moreover, brain cells do not appear to be the best model, since responsive units are restricted to specific areas and, even in culture, only a few cells have been observed to fix the steroids (Toran-Allerand, 1978).

Considerable evidence has been accumulated, using several approaches, that the pituitary gland is one of the first structures to respond to sex steroids. Pituitary cells in culture, therefore, constitute one of the most interesting models for the investigation of the mechanism of action of sex steroids. New evidence has attributed the same neural ridge of the neuroectoderm to be the origin of the pituitary and of the hypothalamus (Pèarse and Takor, 1976), and it has been observed that action potentials are not only a property of neurons but are also detectable in endocrine cells including normal (Taraskevich and Douglas, 1977) and clonal pituitary ones (Dufy et al., 1979b; Kidokoro, 1975).

ELECTROPHYSIOLOGICAL PROPERTIES OF PITUITARY CELLS IN CULTURE

Several authors have studied the electrical properties of dissociated cultures of anterior pituitary cells from normal and tumour tissue (Taraskevich and Douglas, 1977; Kidokoro, 1975). Most of the experiments have been performed with the GH_3 rat prolactin cell line. In these experiments the mean resting membrane potential was about 40 to 50 mV and the input resistance was high, ranging from 40 to 700 MΩ. Under our experimental conditions (Dufy et al., 1979b) about 50% of the cells were found to be excitable and able to display action potentials when depolarized, and 20% were spontaneously active (Figure 2). Experimental manipulations of the ionic composition of the bathing medium showed that the action potentials were calcium (Ca^{2+}) dependent (Figure 2). Action potentials were still recorded in the presence of tetrodotoxin (Taraskevich and Douglas, 1977), a known blocker of sodium (Na^+) spikes, and also in a Na^+-free medium. They were suppressed by cobalt (Co^{2+}), manganese (Mn^{2+}) and D600, a blocker of Ca^{2+} channels (Dufy et al., 1979b; Taraskevich and Douglas, 1977). The phase of repolarization was observed to be much longer when tetraethylammonium (TEA) or 4-amino-pyridine (4-AMP) were ejected on to the cell under investigation (Figure 2). It is therefore likely that the spikes were due to an increase in Ca^{2+} conductance, which corresponds to an entry of calcium into the cell, and terminated with an increase in K^+ conductance.

Thyrotrophin-releasing hormone (TRH) (25 to 125 nmol/l) added to the bathing solution increased the percentage of cells displaying action potentials; this is consistent with the effect of TRH observed with extracellular recording (Taraskevich and Douglas, 1977; Kidokoro, 1975). Ejection of TRH (50 nmol/l, 2 nl) close to the cell evoked a train of action potentials within 1 min (Figure 3). This spiking activity was preceded by a progressive increase of the input resistance without any detectable change in the resting membrane

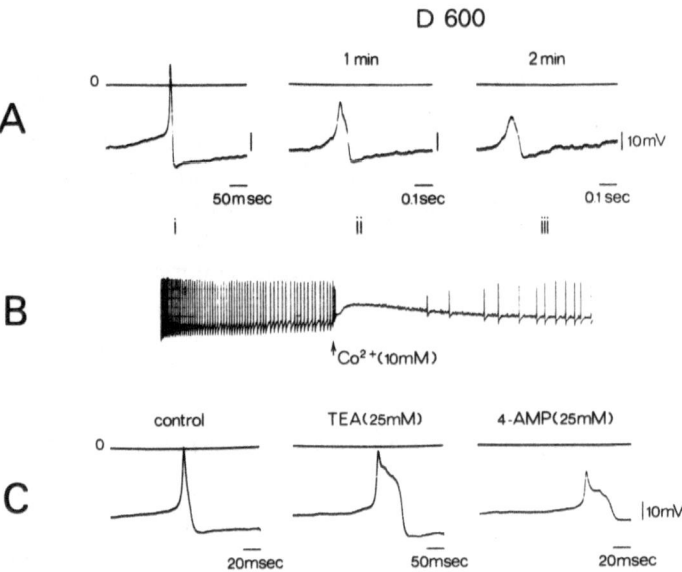

Figure 2   Characteristics of action potentials recorded from $GH_3/B6$ cells. Before being used for electrophysiological studies cells were grown for 5 to 7 days in Ham's F10 solution supplemented with 15% horse serum and 2.5% fetal calf serum. Recordings were taken, using a bathing solution of the following composition (in mmol per litre): NaCl, 142.6; KCl, 5.6; $CaCl_2$, 10; glucose, 5; and Hepes buffer, 5 (pH, 7.4). The substances to be tested were dissolved in the bathing solution and ejected, in the proper concentration, by a pressure ejection system directly on to the cell membrane (Dufy et al., 1979).

A: Effect of D600, a blocker of Ca^{2+} channels, on the shape of action potentials of a spontaneously firing cell.

B: Effects of cobalt (Co^{2+}) ions on a spontaneously firing cell. It should be noted that Co^{2+} ions completely suppressed action potentials and depolarized the cell, which is consistent with an involvement of Ca^{2+} ions in the spiking activity and also the resting membrane polarization.

C: Effects of tetraethylammonium (TEA) and 4-amino-pyridine (4-AMP) on the shape of action potentials of a spontaneously firing cell. Lengthening of the phase of repolarization is to be noted.

polarization, apart from an early hyperpolarization which did not seem to be directly involved in the spiking activity. After 1 to 10 min the cell stopped firing as the resistance returned to the resting level. Once again, the action potentials were reduced or completely abolished by D600. Furthermore, the action potentials were only slightly changed in Na^+-free medium, although no overshoot was observed. These findings are consistent with the observation that Ca^{2+} is essential for the secretion of adenohypophysial hormones (Martin *et al.*, 1973).

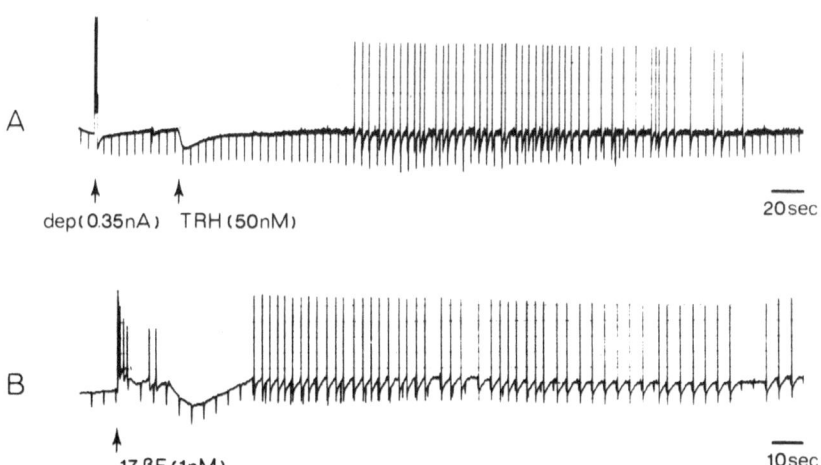

Figure 3   Effects of TRH and 17β-oestradiol (17β-E) on the membrane electrical activity of two GH_3/B6 cells. Both substances were dissolved in the bathing solution. 17β-E was first dissolved in alcohol, the final alcohol concentration being 0.1%.
A: Ejection of TRH (50 nmol/l, 2 nl) into the vicinity of the cell membrane elicits a precocious hyperpolarization followed within 1 min by a sustained spiking activity.
B: Ejection of 17β-E directly on to the membrane of the cell induces an early depolarization followed by the firing of action potential. A measure of the membrane resistance (vertical bars) is obtained by injecting a hyperpolarizing current (0.16 nA). The solvents were ineffective.

EARLY MEMBRANE PERMEABILITY AND CONDUCTANCE CHANGES FOLLOWING ADMINISTRATION OF OESTRADIOL

The experiments reported here were performed on the GH_3/B6 cell line, a sub-clone of the GH_3 rat prolactin clone which secretes prolactin in response to TRH and oestradiol.

We observed that 17β-oestradiol (17β-E) when ejected close to the cell being recorded elicited a series of transient ionic permeability changes beginning within 1 second of the administration of 17β-E (Figure 3). These modifications of passive membrane properties were in two parts: a transient depolarization and a decrease of the overall input resistance which induced a short burst of action potentials, followed, 1 min later, by an increase in the input resistance which led to a sustained discharge of Ca^{2+} dependent action potentials (Figure 3).

When an ejection was successful in eliciting spikes a subsequent ejection of 17β-E 3 to 10 min later was totally ineffective. 17α-Oestradiol had a much weaker effect even at higher doses. Progesterone and testosterone were not able to induce spiking activity.

Our results reveal a rapid effect of 17β-E on the membrane of GH_3/B6 cells. The electrical activity elicited by 17β-E was similar in time course and Ca^{2+} dependence to that induced by TRH. The rapid and specific effect of 17β-E on membrane properties implies recognition sites for the steroid at the membrane surface and probably reflects conformational changes in membrane components. Recent evidence of a membrane site of action for oestrogen has been reported for uterine cells and an early intracellular accumulation of calcium has been clearly demonstrated following oestrogen administration (Pietras and Szego, 1975). The physiological implication of such early effects of oestradiol on the passive membrane properties and excitability of pituitary cells remains unclear. In the case of TRH, which exerts both a short-term effect on PRL release and a long-term effect on PRL synthesis, the TRH-induced electrical activity may be associated with the stimulation of PRL release. 17β-E has been shown to have a long-term effect on PRL synthesis. However, the possibility that PRL release is stimulated within minutes of 17β-E injection, which would be consistent with the Ca^{2+} dependent electrical effect, has not yet been investigated. It is also possible that Ca^{2+} is required to initiate the long-term effect of 17β-E on PRL synthesis. These changes in ionic permeability of the membrane may also initiate other intracellular processes triggered by the steroid, such as growth stimulation and cell division.

MODULATION OF THE INHIBITORY EFFECT OF DOPAMINE BY OESTROGEN

Prolactin (PRL) secreting cells are, at least partially, under the stimulatory influence of TRH and of oestrogen. Nevertheless, they are mainly controlled by inhibitory substances among which dopamine is one of the most potent, *in vivo* as well as *in vitro*. In the GH_3/B6 cell line, DA ejected in the close vicinity of a cell provokes an inhibition of firing within 30 to 60 sec. (Figure 4). Similar results have been observed in teleostean prolactin cells (Taraskevich and Douglas, 1978). Under our experimental conditions (Dufy *et al.*, 1979a), this inhibitory effect is concomitant with a rapid decrease of the input resistance without any detectable change in the resting membrane polarization (Figure 4). In addition, DA inhibits the TRH-induced action potentials (Figure 4). Conversely, the DA antagonists haloperidol (10^{-6} mol) and chlorpromazine

(10^{-6} mol) suppress the inhibitory effect of DA on action potentials when they are administered to a spontaneously firing cell (Figure 4). The DA inhibition of both spontaneous and TRH-induced action potentials may be related to the effect of DA on PRL secretion. It has previously been shown that the DA agonist CB154 decreases TRH-induced PRL release in $GH_3/B6$ cells without modifying the binding of $[^3H]$-TRH.

The fact that DA inhibits both the firing and hormone release supports the hypothesis that Ca^{2+} dependent action potentials are involved in the mechanism of release of anterior pituitary hormones (Taraskevich and Douglas, 1978 and 1977). The mechanism by which DA inhibits the firing of PRL cells is not

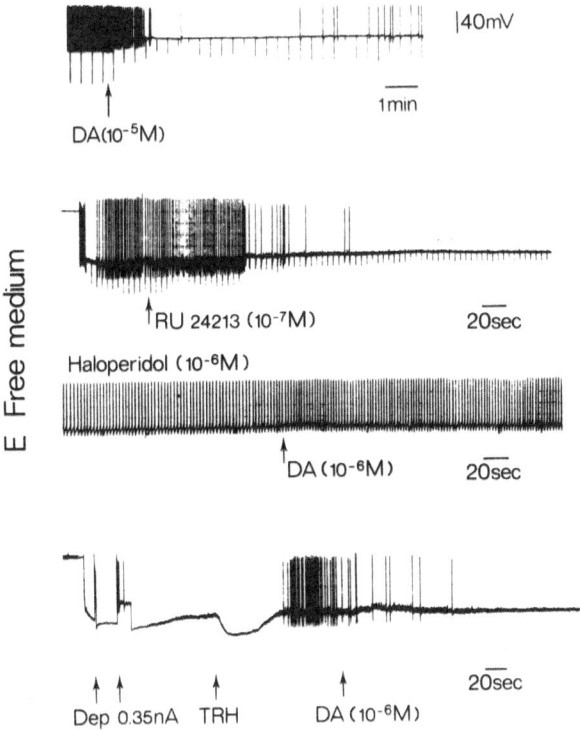

Figure 4 Effects of dopamine (DA), DA agonist and DA antagonists on the firing of action potentials in the $GH_3/B6$ prolactin secreting cell line. Cells were cultured for 24 hours in an oestrogen-free medium obtained by incubating overnight normal medium with activated charcoal (Merck) and dextran (Sigma D4781). DA and RU24213 (DA agonist), obtained respectively from Hoffman–La Roche and Roussel UCLAF, were dissolved in bathing solution. DA and RU24213 depressed the firing of spontaneous action potentials and reduced the membrane resistance. Vertical bars represent a measure of the membrane resistance obtained by injecting a current of 0.16 nA with a bridge amplifier. DA had no effect when haloperidol (Lebrun) or chlorpromazine (Specia) were ejected before the administration of DA on the cell being recorded. DA inhibited the action potential firing induced by TRH. The excitability of the cell was tested by injecting a depolarizing current (Dep.) of 0.35 nA

clearly understood at present. From our experiments this mechanism appears to be different from that already reported for central neurons (Kitai *et al.*, 1976) in that no change in the membrane polarization is observed. We have demonstrated that TRH, which stimulates the secretion of PRL, elicits action potential firing by increasing the membrane resistance without any noticeable depolarization. These data are in agreement with the results presented by Martin *et al.* (1973) showing that although Ca^{2+} ions are necessary for the secretion of pituitary hormones, depolarization is not tightly linked to the release process. Thus, under our experimental conditions, it would appear that DA acts on membrane excitability and resistance of $GH_3/B6$ cells in a way opposite to TRH, though we are not able to determine the exact nature of the mechanism at present.

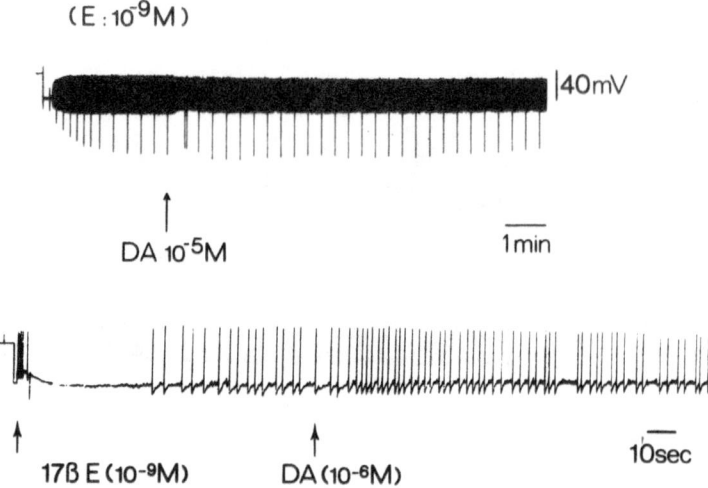

Figure 5 Antagonism between dopamine (DA) and oestrogen. When the bathing medium was supplemented with 17β-oestradiol (1 nmol/l), DA had no effect on action potentials firing nor on membrane resistance, represented by the vertical bars (0.16 nA). DA had no effect on action potentials induced by the ejection of 17β-E (1 nmol/l).

Finally, we have observed that the inhibitory effect of DA on PRL-secreting cells is modulated by oestrogen. In our study the percentage of cells inhibited by DA was different according to the presence or absence of oestrogen in the medium in which the cells were grown. When the cells were grown for at least 24 h in an oestrogen-depleted medium, the percentage of DA-inhibited cells reached 80% ($n = 43$) instead of the 40% in normal medium. When 17β-E (10^{-9} mol) was added to the recording solution, DA did not affect the action potential firing nor the input resistance of any of the cells tested ($n = 30$) (Figure 5). We have reported above that 17β-E, when directly applied to the cell, provoked action potential firing (Dufy *et al.*, 1979b). DA did not inhibit this oestrogen-induced electrical activity (Figure 5). Similarly, Euvrard et al. (1979) antagonized the inhibitory responses of DA in the striatum by applying oestrogen.

CONCLUSIONS

There is a growing amount of data demonstrating an initial interaction of sex steroids with the cell membrane (Dufy et al., 1979b; Szego, 1978; Rao et al., 1976; Milgrom et al., 1973). This interaction elicits rapid changes in ionic membrane permeability and conductance, which lead to modifications of the cell membrane excitability (Dufy et al., 1979b). These early membrane effects do not preclude other biochemical or conformational transformations which cannot be studied by electrophysiological techniques. These early changes in membrane excitability may well explain some of the rapid physiological effects of the steroids, but further work is needed in this field.

In clear contradiction to the conceptual polarization which has been developed between the mechanism of action of sex steroids and those of peptide hormones, we found puzzling similarities between the action of oestradiol and that of TRH. Both substances were able to induce Ca^{2+} dependent action potentials apparently by the same increase in membrane resistance; the only difference was a rapid and temporal desensitization following TRH administration and a complete desensitization following 17β-E administration (Dufy et al., 1979b). Analogies between membrane effects of steroids and peptides have recently been reported (Szego, 1978). From this point of view, it is interesting to note that pre-treatment with oestradiol enhanced the number of cells which were excited by TRH and that, similarly, pre-treatment with TRH increased the number of cells which responded to oestradiol (Dufy et al., 1979b). Such an observation, which at first appeared confusing, may be of the same type of reciprocal interaction as that between steroids and gonadotrophin on the ovary, described recently by Richards et al. (1976).

As expected, DA inhibits action potential firing in prolactin-secreting pituitary cells. This inhibitory effect does not seem to be mediated by a change in membrane polarization and differs therefore from the mechanisms of action of DA previously described (Kitai et al., 1976). However, two classes of DA receptors have recently been described: D1, which increases cyclic AMP synthesis, has been found in the caudate nucleus, and D2, which does not, has been found in nigro-neostriatal neurons and prolactin-secreting cells of the pituitary (Kebabian and Calne, 1979). Therefore, the interaction which we have demonstrated between oestrogen and dopamine in prolactin-secreting cells is highly promising for a better understanding of brain mechanisms. The observations described above suggest a regulatory role of sex steroids in conventional neurotransmission and a new mode for the transfer of information in the nervous system.

Acknowledgements

This work was supported by grants from INSERM (U176 and CRL78-1-2656), CNRS (ERA493), DGRST (77-7-0654) and the University of Bordeaux II. We thank Mr J. B. Seal for his helpful comments and editorial advice.

References

Barker, J. L. (1977). Physiological roles of peptides in the nervous system. In H. Gainer (ed.), *Peptides in Neurobiology*, pp. 295–343. (New York: Plenum Press)

Barraclough, C. and Cross, B. (1963). Unit activity in the hypothalamus of the cyclic female rat: effect of genital stimuli and progesterone. *J. Endocrinol.*, **26**, 339

Dailey, R. A., Tsou, R. C., Tindall, G. T. and Neill, J. D. (1978). Direct hypophysial inhibition of laternizing hormone release by dopamine in the rabbit. *Life Sci.*, **22**, 1491

Dufy, B., Morancé, C., Vincent, J. D., Gourdji, D. and Tixier-Vidal, A. (1979a). Inhibition of action potentials by dopamine in cultured pituitary cells and its modulation by estradiol. Presented at the *Third European Neurosciences Meeting*, September 10–14, Rome

Dufy, B., Partouche, C., Poulain, D., Dufy-Barbe, L. and Vincent, J. D. (1976). Effects of estrogen in the electrical activity of identified and unidentified hypothalamic units. *Neuroendocrinology*, **22**, 38

Dufy, B., Vincent, J. D., Fleury, H., du Pasquier, P., Gourdji, D. and Tixier-Vidal, A. (1979b). Membrane effects of thyrotropin-releasing hormone and estrogen shown by intracellular recording from pituitary cells. *Science*, **204**, 509

Euvrard, C., Labrie, F. and Boissier, J. R. (1979). Effect of estrogen on changes in the activity of striatal cholinergic neurons induced by DA drugs. *Brain Res.*, **169**, 215

Kebabian, J. W. and Calne, D. B. (1979). Multiple receptors for dopamine. *Nature (Lond.)*, **277**, 93

Kelly, M., Moss, R. and Dudley, C. (1977). The effects of microelectrophoretically applied estrogen, cortisol and acetycholine on medial preoptic-septal unit activity throughout the estrus cycle of the female rat. *Exp. Brain Res.*, **30**, 53

Kidokoro, Y. (1975). Spontaneous calcium action potentials in a clonal pituitary cell line and their relationship to prolactin secretion. *Nature (Lond.)*, **258**, 741

Kitai, S. T., Sugimori, M. and Kocsis, J. D. (1976). Excitatory nature of dopamine in the nigrocaudate pathway. *Exp. Brain Res.*, **24**, 351

Krieger, D. T. and Liotta, A. S. (1979). Pituitary hormones in brain: where, how and why? *Science*, **205**, 366

Lincoln, D. and Cross, B. A. (1967). Effects of oestrogen on the responsiveness of neurones in the hypothalamus, septum, and preoptic area of rats with light-induced persistent oestrus. *J. Endocrinol.*, **37**, 191

MacLeod, R. M. and Lehmeyer, J. E. (1974). Studies in the mechanism of the dopamine-mediated inhibition of prolactin secretion. *Endocrinology*, **94**, 1077

Martin, S., York, D. H. and Kraicer, J. (1973). Alterations in trans-membrane potential of adenohypophysial cells in elevated potassium and calcium-free media. *Endocrinology*, **92**, 1084

McEwen, B. (1978). Specificity, mechanisms and functional consequences of steroid-receptor interactions in the CNS. In J. D. Vincent and C. Kordon (eds.), *Cell Biology of Hypothalamic Neurosecretion*, pp. 239–265. (Paris: CNRS)

Milgrom, E., Atger, M. and Baulieu, E. E. (1973). Studies on estrogen entry into uterine cells and on estradiol receptor complex attachment to the nucleus. Is the entry of estrogen into uterine cells a protein-mediated process? *Biochim. Biophys. Acta (Amst.)*, **320**, 267

Pearse, A. G. E. (1968). Common cytochemical and ultra-structural characteristics of cells producing polypeptide hormones (the APUD series) and their relevance to thyroid and ultimobranchial C cells and calcium. *Proc. R. Soc. B.*, **170**, 71

Pearse, A. G. E. and Takor, T. (1976). Neuroendocrine embryology and the APUD concept. *Clin. Endocrinol.*, **5**, 229S

Pietras, R. J. and Szego, C. M. (1975). Endometrial cell calcium and oestrogen action. *Nature (Lond.)*, **253**, 357

Rao, G. S., Schulze-Hagen, K., Rao, M. L. and Breuer, H. (1976). Kinetics of steroid transport through cell membranes: comparison of the uptake of cortisol by isolated rat liver cells with binding of cortisol to rat liver cytosol. *J. Steroid Biochem.*, **7**, 1123

Richards, J. S., Ireland, J. J., Rao, M. L., Bernath, G. A., Midgley, A. R. and Reichert, L. E. (1976). Ovarian follicular development in the rat: hormone receptor regulation by estradiol, follicle stimulating hormone and luteinizing hormone. *Endocrinology*, **99**, 1562

Scharrer, E. and Scharrer, B. (1940). Secretory cells within the hypothalamus. In E. Scharrer and B. Scharrer (eds.), *The Hypothalamus and Central Levels of Autonomic Formation*, pp. 170–194. (Baltimore: Williams and Wilkins)

Szego, C. M. (1978). Parallels in the modes of action of peptide and steroid hormones: membrane effects and cellular entry. In K. W. McKerns (ed.), *Structure and Function of the Gonadotropins*, pp. 431–472. (New York: Plenum Press)

Taraskevich, P. S. and Douglas, W. W. (1978). Catecholamines of supposed inhibitory hypophysiotropic function suppress action potentials in prolactin cells. *Nature (Lond.)*, **276**, 832

Taraskevich, P. S. and Douglas, W. W. (1977). Action potentials occur in cells of the normal anterior pituitary gland and are stimulated by the hypophysiotropic peptide thyrotropin-releasing hormone. *Proc. Natl. Acad. Sci. (Wash.)*, **74**, 4064

Tischler, A. S., Dichter, M. A., Biales, B., Delellis, R. A. and Wolfe, H. (1976). Neural properties of human endocrine tumor cells of proposed neural crest origin. *Science*, **192**, 902

Toran-Allerand, C. (1978). Culture of hypothalamic neurons: organotypic culture. In J. D. Vincent and C. Kordon (eds.), *Cell Biology of Hypothalamic Neurosecretion*, pp. 759–776. (Paris: CNRS)

Warembourg, M. (1978). Distribution of steroid receptors in the CNS. In J. D. Vincent and C. Kordon (eds.), *Cell Biology of Hypothalamic Neurosecretion*, pp. 221–237. (Paris: CNRS)

Yagi, K. (1973). Changes in firing rates of single preoptic and hypothalamic units following an intravenous administration of estrogen in the castrated female rat. *Brain Res.*, **53**, 343

Address for correspondence

Dr B. Dufy, Maître de Recherche CNRS, Institut National de la Santé et de la Recherche Médicale, Unité de Neurobiologie des Comportements, U.176, Rue Camille Saint-Säens, 33077 Bordeaux, France

1.4
Changing concepts about neuroregulation: neurotransmitters and neuromodulators

G. R. ELLIOTT and J. D. BARCHAS

ABSTRACT

Recently, discoveries of an astounding number of endogenous sub-stances which affect interneuronal communication, and advances in our understanding of mechanisms by which it is controlled, have created a growing need for a better classification of compounds which are involved in neuronal transmission. In this paper we describe a nomenclature based on the common ability of such neuroactive substances to regulate neuronal communication.

We suggest that 'neuroregulator' is a good generic term, since it focuses on the relevant activity. This can be further subdivided according to function. Thus, a 'neurotransmitter' would correspond to the classical concept of a substance which conveys a transient and unilateral signal across a specialized synapse. In contrast, a 'neuro-modulator' would alter neuronal activity by mechanisms which might or might not involve a synapse. Two types of neuro-modu-lators might be: *hormonal* neuromodulators, providing direct short- or long-lasting modulation of neurons far from the release site, and *synaptic* neuromodulators, acting indirectly by modulating neuro-transmitter function. Preliminary criteria for classifying neuroregu-lators are described.

As discussed in the paper, introduction of a nomenclature for neuroregulators could have several salutary effects. For example, it should facilitate discussions about substances which are presently referred to by a variety of confusing and poorly defined terms. Also, it may suggest new kinds of potentially valuable research into mechanisms of neuronal modulation. We believe that this nomenclature provides the necessary balance between specificity and generalizability.

INTRODUCTION

It sometimes is easy to forget that the role of chemicals in transmitting signals between peripheral neurons was firmly established only 60 years ago and difficult to believe that it has been accepted as the principal means of communication among neurons in the central nervous system for less than 25 years. During that time technical advances have expanded enormously the ability of scientists to examine and manipulate the electrical and chemical properties of brain cells. Many of the resulting data have confirmed that certain compounds do convey signals between neurons. However, as amply demonstrated by some of the papers presented at this conference, evidence also has amassed that argues forcefully for the need to reconsider the ways in which endogenous substances might regulate neuronal activity. We would like first to examine briefly the historical context of our current nomenclature for endogenous neuroactive compounds and then to propose a modified nomenclature which appears to fit better with our current knowledge about such substances.

HISTORICAL PERSPECTIVE ON NEUROTRANSMISSION

In 1904 a Cambridge graduate student, T. R. Elliott, proposed that the systemic effects of stimulating a peripheral autonomic nerve might result from the release of tiny amounts of a chemical which then could act on specific target organs (Elliott, 1904). This novel idea was shaped into a theory of chemical neurotransmission by the elegant studies of Loewi (1921) and of Cannon and Uridil (1921), whose pioneering work on parasympathetic and sympathetic nervous systems, respectively, led eventually to the identification of acetylcholine and norepinephrine and to the elucidation of their role in autonomic neuronal activity.

Extrapolation of these important findings in peripheral nerves to the central nervous system proved to be difficult. For many years scientists argued convincingly that only electrical processes could provide the rapid transfer of information among neurons needed in the brain (Eccles, 1948). However, two discoveries in the early 1950s provided compelling evidence for chemical, rather than electrical, neurotransmission in the brain. First, newly developed techniques for single-cell electrical recordings (Fatt and Katz, 1951) and for microiontophoretic application of substances on to single neurons (Curtis and Eccles, 1958) yielded results which were incompatible with purely electrical neuronal junctions. Second, the discovery that norepinephrine was present in brain (von Euler, 1956), along with the subsequent demonstration that changes in its brain concentrations reflect changes in brain function (Vogt, 1954), clearly implied a crucial role for chemical transmission in the brain.

By any standards, the effects of these discoveries have been phenomenal (Barchas *et al.*, 1978). They have led to the creation of a variety of new scientific subspecialties, such as neurohistochemistry, neuropharmacology and behavioural neurochemistry, as well as to the development of many new drugs which can alter brain function selectively. But in addition they have resulted in the discovery of a number of intriguing brain substances whose functions do not appear to fit within a simple model of neurotransmission.

THE CONCEPT OF NEUROREGULATION

In the past few years many neuroscientists have become increasingly aware of the need for a new nomenclature with which to categorize the burgeoning array of endogenous neuroactive compounds, many of which appear not to act as neurotransmitters. Such a system must be discriminative enough to exclude substances which are important for intraneuronal maintenance but not for interneuronal interactions and yet be sufficiently general to include as many appropriate substances as possible, even when precise mechanisms of action remain to be established.

Most endogenous neuroactive compounds have been named either for their biological activity or for their tissue source. Thus, when 5-hydroxytryptamine was isolated from body tissues by two groups in the 1950s, one group called it 'serotonin', to denote its effect on blood vessels, while the other named it 'enteramine', for the enterochromaffin cells from which they extracted it. Of more direct relevance to this conference are the endogenous opioid peptides. The first of these peptides were called 'enkephalins', because they were extracted from brain; but the compounds as a class are 'endorphins', indicating their morphine-like activity. The subsequent discovery of enkephalins in tissues other than brain makes clear the difficulties of a nomenclature based on organ of origin and suggests the utility of nomenclature based upon function.

We believe that function is a good basis for developing a new nomenclature for the entire group of endogenous neuroactive agents (Table 1). Focusing on the ability of these compounds to regulate communication among nerve cells, we have proposed the generic term 'neuroregulators' (Barchas *et al.*, 1978). Neuroregulators then can be subdivided further into neurotransmitters, which correspond to the classical concept of compounds conveying signals between two neurons across a specialized structure, and neuromodulators, which include many of the more recently discovered substances that may play critical functions in neuronal communication but through mechanisms other than neurotransmission.

Table 1   A suggested nomenclature for substances involved in interneuronal communication

Neuroregulators are any members of the entire class of substances involved in the regulation of interneuronal communication

    Neurotransmitters act within a neuronal synapse to transmit a presynaptic signal to a post-synaptic neuron

    Neuromodulators alter interneuronal communication through mechanisms other than synaptic transmission

        Hormonal neuromodulators alter neuronal activity at relatively great distances from the site of release, possibly at many targets simultaneously; they exert their effects either via specific membrane receptors or by selectively interfering with some aspect of neurotransmission

        Synaptic neuromodulators affect neuronal function locally by altering neurotransmitter activity in a single synapse through a specific site which may or may not be a membrane receptor

Neurotransmission

Concepts of synaptic transmission continue to draw heavily from studies of peripheral nervous systems. Although it is possible that synapses in the central nervous system differ in some important respects which remain to be defined, available information does permit formulation of a reasonably precise set of criteria by which to identify a brain neurotransmitter (Table 2). A brief review of an idealized synapse will illustrate the salient aspects of our present conception of neurotransmission.

Table 2   Criteria for establishing the identity of a neurotransmitter in the central nervous system

- The substance must be present in presynaptic elements of a neuronal synapse
- Precursors and synthetic enzymes must be present in the neuron, probably in close proximity to the site of action
- Stimulation of neuronal afferents should cause release of the substance in physiologically significant amounts
- Stimulation of afferents and direct application of the substance to the synapse should produce identical effects
- Specific receptors for the substance must be present on the postsynaptic membranes and may be present presynaptically
- Interaction of the substance with its postsynaptic receptor must produce changes in membrane permeability which lead to either excitatory or inhibitory postsynaptic potentials
- Specific inactivating mechanisms should exist which stop interactions of the substance with its receptor in a physiologically reasonable timeframe
- Stimulation of afferents and direct application of the substance should be equally responsive to and similarly affected by interventions involving postsynaptic sites or inactivating mechanisms

Modified from Barchas *et al.*, 1978

Figure 1 highlights essential features of the current model for dopaminergic synapses (Cooper *et al.*, 1978). In the presynaptic terminal, the neurotransmitter, dopamine, is synthesized in two steps from its amino-acid precursor tyrosine. Tyrosine hydroxylase is the first, rate-limiting step in this conversion; the enzyme also is present in neurons which contain the catecholamines epinephrine and norepinephrine. Dopa decarboxylase, which completes the synthesis of dopamine, is found in many cells and catalyses the decarboxylation of several important amino acids. The precise milieu in which synthesis occurs remains to be established; but it may be associated in some manner with membranes of the presynaptic vesicles, or granules, in which dopamine is stored after its synthesis.

IDEALIZED MODEL OF A DOPAMINERGIC SYNAPSE

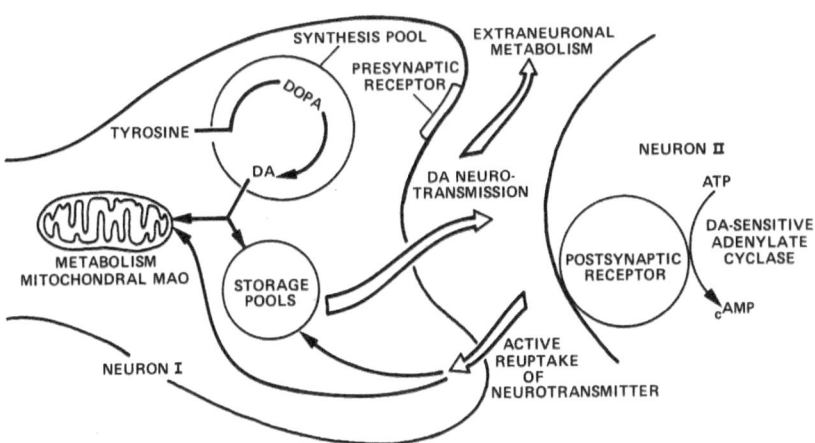

Figure 1   Idealized representation of a dopaminergic synapse. Dopamine (DA) is synthesized in two steps from the amino acid tyrosine and then stored in synaptic vesicles. An action potential depolarizes the presynaptic membrane, resulting in the release of dopamine into the synaptic cleft. The neurotransmitter then interacts with specific postsynaptic receptors, initiating a series of complex events which include changes in membrane permeability to specific ions and cyclic AMP formation. The latter, in turn, facilitates other intracellular processes. There also is some evidence for presynaptic receptors, which may alter dopamine synthesis as a function of synaptic activity. The neuronal signal is terminated when dopamine is cleared from the synaptic cleft, primarily through an active re-uptake mechanism which returns it to the presynaptic terminal, where it is either metabolized by monoamine oxidase (MAO) or restored in vesicles for future use
(Barchas *et al.*, 1978; reproduced with permission)

Electrical depolarization of the presynaptic membrane starts a chain of events which results in the release of dopamine into the synaptic cleft, where the transmitter interacts with specific membrane receptors in a 'lock-and-key' fashion. Interaction with postsynaptic receptors is thought to produce conformational changes in the receptor. These, in turn, affect membrane ion permeability to cause either depolarization or hyperpolarization, thus altering the electrical activity of the postsynaptic neuron. For dopamine, receptor activation also initiates a complex series of intracellular events which are mediated by the synthesis of cyclic adenosine monophosphate (cyclic AMP) (Greengard, 1976). The purpose of many of these events remains to be determined. There also appear to be presynaptic receptors for dopamine which probably are part of a feedback loop to regulate neuronal activity.

Signal termination requires removal of the transmitter from the synaptic cleft. This occurs partially as a result of passive diffusion out of the cleft and of extraneuronal metabolism. But, as is true for several other neurotransmitters, dopamine also has a specific re-uptake mechanism in the presynaptic membrane which rapidly returns most of the transmitter back to the presynaptic terminal. It then is either stored again in vesicles for later re-use or destroyed enzymatically.

Neuromodulation

The concept of neuromodulation is relatively new and remains difficult to define precisely. As noted earlier, it arises from the discovery of an increasing number of endogenous neuroactive substances which do not seem to satisfy the criteria described for a neurotransmitter. Their existence clearly suggests the possibility that the brain utilizes compounds which do not act by conveying a signal from a pre- to a postsynaptic neuron but which nevertheless profoundly and specifically affect neuronal function. Table 3 lists a preliminary set of criteria by which such substances might be identified.

Table 3   Criteria for establishing the identity of a neuromodulator in the central nervous system

- The substance must permit sensitive and specific modulation of *inter*neuronal signals, rather than being involved mainly in an *intra*neuronal process such as cell catabolism or ion balance
- The substance must be present in physiological fluids and must have access to the presumed modulatory site in physiologically relevant concentrations
- Both direct application of the substance and alteration of its endogenous concentration should affect neuronal activity consistently and predictably
- The substance should have one or more specific sites of action through which it can alter neuronal activity incrementally as a function of its concentration
- Inactivating mechanisms should account for the time course of neuronal effects produced by endogenously or exogenously induced changes in concentrations of the substance
- Interventions which alter the neuronal effects of increasing the endogenous concentrations of the substance also should alter the neuronal effects of its exogenous administration
- A neuromodulator may be either hormonal or synaptic, as defined in Table 1

Modified from Barchas *et al.*, 1978

We suggest the term 'hormonal neuromodulators' for those substance which regulate neuronal activity at locations that are relatively distant from their release site. An hormonal neuromodulator might be released from neurons, glia, true secretory cells, or other tissue sources; and it might have widespread effects throughout the brain, either via specific synaptic or non-synaptic receptors or at specific steps in neurotransmitter regulation (Figure 2). In contrast to the short action of neurotransmitters, the effects of an hormonal neuromodulator might be quite prolonged, altering the baseline activity of spontaneously firing neurons or affecting responses to other neuronal input. Such a system could provide precise modulation of the activity of an entire neuronal system. Recent descriptions of corticosteroid receptors (McEwen and Micco, 1980) suggest that, among other functions, adrenal steroids might have a role as hormonal neuromodulators. Similarly, both the wide distribution of its receptors within the brain and the long-lasting effects which follow its intraventricular injection would be consistent with such a role for *beta*-endorphin (Watson and Akil, 1980).

Synaptic neuromodulators may represent another important group of neuroactive compounds. These substances could affect neuronal function indirectly by modulating the activity of a neurotransmitter. Such neuromodulators need not have specific membrane receptors: neurotransmitter synthesis, release, receptor interactions, re-uptake and metabolism all provide

POTENTIAL SITES FOR NEUROMODULATION

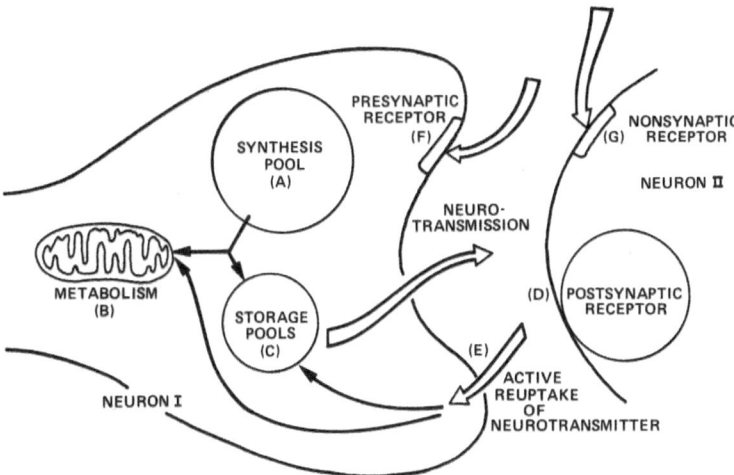

Figure 2 Possible sites of action for neuromodulators. Each letter indicates a potential site for synaptic or hormonal neuromodulation of neuronal activity:

A) Inhibition or stimulation of neurotransmitter synthesis
B) Blockade or induction of neurotransmitter metabolism
C) Interference with neurotransmitter storage, possibly by replacing it with a less active analogue, i.e. a 'false transmitter'
D) Competitive or non-competitive inhibition at postsynaptic neurotransmitter receptor sites
E) Blockade of re-uptake mechanisms
F) Competitive or non-competitive inhibition at presynaptic neurotransmitter receptor sites
G) Interaction with specific non-synaptic receptors which either affect basal neuronal activity or alter neuronal responsiveness to other neuronal input

potential sites of action (Figure 2). Although we know of no clear example of a synaptic neuromodulator at this time, it is interesting that some neurons do appear to contain more than one neuroregulator, an apparent violation of Dale's Principle (Watson and Akil, 1980; Brownstein *et al.*, 1974). Perhaps only one of those substances is a neurotransmitter, while the others are synaptic or hormonal neuromodulators.

CONCLUSIONS

Few would debate either the hardiness or the fruitfulness of the concept that chemical neurotransmitters mediate neuronal communication. It has provided impetus for the development of pharmacological agents which powerfully and selectively alter specific aspects of brain function. In addition, it provides a paradigm from which a variety of interesting and challenging hypotheses about possible biochemical causes of severe mental disorders have developed (de Wied, 1980; Berger, 1978). For that reason, it is reasonable to ask why one would wish to modify that concept. We believe that there are at least two compelling reasons to propose such a modification.

First, the increasing number of endogenous substances which appear not to be classical neurotransmitters and yet markedly affect neuronal activity strongly argue the need for a broader nomenclature. We still know distressingly little about most of these compounds, although improvements in research technologies continue to enhance our ability both to study their synthesis, distribution, release and catabolism and to examine their relationship to behaviour. A clearly defined nomenclature, based on possible functions of such compounds, should facilitate discussion about them and focus research efforts on ways to enhance our understanding of the mechanisms by which they contribute to the regulation of brain activity.

Second, it is at least possible that preoccupation with the importance of neurotransmission has tended to overshadow other potentially valuable avenues of research. Thus, we already have mentioned Dale's Principle, which proposes that a single neuron contains, at most, one neurotransmitter. The broader concept of neuroregulation suggests an interesting new dimension to that postulate. For example, suppose that a neurotransmitter and a long-acting hormonal neuromodulator could co-exist in neurons of a specific neuronal tract. With sporadic firing, the activity of the neurotransmitter would predominate. But, with frequent or prolonged firing, the neuromodulator could begin to accumulate and spread throughout the neuronal tract, where it might interact with its receptors to alter the reactivity of the entire system to subsequent input. Thus, without violating Dale's Principle, one can suggest a mechanism by which brief and prolonged neuronal firing could produce exactly opposite effects. To date, no-one has demonstrated that such a dual system exists, but previously cited examples of multiple neuroregulators within a single neuron at least are consistent with such a possibility.

Thus, we suggest that the adoption of a new nomenclature for the many neuroregulators in the brain might be both practical and heuristic. On the one hand, by defining substances according to function, the system emphasizes the wide variety of mechanisms by which neuroregulators can affect inter-neuronal communication. On the other hand, by postulating that neuro-transmitters and neuromodulators have distinct but interlocking functions, it raises the possibility that attempts to characterize a neuronal system cannot be restricted to studies of a single neuroregulator. Instead, it may be necessary to examine several neuroregulators simultaneously, particularly when attempt-ing to identify the neuronal substrates of the complex events which underlie normal behavioural or mental disease. Such studies will test the limits of available technology and often may require further refinements in data acquisition and interpretation. However, the wealth of new information which should result will offer a rich milieu for continuing efforts to understand both normal and abnormal brain function.

Acknowledgements

We would like to thank Drs Huda Akil, Philip A. Berger, R. Bruce Holman and Stanley Watson for helpful discussions about this topic. We are most appreciative of the gracious encouragement we received from Professor David de Wied in the preparation of this paper. Our work has been primarily supported by NIMH Program-Project MH23861.

References

Barchas. J. D., Akil, H., Elliott, G. R., Holman, R. B. and Watson, S. J. (1978). Behavioral neurochemistry: neuroregulators and behavioral states. *Science*, **200**, 964

Berger, P. A. (1978). Medical treatment of mental illness. *Science*, **200**, 974

Brownstein, M. J., Saavedra, J. M., Axelrod, J., Zehman, G. H. and Carpenter, D. O. (1974). Coexistence of several putative neurotransmitters in single identified neurons of Aplysia. *Proc. Natl. Acad. Sci. USA*, **71**, 4662

Cannon, W. B. and Uridil, J. E. (1921). Studies on the conditions of activity in endocrine glands. VIII. Some effects on the denervated heart of stimulating the nerves of the liver. *Am. J. Physiol.*, **58**, 353

Cooper, J. R., Bloom, F. E. and Roth, R. H. (1978). *The Biochemical Basis of Neuro-pharmacology*. 3rd Edn. (New York: Oxford University Press)

Curtis, D. R. and Eccles, R. M. (1958). The effect of diffusional barriers upon the pharmacology of cells within the central nervous system. *J. Physiol. (Lond.)*, **141**, 446

Eccles, J. C. (1948). Conduction and synaptic transmission in the nervous system. *Ann. Rev. Physiol.*, **10**, 93

Elliott, T. R. (1904). On the action of adrenalin. *J. Physiol. (Lond.)*, **31**, 20

von Euler, U. S. (1956). *Noradrenalin: Chemistry, Physiology, Pharmacology, and Clinical Aspects*. (Springfield: Charles C. Thomas)

Fatt, P. and Katz, B. (1951). An analysis of the end-plate potential recorded with an intra-cellular electrode. *J. Physiol. (Lond.)*, **115**, 320

Greengard, P. (1976). Possible role for cyclic nucleotides and phosphorylated membrane proteins in postsynaptic actions of neurotransmitters. *Nature (Lond.)*, **260**, 101

Loewi, O. (1921). Ueber humorale Uebertragbarkeit der Herznervenwirkung. *Arch. Gen. Physiol.*, **189**, 239

McEwen, B. S. and Micco, D. J. (1980). Toward an understanding of the multiplicity of glucocorticoid actions on brain function and behaviour. In D. de Wied and P. A. van Keep (eds.), *Hormones and the Brain*. (Lancaster: MTP Press)

Vogt, M. (1954). The concentration of sympathin in different parts of the central nervous system under normal conditions and after administration of drugs. *J. Physiol. (Lond.)*, **123**, 451

Watson, S. J. and Akil, H. (1980). On the multiplicity of active substances in single neurons: β-endorphin and α-melanocyte stimulating hormone as a model system. In D. de Wied and P. A. van Keep (eds.), *Hormones and the Brain*. (Lancaster: MTP Press)

de Wied, D. (1980). Peptides and adaptive behaviour. In D. de Wied and P. A. van Keep (eds.), *Hormones and the Brain*. (Lancaster: MTP Press)

Address for correspondence

Dr J. D. Barchas, Nancy Friend Pritzker Professor, Department of Psychiatry and Behavioral Sciences, Stanford University School of Medicine, Stanford, CA 94305, USA

1.5
Cholecystokinin and bradykinin: putative peptide neurotransmitters

R. B. INNIS and S. H. SNYDER

ABSTRACT

Cholecystokinin (CCK) and bradykinin are two peptides which have joined the rapidly expanding group of putative peptide neurotransmitters. CCK, originally identified as an intestinal hormone, is found in mammalian brain in high concentrations. Immunofluorescence staining of rat brain shows an extensive distribution of CCK-8-like immunoreactivity. Particularly dense collections of positively stained cell bodies occur in dorsal and perirhinal cortices, hippocampus, hypothalamus and periaqueductal grey. One can speculate that CCK's role in feeding is mediated by the neuronal systems in the hypothalamus. Bradykinin is a nonapeptide first found in mammalian blood and subsequently shown to be involved in inflammation and pain generation. Bradykinin-like immunoreactivity in rat brain was found in neuronal cell bodies only in the hypothalamus or closely adjacent regions. Positively stained fibres in the lateral septal area may mediate the hypertensive response elicited by the intracerebroventricular administration of bradykinin. Similarly, fibres in the periaqueductal grey may mediate the analgesic effect of centrally administered bradykinin.

INTRODUCTION

The identification first of opiate receptors and subsequently of opioid peptides in brain stimulated an already developing interest in peptides as neurotransmitters or modulators of information transfer in the brain. The number of putative peptide neurotransmitters has been increasing at an almost bewildering rate. In this paper we shall deal with cholecystokinin and bradykinin, which have been the subjects of recent investigation in our laboratory.

CHOLECYSTOKININ

Cholecystokinin (CCK) is an intestinal hormone which causes contraction of the gallbladder and secretion by the pancreas. It was originally found by Ivy *et al.* (1930) in extracts from duodenal mucosa as a substance which caused contraction of the gallbladder and was called cholecystokinin. Harper and Raper (1943) independently discovered a substance which caused secretion by the pancreas and called the substance pancreozymin. From analysis of their common biological actions and co-migration in all purification steps, Mutt and Jorpes (1968) correctly suggested that CCK and pancreozymin were, in fact, just one hormone. CCK is the more commonly used name. It has been isolated from porcine intestine as a triacontatriapeptide, CCK-33, which has been sequenced and synthesized (Ondetti *et al.*, 1970).

Vanderhaeghen *et al.* (1975) discovered a peptide from boiling water extracts of vertebrate brain which reacted with antigastrin antibodies. Dockray (1976) was the first to recognize that this immunoreactivity is actually due to CCK and that the cross-reactivity derives from the identical C-terminal pentapeptide sequence shared by both gastrin and CCK. Muller, Straus and Yalow (1977) found two components in porcine cerebral cortex: one resembling intact CCK-33 and the other resembling the C-terminal octapeptide of CCK (CCK-8). Using several different antisera, Rehfeld (1978) has studied the distribution of the molecular forms of CCK in the central nervous system and small intestine of man. In both tissues the predominant molecular form is CCK-8 (80% of cerebral immunoreactivity and 60% of intestinal immunoreactivity is due to CCK-8). The second most abundant form corresponds to the C-terminal tetrapeptide, with only a small percentage of immunoreactivity due to CCK-33. Only the posterior pituitary contains any immunoreactive gastrin. Among different brain regions, the cerebral cortex contains by far the highest concentration of CCK-8 (200–2300 pmol/g tissue). Considering the large size of human cerebral cortex one can make the startling calculation that the human brain contains 1–2 mg CCK-8, whereas other hormonal peptides are often present in microgram amounts.

Pinget, Straus and Yalow (1978) have found with subcellular fractionation of rat cerebral cortex immunoreactive CCK in the pellet identified by electron

microscopy as containing a high proportion of synaptic vesicles. Straus *et al.*
(1977) have also demonstrated by peroxidase-antiperoxidase immunohistochemistry the presence of CCK-8-like immunoreactivity in rabbit cerebral
cortex. Their photomicrographs lack enough clarity to say whether neurons
and/or glia show positive staining. In addition, important control experiments
(for example, preadsorption of the antisera with CCK-8) were not reported.
Innis *et al.* (1979) have used the indirect immunohistofluorescence technique
to study the distribution of CCK-8 in the rat brain. The details of the
technique have been described elsewhere (Innis *et al.*, 1979). Basically, 15 μm
cryostat sections of formaldehyde fixed rat brain are sequentially incubated
first with a rabbit anti-CCK-8 antiserum and then with a fluorescein con-
jugated guinea-pig anti-rabbit IgG. The antiserum which is not bound to
CCK-8 fixed in the tissue section is washed away. One may then observe the
distribution of staining under a fluorescence microscope.

By far the most important question with regard to the technique of
immunohistochemistry is that of specificity. One can never prove that the
staining results from the target antigen. However, the specificity of staining
can be supported by a variety of criteria. First, the staining we observe is
localized to neuronal cell bodies, fibres and apparent terminal varicosities.
The staining is not due, therefore, to cross-reactivity to a substance diffusely
present in rat brain. Secondly, two different antisera to CCK-8 give virtually
identical results. Thirdly, preadsorption of the primary antisera with a wide
variety of unrelated peptides (bradykinin, neurotensin, met-enkephalin, leu-
enkephalin, angiotensin II, Substance P, secretin or bovine serum albumin) up
to 400 μmol/l does not eliminate the staining. Fourthly, preadsorption of the
primary antiserum with CCK-8 at 10–400 μmol/l overnight at 4°C almost
totally eliminates the staining. Because gastrin shares the same C-terminal
pentapeptide sequence with CCK-8, preadsorption with gastrin or penta-
gastrin (10–400 μmol/l) also eliminates the immunofluorescence. The evidence
that this staining reflects cholecystokinin rather than gastrin derives from the
elegant work of Muller, Straus and Yalow (1977) and Rehfeld (1978). They
have shown with several different antisera and gel filtration techniques that
the vast majority of immunoreactivity in brain is due to CCK-8. Nevertheless,
the positive staining could be due to precursors or other closely related
antigens. Although we should speak of CCK-8-like immunoreactivity, we will
merely refer to it as CCK-8. Throughout the rat brain we and others have
localized CCK-8 to neuronal cells, fibres and terminals (Larsson and Rehfeld,
1979; Loren *et al.*, 1979). Pretreatment of rats with colchicine to block axonal
flow facilitated detection of CCK-8 in neuronal cells.

We failed to detect CCK-8 in the spinal cord, cerebellar cortex and nuclear
regions, pituitary, pineal gland or medulla oblongata-pons, although Loren *et
al.* (1979) have noted apparent CCK fibres concentrated in the parabrachial
nuclei, and the gracilis, cuneate and solitary nuclei. In the metencephalon, a
dense group of CCK-8 cells occurred in the midline of the caudal dorsal raphe

nucleus and extended laterally for a short distance just ventral to the dorsal tegmental nucleus of Gudden. Fibres emerging from these cells passed over the medial longitudinal fasciculus. Fibres at this level were also noted in the ventral boundary of the midbrain.

The most densely packed collection of CCK-8 cells occurred in the peri-aqueductal grey, especially at the level of the exit of cranial nerve III (Figure 1). Somewhat ventral to this zone, a group of cells occurred overlying the interstitial nucleus of the ventral tegmental decussation.

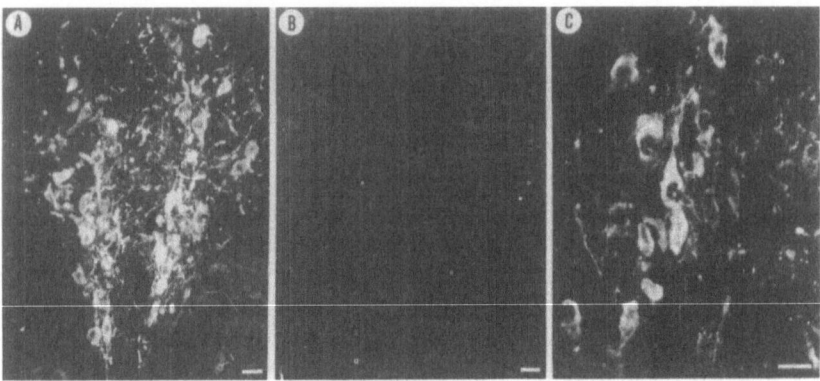

Figure 1   Immunohistofluorescence micrographs of CCK-8 cells and fibres in the ventral peri-aqueductal area. (A and B) The anatomical midline is located vertically in the centre of the picture with the aqueduct above the photographic field. These are serial sections, but in B the primary antiserum was preadsorbed with CCK-8. (C) Higher power magnification of the cluster. Bars = 20 μm

Within the hypothalamus, cells with associated fibres were concentrated in the dorsomedial nucleus. Cells were also detected in the periventricular nucleus from which dense fibres projected both ventrally and dorsally.

One of the most striking features of CCK-8 and vasoactive intestinal peptide (VIP) is their high concentration in the cerebral cortex, where most other peptides occur only in low levels. We observed CCK-8 cells most prominently in the pyriform cerebral cortex in the vicinity of the rhinal sulcus and in dorsal cerebral cortex (Figure 2; Table 1). The cells were noted throughout layers II–VI, but were most concentrated in layers II and III. Fibres emerging from these cells were oriented radially with respect to the surface of the cerebral cortex. CCK-8 cells and fibres were also noted in the hippocampus. The cells were confined to a narrow band in the pyramidal cell layer. The dentate gyrus appeared devoid of CCK-8.

Within the amygdala, fibres of considerable density were ubiquitous. However, the highest density of fibres was localized to the central nucleus. Interestingly, though the central nucleus is one of the smallest subdivisions of the amygdala it has the highest concentration of enkephalin and neurotensin as well as CCK-8 and also receives a uniquely dense projection of dopamine nerve terminals. Despite the considerable numbers of CCK-8 fibres in the amygdala, no cells were detected.

While the concentration of CCK-8 in the amygdala resembles the distribution of enkephalin, CCK-8 could not be detected in the basal ganglia, where high concentrations of enkephalin exist. Loren et al. (1979) did observe CCK fibres in the rat caudate. A moderate amount of CCK-8 fibres was observed in the lateral septal area and more ventrally in the diagonal tract of Broca.

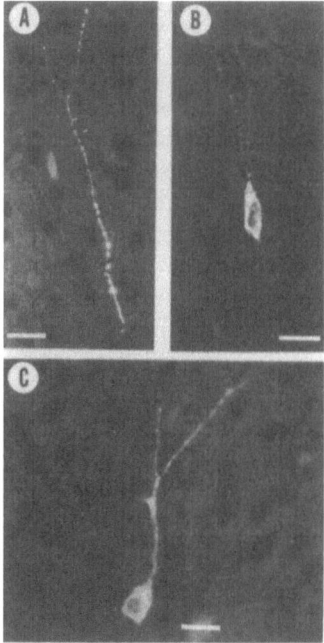

Figure 2 Fluorescence micrographs of CCK-8 cells and fibres from the telencephalon. (A) Varicose fibre oriented radially to the surface of the brain, traversing cortical layer III and then branching in layer II. (B) Typical radially oriented cortical neuron. There is a single inferior process, and the superior process branches close to its contact with the cell body. (C) Cortical neuron from layer III of anterior cingulate cortex. Bars = 20 μm

Table 1 **Areas of rat CNS enriched in cholecystokinin immunoreactivity**

	Cell bodies	Fibres
Cortex (perirhinal, dorsal)	+ +	+ +
Amygdala (central nucleus)	—	+ + +
Hippocampus	+ +	+
Hypothalamus (dorsomedial and periventricular n.)	+ + +	+ +
Periaqueductal grey	+ + +	+ +
Pons (caudal dorsal raphe)	+ +	+

It is unclear just what functions may be served by CCK-8 neurons. One can speculate that the cells in the periaqueductal grey are involved in pain perception, a function associated with this region of the brain. CCK has been implicated in feeding behaviour and conceivably the CCK-8 neurons in the medial hypothalamus, a well known 'feeding centre', might be related to such a role. Perhaps the CCK-8 in the amygdala and parts of the cerebral cortex related to the limbic system play a role in emotional regulation.

BRADYKININ

Bradykinin is a 9-amino acid peptide, first found in mammalian blood and subsequently shown to be involved in several pathophysiological conditions, including inflammation, pain generation, cardiovascular shock and hypertension. A variety of evidence suggests possible roles for bradykinin-like systems in mammalian brain. Bradykinin injections into highly specific areas produce a variety of marked autonomic alterations. Injections of bradykinin into the lateral ventricle of rats raise blood pressure, and these effects are abolished by lateral septal lesions and reproduced by injections directly into the lateral septal area (Correa and Graeff, 1976). Injections of bradykinin close to the periaqueductal grey elicit analgesia (Ribeiro et al., 1971). Moreover, injection of bradykinin in the medial and anterior hypothalamus is associated with hyperthermia (unpublished observations). Bioassay had suggested the existence of bradykinin-like substances in mammalian brain. Recently, using bradykinin antisera of high titre, we have obtained evidence from immunohistochemical studies visualizing bradykinin-like immuno-reactivity in the brain (Correa et al., 1979). Antisera were raised in rabbits to bradykinin coupled to hemocyanin with glutaraldehyde. The antiserum has a high titre in radioimmunoassay, binding about 30% of ^{125}I-tyr$_8$-bradykinin at 1:12,800 dilution. The radioimmunoassay is quite sensitive, eliciting 50% displacement of ^{125}I-tyr$_8$-bradykinin binding at 1 nmol/l unlabelled brady-kinin. The antiserum is highly specific. Lysyl-bradykinin and methionyl-lysyl-bradykinin are 25–50% as potent as bradykinin itself in competing for binding, while a large number of other peptides have no effect in concentrations as high as 10 μmol/l. Brain extracts fractionated by a variety of procedures display material which reacts with bradykinin antisera, elicits effects upon smooth muscle preparations essentially the same as does authentic bradykinin, and migrates in various column chromatographic procedures similarly to bradykinin (unpublished observations).

Besides the biochemical evidence for endogenous bradykinin in the brain, immunohistochemical studies reveal a system of bradykinin containing neurons (Correa et al., 1979) (Table 2). Pretreatment of rats with colchicine permits localization of bradykinin containing cells as well as fibres and terminals. All observed specific bradykinin fluorescence is abolished by preadsorption with bradykinin but not by preadsorption with a variety of other peptides (Figure 3). Identical histochemical patterns are observed with two different bradykinin antisera which have different relative affinities for bradykinin and bradykinin analogues.

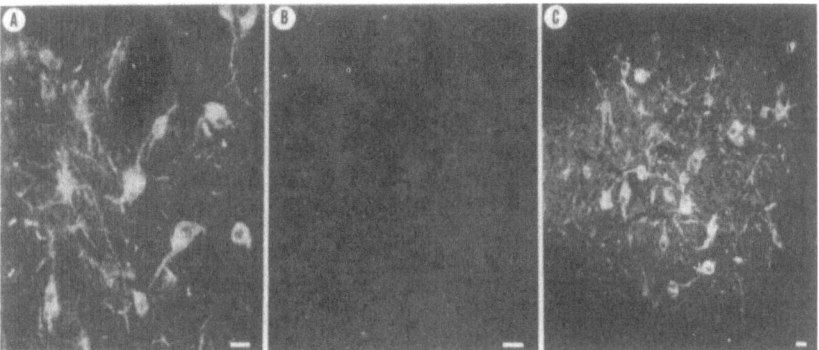

Figure 3 Immunofluorescence micrographs of bradykinin fibres and cell bodies in the dorsomedial nucleus of the hypothalamus. (A) Immunofluorescence located in the cytoplasm of cells and extending in fibres from the perikarya. (B) The almost complete elimination of fluorescence when the primary antiserum has been preadsorbed with 15 μM bradykinin. (C) Bradykinin-positive cells and fibres just lateral to the dorsomedial nucleus of the hypothalamus. Bars = 20 μm

Table 2 **Distribution of bradykinin-like immunohistofluorescence in rat CNS**

Area	Fibres	Cell bodies
Spinal cord	—	—
Medulla	—	—
Mesencephalon	+	—
Hypothalamus		
(i) posterior	+	+
(ii) medial	+ + + +	+ + +
(iii) lateral/z. incerta	+	+ +
(iv) anterior	+ +	+
Thalamus	+	+
Lateral septal area	+ +	—
Caudate/pallidum	+	—
Cortex	+ + +	—

Unlike neurotensin and enkephalin, no bradykinin fluorescence is observed in the spinal cord or lower brainstem. In the pons and midbrain over the entire length of the periaqueductal grey, modest numbers of bradykinin fibres are observed. The only bradykinin containing cells in the central nervous system are contained in the hypothalamus (Figures 3 and 4). The highest density of bradykinin cells is in the medial hypothalamus close to the midline. Fibres pass from the hypothalamus to localize over the ventrolateral border of the medial forebrain bundle, the pyriform cortex and the cingulate gyrus. More anteriorly, fibres occur near the midline of the preoptic area as well as over the lateral portion of the medial forebrain bundle and the most ventral portion of the globus pallidus. At precommissural levels, fibres pass throughout the lateral septal area. A few fibres are also observed in the ventral portion of the caudate-putamen.

Though the localization of bradykinin does not involve as many structures associated with pain perception as is the case for neurotensin and enkephalin, the region of the periaqueductal grey might represent an area where brady-kinin could be involved in pain integration. It is at the periaqueductal grey that bradykinin injection elicits analgesia. It is conceivable that the bradykinin neurons in the lateral septum play a role in blood pressure regulations, since bradykinin injection in this area specifically elevates blood pressure.

In summary, there is evidence that a variety of peptides in the brain play a role in integrating information about pain. Substance P and enkephalin are

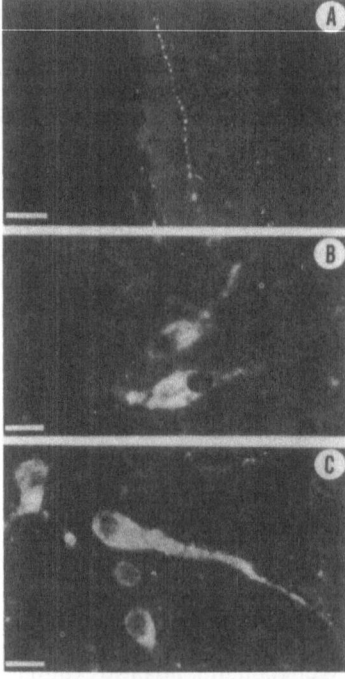

Figure 4   Immunofluorescence micrographs of bradykinin. (A) A varicose fibre in layer I of perirhinal cortex. The varicosities are large and prominent with short intervaricose segments. (B) Two positively stained perikarya from lateral hypothalamus. (C) A positively stained neuron in the lateral hypothalamus with fluorescence extending into a wide and long process. Bars = 20 μm

the most clear-cut candidates. However, neurotensin seems as likely to be involved as enkephalin. Indeed, one might suggest that drugs mimicking neurotensin would afford potent analgesic actions. We do not know whether tolerance develops to the analgesic effects of neurotensin. However, the fact that neurotensin analgesia is not blocked by naloxone indicates that it is not associated with the opiate-like addictive system. The evidence for a role of bradykinin in pain perception is weaker than for the other peptides. Interestingly, in the periphery bradykinin is an extraordinarily potent pain stimulus. Perhaps the economy of nature results in bradykinin also playing a role in pain processing in the central nervous system. Analogously, norepinephrine is a transmitter of the peripheral sympathetic nervous system and in the brain seems to be involved in similar functions.

Acknowledgements

Supported by USPHS grant DA-00266 and a grant of the McKnight Foundation. Collaborators in these studies were Fernando M. A. Correa, George Uhl and Bruce Schneider. Robert B. Innis is the recipient of a stipend from The Insurance Medical Scientist Scholarship Training Fund sponsored by Mutual of Omaha.

References

Correa, F. M. A. and Graeff, F. G. (1976). On the mechanism of the hypertensive action of intraseptal bradykinin in the rat. *Neuropharmacology*, **15**, 713

Correa, F. M. A., Innis, R. B., Uhl, G. R. and Snyder, S. H. (1979). Bradykinin-like immunoreactive neuronal systems localized histochemically in rat brain. *Proc. Natl. Acad. Sci., USA*, **76**, 1489

Dockray, G. J. (1976). Immunochemical evidence of cholecystokinin-like peptides in brain. *Nature*, **264**, 568

Harper, A. A. and Raper, H. S. (1943). Pancreozymin, a stimulant of the secretion of pancreatic enzymes in extracts of the small intestine. *J. Physiol.*, **102**, 115

Innis, R. B., Correa, F. M. A., Uhl, G. R., Schneider, B. and Snyder, S. H. (1979). Cholecystokinin octapeptide-like immunoreactivity: histochemical localization in rat brain. *Proc. Natl. Acad. Sci., USA*, **76**, 521

Ivy, A. C., Kloster, H. M., Lueth, H. C. and Drewyer, G. E. (1930). On the preparation of cholecystokinin. *Am. J. Physiol.*, **91**, 336

Larsson, L. I. and Rehfeld, J. F. (1979). Localization and molecular heterogeneity of cholecystokinin in the central and peripheral nervous system. *Brain Res.*, **165**, 201

Loren, L. I., Alumets, J., Hakanson, R. and Sundler, F. (1979). Distribution of gastrin and CCK-like peptides in rat brain. *Histochemistry*, **59**, 249

Muller, J. E., Straus, E. and Yalow, R. S. (1977). Cholecystokinin and its COOH-terminal octapeptide in the pig brain. *Proc. Natl. Acad. Sci., USA*, **74**, 3035

Mutt, V. and Jorpes, S. E. (1968). Structure of porcine cholecystokinin-pancreozymin. *Eur. J. Biochem.*, **6**, 156

Ondetti, M. A., Pluscec, J., Sabo, E. F., Sheehan, J. T. and Williams, M. (1970). Synthesis of cholecystokinin-pancreozymin. *J. Am. Chem. Soc.*, **92**, 195

Pinget, M., Straus, E. and Yalow, R. S. (1978). Localization of cholecystokinin-like immuno-reactivity in isolated nerve terminals. *Proc. Natl. Acad. Sci., USA*, **75**, 6324

Rehfeld, J. F. (1978). Immunochemical studies on cholecystokinin. *J. Biol. Chem.*, **253**, 4016

Ribeiro, S. A., Corrado, A. P. and Graeff, F. G. (1971). Antinociceptive action of intraventricular bradykinin. *Neuropharmacology*, **10**, 725

Straus, E., Muller, J. E., Choi, H., Paronetto, F. and Yalow, R. S. (1977). Immunohistochemical localization in rabbit brain of a peptide resembling the COOH-terminal octapeptide of cholecystokinin. *Proc. Natl. Acad. Sci., USA*, **74**, 3033

Vanderhaeghen, J. J., Signeau, J. C. and Gepts, W. (1975). New peptide in the vertebrate CNS reacting with antigastrin antibodies. *Nature*, **257**, 604

Address for correspondence

Dr R. B. Innis, The Johns Hopkins University School of Medicine, Department of Pharmacology and Experimental Therapeutics, 725 North Wolfe Street, Baltimore, MD 21205, USA

1.6
Growth hormone dependent polypeptides and the brain

V. R. SARA, K. HALL and L. WETTERBERG

ABSTRACT

Brain growth appears to be regulated by a growth hormone dependent growth factor called BGA (brain growth-promoting activity). A family of growth hormone dependent growth-promoting polypeptides has recently been isolated from serum. These hormones, the somatomedins, are believed to develop from a common embryonic form to the slightly different polypeptides found in the adult circulation. BGA appears to be the embryonic somatomedin and, until its isolation is complete, one of the adult forms, somatomedin A (SMA), has been used. SMA has a direct growth-promoting action on cultured fetal brain cells. Specific SMA binding sites are found in both human and rat brain. In the human fetus, there is an increase in specific SMA binding to brain plasma membranes during the rapid growth phase. In the rat, the concentration of SMA binding sites is increased in the growing fetal brain. Animal studies reveal a significant relationship between circulating levels of BGA and brain growth *in vivo*. The presence of specific SMA binding sites on mature brain tissue indicates a role in adult brain function. Significant amounts of BGA are found in cerebrospinal fluid. Administration of SMA to hypophysectomized rats stimulates labelled amino acid uptake into brain protein. Such findings led to the proposal that BGA is the growth and maintenance hormone for the brain.

The development of the nervous system follows a complex pattern leading to the formation of an intricate network of connections between billions of cells. The maintenance of these cells and their pattern of connectivity provides one of the most crucial functions throughout life. It has become apparent that the formation of the nervous system is guided by trophic factors which interact with the genetic information. The pioneering work of Levi-Montalcini led to the identification of the first such neurotrophin, nerve-growth factor (NGF), which appears to be the growth and maintenance factor for the sympathetic nervous system (Levi-Montalcini and Calissana, 1979). Apart from embryonic sensory ganglion cells, NGF has a selective action on sympathetic neurones and does not appear to be involved in the development of any other neural tissue. It is likely that there are several neurotrophins which have specific neural targets.

The existence of a specific brain trophin was first suggested as a mechanism to explain the stimulation of fetal brain growth following maternal growth hormone administration (Sara *et al.*, 1974). Cultured rat or human fetal brain cells, consisting of dividing stem cells and neuroblasts in varying stages of differentiation, have been used to identify this trophic factor (Sara *et al.*, 1976). Brain cell proliferation is stimulated by a serum factor which is heat stable and non-dialysable. This effect is not due to any available hormone, such as growth hormone, insulin, thyroid or steroid hormones, or to any growth factor, such as NGF, fibroblast growth factor or epidermal growth factor, as their addition to the medium does not evoke a proliferative response. The brain trophin is operationally defined as brain growth-promoting activity (BGA) until it can be completely characterized. The serum concentration of BGA can be determined by bioassay and recently by radioreceptor assay. Although growth hormone has no direct effect on the brain cells, serum BGA is growth hormone dependent in adults. The low serum values found after hypophysectomy, or in growth hormone deficiency, can be restored by growth hormone administration. Elevated serum values are found in acromegalic patients.

In recent years a group of growth-promoting polypeptides which are growth hormone dependent has been purified from human plasma. This family of multitargetal polypeptides is termed the somatomedins (Hall *et al.*, 1979). The somatomedins stimulate glucose and amino acid uptake, protein, RNA and DNA synthesis, and cell proliferation in their target cells. At present four such polypeptides with molecular weights of approximately 7000–8000 have been purified: somatomedin A (SMA), somatomedin C (SMC), insulin-like growth factor 1 (IGF 1) and insulin-like growth factor 2 (IGF 2). A similar group of polypeptides, termed multiplication stimulating activity (MSA), has been purified from rat liver cell-conditioned medium. The somatomedins probably contain a common biologically active sequence, as each polypeptide can compete with the others for their binding sites on the plasma membrane.

It is proposed that the somatomedins develop from a common embryonic form and differentiate to slightly different chemical structures which display preferential target tissues (Hall *et al.*, 1979). A parallel development in receptor specificity would be expected as the cell differentiates (Figure 1). Current studies are aimed at identifying BGA. Brain growth occurs rapidly during fetal development and thus BGA is probably the embryonic form of the somatomedins. Fetal serum is required as the source for BGA isolation. Until this is achieved, SMA, purified from adult human plasma, is used to give an indication of somatomedin action on the brain. SMA acts as a potent mitogen for fetal brain cells *in vitro* (Sara *et al.*, unpublished observation). The addition of an impure SMA preparation to the culture medium stimulates DNA synthesis in brain cells taken from fetal rats at day 18 of gestation.

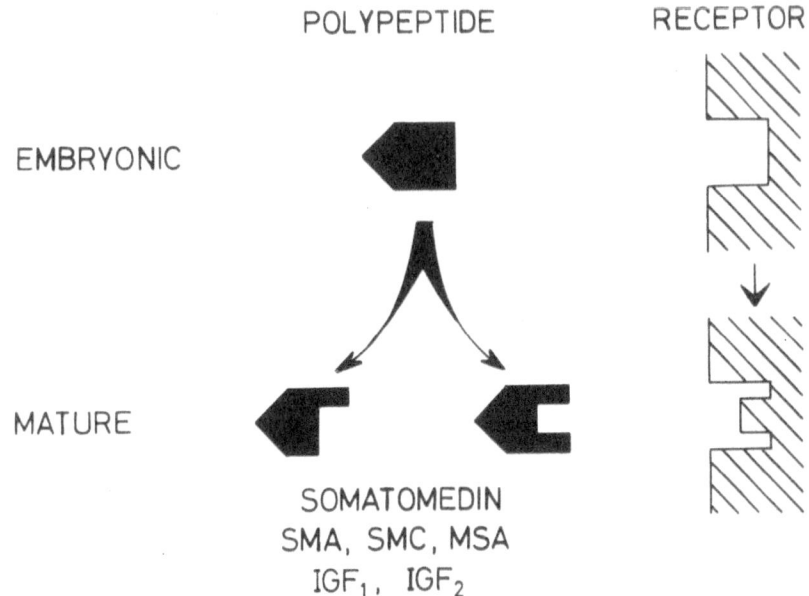

POLYPEPTIDE   RECEPTOR

EMBRYONIC

MATURE

SOMATOMEDIN
SMA, SMC, MSA
IGF_1, IGF_2

Figure 1 Hypothetical development of the somatomedins and their receptors from a common embryonic form

A significant stimulation of tritiated thymidine uptake into DNA is found with a concentration of 20 ng/ml. A similar stimulation has been observed in brain cells from human fetuses between 12–24 weeks of gestational age. SMA is the only polypeptide used which has stimulated fetal brain cell proliferation. During purification from adult human plasma, BGA is found in only the fraction containing SMA and similarly sized polypeptides with a neutral iso-electric point.

The first stage in the biological action of a polypeptide hormone is its binding to specific receptor sites on the plasma membrane of the target cell.

Specific binding sites for SMA have been shown to exist in the brain of both man and rat (Sara *et al.*, unpublished observation). Human fetuses have been obtained after legal prostaglandin abortion. Particulate plasma membranes were prepared from the brains by stepwise ultracentrifugation. The SMA used for labelling and displacement was pure according to gel chromatography, electrophoresis and *N*-terminal analysis (Fryklund *et al.*, 1978). SMA was labelled by the lactoperoxidase method. Labelled SMA was bound to human fetal brain membranes and was readily displaced by pure SMA in concentrations between 3 and 100 ng/ml (Figure 2). A less pure SMA preparation was

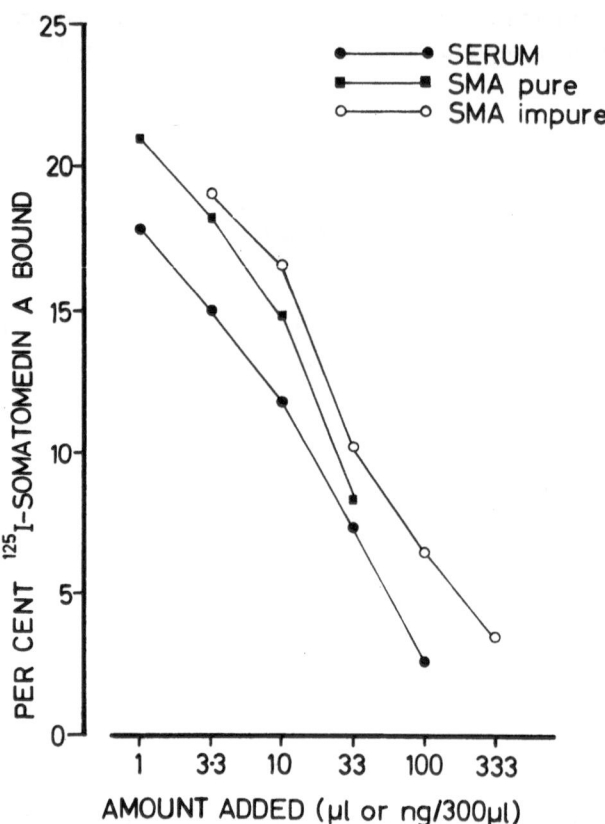

Figure 2   Displacement of ^{125}I-SMA bound to human fetal brain plasma membrane by the polypeptide SMA and a less pure SMA preparation. Displacement by human reference serum is shown

used at higher concentrations. Normal human serum causes a parallel dose-dependent displacement of ^{125}I-SMA bound to the brain membrane and is used as a reference due to the lack of stability displayed by pure SMA. Of all hormones examined, including NGF, only MSA competed with SMA for its binding sites. High unphysiological concentrations of insulin and proinsulin caused some degree of displacement. Human fetal brain membrane is now used as the matrix and SMA as the ligand in a radioreceptor assay to detect BGA.

The age-dependent variation in ^{125}I-SMA binding to human fetal brain plasma membrane is shown in Figure 3. The total specific binding of ^{125}I-SMA rose between 16 and 19 weeks and had declined at 26 weeks gestational age. This pattern corresponds to the early brain growth spurt described in the human by Dobbing and Sands (1973) as a period of rapid neuronal multiplication occurring between 10 and 18 weeks gestational age. In the rat, the total specific binding of ^{125}I-SMA is higher in the fetus at day 20 of gestation as compared to 50-day-old adults (Sara *et al.*, unpublished observation).

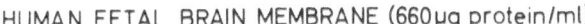

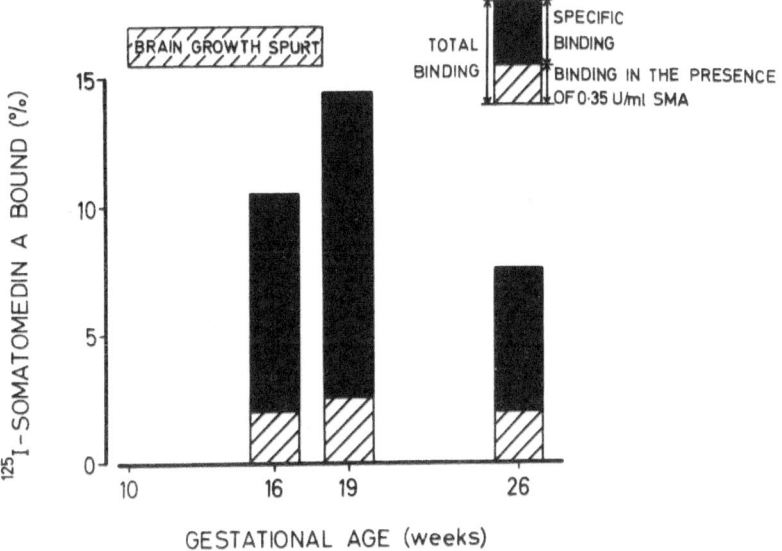

Figure 3 The binding of ^{125}I-SMA to brain plasma membranes prepared from human fetuses at different gestational ages. The period of rapid neuronal multiplication is indicated

Scatchard plots revealed the presence of at least two binding sites. There is no change in the affinity constant during development, but a greater concentration of SMA binding sites occurs in the fetus when brain growth is rapid. The high percentage binding of ^{125}I-SMA and its displacement by physiological amounts of SMA indicates the presence of receptors for SMA or a closely related polypeptide in the brain. These findings delineate the brain as a target organ for the somatomedins.

The presence of SMA binding sites in the adult brain suggests a much more extensive role in brain function. BGA may not only regulate brain development but may act as a maintenance factor for mature cells. Brain protein synthesis is reduced after hypophysectomy (Reith *et al.*, 1978). An impure SMA preparation produced a potent and rapid stimulation of labelled amino acid uptake into brain protein when given to hypophysectomized rats (Sara *et al.*, unpublished observation). Significant amounts of BGA are found in cerebrospinal fluid from adults. In patients with the 'empty sella' syndrome, the concentration of BGA determined by the human fetal brain radioreceptor assay was approximately 18% that found in normal adult human serum (Figure 4). These findings indicate that BGA is available to mature brain tissue, although the source of cerebrospinal fluid BGA has yet to be identified. The relationship between levels in blood, cerebrospinal fluid and brain tissue is not known.

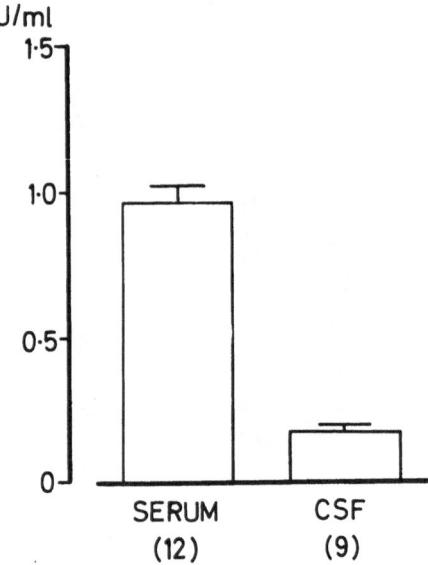

Figure 4   The BGA levels determined by the human fetal brain radioreceptor assay in serum from 12 healthy adult humans and cerebrospinal fluid from nine patients with the 'empty sella' syndrome. Results are given as the mean and standard error of the mean

The limited availability of pure somatomedins has restricted studies of their action *in vivo*. An alternative approach is provided by the use of experimental conditions which are known to alter somatomedin production. Several factors influence somatomedin levels in serum. In adults, the somatomedins are growth hormone dependent, but their production is also regulated by several other factors such as nutrition and possibly insulin (Hall *et al.*, 1979). During pregnancy, placental lactogen appears to replace growth hormone. In pregnant rats, normal somatomedin levels are maintained after hypophysectomy (Daughaday and Kapadia, 1978), although growth hormone still retains the ability to elicit a somatomedin response (Sara *et al.*, 1979b). In early life, the somatomedins are believed to be independent of growth hormone and to be regulated primarily by nutritional factors (Hall and Sara, 1978).

In animal studies, both growth hormone and nutrition have been used to examine the relationship between BGA and the brain. Daily administration of growth hormone to rats throughout the last trimester of pregnancy resulted in a threefold increase in bioassayable BGA (Sara *et al.*, 1979b). Fetuses removed from these mothers showed a significant increase in brain weight and cell proliferation when compared to those whose mothers received saline during gestation. Earlier results reported a similar enhancement of brain growth following maternal growth hormone administration for the last two trimesters of pregnancy (Sara and Lazarus, 1974; Sara *et al.*, 1974; Zamenhof *et al.*, 1971). When adult, these offspring displayed significant decrements in the number of trials taken to reach a learning criterion on a series of conditional discrimination tasks (Sara and Lazarus, 1974). It is difficult to attribute this increase in performance to motivational variables as neither latency measures nor the corticosterone response to stress was altered. Instead, it is suggested that the improved learning performance results from structural changes following BGA stimulation during the critical period of brain growth. A significant correlation between fetal brain cell proliferation and circulating levels of BGA during pregnancy has been obtained (Sara *et al.*, 1979b). Selective growth hormone deficiency induced by neonatal growth hormone antiserum administration results in impaired myelination and cell deficits in the adult brain (Williams Pelton *et al.*, 1977). Nutritional restrictions during early life impair brain development and later behaviour. Serum levels of immunoreactive SMA are reduced in the undernourished animals (Sara *et al.*, 1979a). Zamenhof has reported that the deficiencies resulting from maternal malnutrition may be prevented by the concomitant administration of growth hormone (Zamenhof *et al.*, 1966).

Few clinical studies have been concerned with the relationship between growth hormone and behaviour. No major behavioural abnormalities have been reported in patients with acromegaly or growth hormone deficiency. Critical psychological studies are required to examine the relation between adult somatomedin levels and behaviour. Gross behavioural disturbances arising from impaired brain development are not to be expected in such patients. Growth hormone regulation of somatomedin production begins some time after birth. Adequate BGA is presumably available during the critical brain growth period in fetal and early postnatal life. Laron dwarfs, on the other hand, fail to generate somatomedin in response to growth hormone and could be BGA deficient during the critical time of brain growth (Laron *et al.*, 1971). Reduced IQ scores have been reported in Laron dwarfs when compared to their normal siblings. The observed relationship between mental retardation and short stature supports the existence of some common mechanism (Mosier *et al.*, 1965).

The trophic factor for the brain has been identified and called BGA. Whether BGA's action is restricted to the central nervous system remains to be determined. The chemical nature of BGA has not yet been completely established, but appears to be either identical to SMA or to be a closely related polypeptide. Consequently, SMA may be used as ligand to detect BGA receptors on brain tissue. *In vitro* mitotic action, numerous receptor sites which relate to periods of rapid brain growth, and *in vivo* correlation with altered brain development after growth hormone administration or under-nutrition, provide evidence that BGA is the growth factor for the brain. However, the finding of binding sites on mature brain tissue, together with its presence in cerebrospinal fluid and biological action on amino acid uptake, suggests that BGA also plays a significant role in adult brain function.

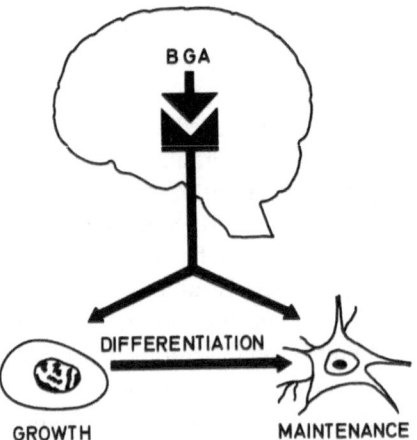

Figure 5 Schematic representation of the hypothesized role of BGA as the growth and maintenance factor for the brain.

Various pituitary hormones, particularly ACTH and vasopressin, have been demonstrated to influence adult brain function (de Wied, 1977). Growth hormone and its dependent polypeptides have not been implicated in these effects, but their ability to shift the dose-response curve of other hormones has not been examined. There is evidence that an anabolic polypeptide hormone, like the somatomedins, changes the plasma membranes to a more coupled state (Löw *et al.*, 1979). Consequently, the somatomedins should change cell sensitivity to cAMP-stimulating hormones such as ACTH. Presumably BGA acts in a similar way on mature brain cells and regulates their sensitivity to impinging neuroregulators. This suggests a new class of neuroactive substance which is not directly involved in the communication between nerve cells, but regulates the threshold of response and is essential for cell metabolism and survival. Such substances may be termed maintenance factors. NGF appears to be a maintenance factor for the sympathetic nervous system and it is suggested that BGA fulfils a similar function in the central nervous system. As schematically shown in Figure 5, we propose that BGA is the growth and maintenance factor for the brain. The elicited response will vary according to the state of differentiation of the brain target cell. In other tissues, like muscle and cartilage, the somatomedins act as mitotic factors on dividing cells, but as the cell differentiates they act as maintenance factors stimulating glucose and amino acid uptake and protein synthesis (Hall *et al.*, 1979).

Although BGA has not been completely characterized and its chemical structure determined, available evidence points to its inclusion in the somatomedin family of growth hormone dependent polypeptides. Two members of the somatomedin family, namely IGF 1 and IGF 2, share features of structural similarity with proinsulin (Blundell *et al.*, 1978). NGF also displays a structural homology with proinsulin. Possibly all these factors evolved from a common ancestral gene. BGA is a polypeptide which appears closely related, if not identical, to SMA. In all likelihood there are two forms of BGA—one embryonic form which is common to the somatomedin family and regulates growth, and one more differentiated form which occurs later and displays preferential specificity for brain tissue.

Acknowledgements

This work was supported by grants from the Swedish Medical Research Council (4224 and 5669). We are grateful to Dr Linda Fryklund, AB Kabi, for the purification of SMA.

References

Blundell, T. L., Bedarkar, S., Rinderknecht, E. and Humbel, R. E. (1978). Insulin-like growth factor: a model for tertiary structure accounting for immunoreactivity and receptor binding. *Proc. Natl. Acad. Sci., USA*, **75**, 180

Daughaday, W. H. and Kapadia, M. (1978). Maintenance of serum somatomedin activity in hypophysectomized pregnant rats. *Endocrinology*, **102**, 1317

Dobbing, J. and Sands, J. (1973). Quantitive growth and development of human brain. *Arch. Dis. Child.*, **48**, 757

Fryklund, L., Skottner, A. and Hall, K. (1978). Chemistry and biology of the somatomedins. In K. W. Kastrup and J. H. Nielsen (eds.), *Proc. 11th FEBS Meeting: Growth Factors*, **48**, p. 55. (Oxford: Pergamon Press)

Hall, K. and Sara, V. R. (1978). Significance of growth factors for fetal growth. In F. Naftolin (ed.), *Abnormal Fetal Growth: Biological Bases and Consequences*, p. 121. (Berlin: Dahlem Konferenzen)

* Hall, K., Sara, V., Enberg, G. and Fryklund, L. (1979). Somatomedins. *Proceedings 10th Congress of Int. Diabetes Fed. 1979*. (In press)

72

RECEPTORS AND PEPTIDERGIC PATHWAYS

Laron, Z., Pertzelan, A. and Frankel, J. (1971). Growth and development in the syndromes of familial isolated absence of hGH or pituitary dwarfism with high serum concentration of an immunoreactive but biologically inactive hGH. In M. Hamburgh and E. J. W. Barrington (eds.), *Hormones in Development*, p. 573. (New York: Appleton Century Crofts)

Levi-Montalcini, R. and Calissana, P. (1979). The nerve-growth factor. *Sci. Am.*, **240**, 44

Löw, H., Crane, F. L., Grebing, C., Hall, K. and Tally, M. (1979). Metabolic milieu and insulin action. *Proceedings 10th Congress of Int. Diabetes Fed.* (In press)

Mosier, H. D., Jr, Grossman, H. J. and Dingman, H. F. (1965). Physical growth in mental defectives: a study in an institutionalized population. *Pediatrics*, **36**, 465

Reith, M. E. A., Schotman, P. and Grispen, W. H. (1978). Measurements of *in vivo* rates of protein synthesis in brain, spinal cord, heart and liver of young versus adult rats, intact versus hypophysectomized rats. *J. Neurochem.*, **30**, 587

Sara, V. R. and Lazarus, L. (1974). The prenatal action of growth hormone on brain and behaviour. *Nature*, **250**, 257

Sara, V., Hall, K., Sjögren, B., Finnson, K. and Wetterberg, L. (1979a). The influence of early nutrition on growth and the circulating levels of immunoreactive somatomedin A. *J. Dev. Physiol.* (In press)

Sara, V. R., Hall, K., Wetterberg, L., Fryklund, L., Sjögren, B. and Skottner, A. (1979b). Fetal brain growth: the role of the somatomedins and other growth-promoting peptides. *Proceedings of Int. Symp. on Somatomedins and Growth.* (In press)

Sara, V. R., King, T. L., Stuart, M. C. and Lazarus, L. (1976). Hormonal regulation of fetal brain cell proliferation: presence in serum of a trophin responsive to growth hormone stimulation. *Endocrinology*, **99**, 90

Sara, V. R., Lazarus, L., Stuart, M. C. and King, T. (1974). Fetal brain growth: selective action by growth hormone. *Science*, **186**, 446

de Wied, D. (1977). Peptides and behaviour. *Life Sci.*, **20**, 195

Williams Pelton, E., Grindeland, R. E., Young, E. and Bass, N. H. (1977). Effects of immunologically induced growth hormone deficiency on myelinogenesis in developing rat cerebrum. *Neurology*, **27**, 282

Zamenhof, S., van Marthens, E. and Grauel, L. (1971). Prenatal cerebral development: effect of restricted diet, reversal by growth hormone. *Science*, **174**, 954

Zamenhof, S., Mosley, J. and Schuller, E. (1966). Stimulation of the proliferation of cortical neurons by prenatal treatment with growth hormone. *Science*, **152**, 1396

Address for correspondence

Dr V. R. Sara, Karolinska Institute, Department of Psychiatry, St Göran's Hospital, Box 12500, S-112 81 Stockholm, Sweden

1.7
On the multiplicity of active substances in single neurons: β-endorphin and α-melanocyte stimulating hormone as a model system

S. J. WATSON and H. AKIL

ABSTRACT

This paper emphasizes the problems associated with neuronal systems which contain two or more active substances (transmitters or modulators) within the same cell. The main focus will be on the arcuate neurons which contain the 31K Dalton precursor of adrenocorticotrophic hormone (ACTH) and β-endorphin. These neurons actually produce β-endorphin (β-END) and α-melanocyte stimulating hormone (α-MSH) as active substances in brain. This neuronal system is the most carefully studied of the systems with two or more potentially active substances in them. A great deal is known about the biosynthesis, anatomy, release receptor pharmacology and behaviour associated with this 31K system. Several topics are reviewed in order to more clearly explain the key control points and problems in multiple transmitter systems. In the final section of the paper, future problems and implications associated with multiple active substances are presented. Special attention is paid to biosynthesis and packaging, multiple forms, metabolism and regulation, receptors and, finally, physiological function and pharmacology.

INTRODUCTION

In this paper we shall describe some of the current evidence for the occurrence of multiple active substances within the same neuronal pool in brain. We shall then discuss the physiological and conceptual issues related to the co-existence of two neuromodulators within the same neurons. The system we shall focus on is the β-endorphin/α-melanocyte stimulating hormone (β-END/α-MSH) neuronal system in the arcuate nucleus of hypothalamus. This is the most carefully studied of the systems reported to contain several active materials, and since relatively more is known about its biochemical, synthetic and release properties, it is useful in indicating the types of problems we are likely to face as we study neuronal pathways containing more than one putative neuro-transmitter. In this chapter we shall specifically describe the immunocyto-chemical anatomy, biosynthesis, release, receptors and physiology of the β-END/α-MSH system, while attempting to highlight the key questions concerning its feedback mechanisms and overall function.

THE β-END/α-MSH SYSTEM: ANATOMY AND BIOSYNTHESIS

Over the past several years a great deal of work has led to the discovery of three endogenous opioid peptides in brain. Two of them, methionine enkeph-alin (met-enkephalin) and leucine enkephalin (leu-enkephalin), were the first to be described in brain (Simantov and Snyder, 1976; Hughes et al., 1975). Soon thereafter, several laboratories reported the occurrence of β-END or the C fragment of β-lipotrophin (β-LPH) in pituitary of several species (Rubin-stein et al., 1977; Bradbury et al., 1976; Chretien et al., 1976; Goldstein, 1976; Guillemin et al., 1976; Li and Chung, 1976). As the discovery of β-END had followed that of met- and leu-enkephalin, a great number of questions arose concerning the relationship between met-enkephalin and β-END. Since met-enkephalin was found to consist of the first five amino acids of $\beta\text{-LPH}_{61-91}$ (Hughes et al., 1975), it was suggested that there might be a synthetic or precursor/product relationship between these two peptides. Much speculation occurred around the issue of whether met-enkephalin was 'merely' a break-down product of β-END or whether β-END was 'just' the precursor for met-enkephalin. Alternatively, it was possible to conceive of enkephalins as brain neurotransmitters and of β-END as a pituitary hormone.

Early on, immunocytochemical studies using anti-enkephalin antibodies showed that met- and leu-enkephalin were stored in cell bodies and in fibres in such a way that it would be very difficult for the enkephalins to be breakdown products of β-END (Bloom et al., 1978a; Cuello and Paximos, 1978; Uhl et al., 1978; Hökfelt et al., 1977a; Simantov et al., 1977; Watson et al., 1977a; Elde et al., 1976). Subsequent immunohistochemical studies using anti-β-

END and anti-β-LPH antibodies revealed that these two peptides were also located in cell bodies and fibres in the central nervous system (Nilaver et al., 1979; Sofroniew, 1979; Akil et al., 1978b; Bloch et al., 1978; Bloom et al., 1978a; Pelletier et al., 1978; Watson et al., 1978a and 1977b; Zimmerman et al., 1978). However, the distribution of the enkephalins in brain was quite different from β-END, as indicated by radioimmunoassay, lesion and immunohistochemical studies (Akil et al., 1978b; Bloom et al., 1978a; Watson et al., 1978a; Rossier et al., 1977). The enkephalin system occupied many small cell groups throughout the neuraxis, from spinal cord up to rostral limbic structures, with fine, probably interneuronal, fibre systems (cf. above). In contrast, β-END and β-LPH were found in a single cell group in the arcuate nucleus of hypothalamus with very long fibre paths, through limbic structures and thalamus, descending to the level of the locus coeruleus (cf. above); there were no β-END fibres reported in the spinal cord. Thus, based on several types of studies, it became apparent that there are at least two distinct opiate peptide systems in brain, the enkephalin system and the β-END system.

Soon after the anatomical localization of β-END and β-LPH, an interesting biochemical finding related β-END to ACTH. The early studies (Moon et al., 1973) demonstrating the localization of β-LPH in pituitary showed that β-LPH was located in the corticotrophs in anterior lobe and in all of the intermediate lobe cells. Bloom and co-workers (1977) later showed β-END to exist in those same pituitary cells. Both of these pituitary cell types are known to produce adrenocorticotrophic hormone (ACTH) or ACTH-like peptides (α-MSH and CLIP), suggesting a physiological relationship between β-END and ACTH. The elegant work of Mains, Eipper and Ling (1977) and of Roberts and Herbert (1977) demonstrated that β-END, β-LPH and ACTH derive from a common 31 000 mol. wt. precursor protein now termed pro-opiocortin. Using mouse tumour and normal rat pituitary, Mains et al. (1977) studied the biosynthesis of β-END, β-LPH and ACTH and demonstrated that these peptides were cleaved free from pro-opiocortin and released in a co-ordinate fashion from pituitary cells. Since ACTH had been so intimately linked with β-END in pituitary, and since β-END had been demonstrated in brain, we then attempted to localize ACTH in brain (Watson et al., 1978b). Using several different antisera against ACTH, our group and others were able to visualize immunoreactive ACTH in the same neurons that contained β-END and β-LPH in rat arcuate nucleus (Nilaver et al., 1979; Pelletier, 1979; Sofroniew, 1979; Bloch et al., 1978; Watson et al., 1978a). Radioimmuno-assay studies by Krieger and co-workers (1977) also indicated the presence of ACTH in brain.

Biosynthetic work on the 31K precursor revealed that anterior and inter-mediate lobes of pituitary had quite different synthetic routes (Gianoulakis et al., 1979; Eipper et al., 1976). The anterior pituitary cells (corticotrophs) produce $ACTH_{1-39}$ and β-LPH almost totally. However, the intermediate lobe cells of rat pituitary have been shown to process ACTH one step further to α-MSH and CLIP, and to process β-LPH one step further to β-END and γ-LPH. Thus, the question arose as to the nature of the brain β-END system, when compared to pituitary. Does the brain produce β-LPH and ACTH like the anterior lobe, or does it produce α-MSH and β-END, like the intermediate lobe? Or is it some combination of the two? In an extensive set of studies using α-MSH antisera, we have been able to conclude that all β-END cells in the arcuate nucleus contain α-MSH (Watson and Akil, unpublished). It therefore seems probable that brain processes the 31K precursor, like the intermediate lobe, and does not seem to produce great quantities of β-LPH and ACTH proper. We were able further to confirm that brain contains a 31K pro-opiocortin system by the use of an antibody against the 16K N-terminus fraction of the 31K precursor. Antisera, directed against the 16K peptide, stained the same arcuate cells that contained α-MSH, γ-LPH and β-END (Watson, unpublished observation).

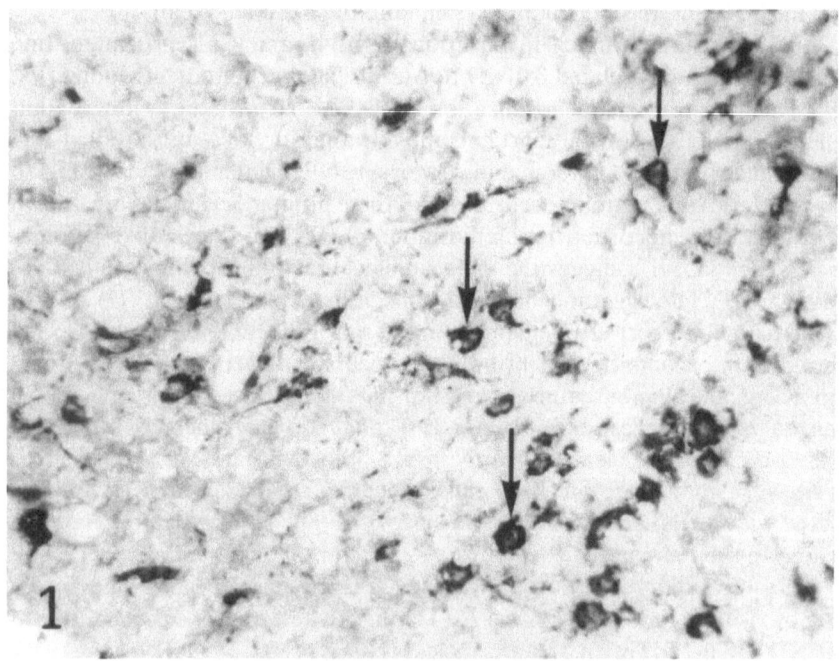

Figure 1   α-MSH stained cells in the arcuate nucleus of rat hypothalamus, after colchicine pretreatment. These cells can be stained by all 31K related antisera (arrow indicates cells, × 860)

As an interesting aside, it should be noted that not only was α-MSH detected in the β-END cells of the arcuate nucleus, but also in cells outside of the arcuate nucleus (Watson and Akil, 1979). As of this writing, these extra-arcuate cells do not appear to contain portions of the 31K precursor.

It seems clear from the above-mentioned anatomical and biosynthetic studies that the brain β-END system is separate from the enkephalin system, contains two substances that are potentially active (α-MSH and β-END) and would appear to share the same synthetic chemistry as the pituitary. The question then arises as to whether these immunoreactivities are associated with free peptide or merely the long precursor, pro-opiocortin. In radio-immunoassay and sizing studies, β-END has been found to be approximately

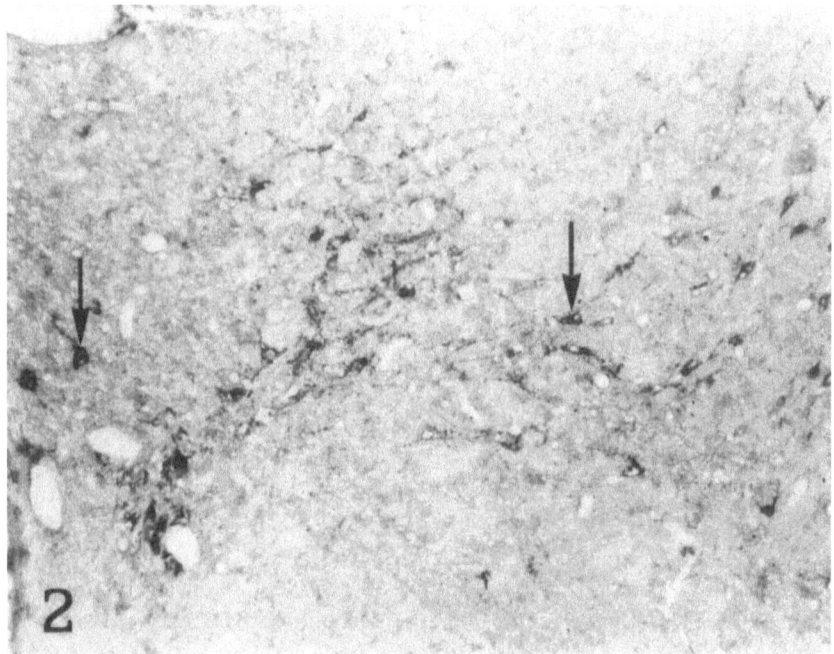

Figure 2 α-MSH positive cells in the lateral hypothalamus near the optic tract, after colchicine pretreatment. These cells do not stain with other 31K antisera (arrow indicates cells, × 530)

80% of the endorphin-like immunoreactivity in rat brain (Rossier *et al.*, 1977). It therefore appears that lipotrophin and the 31K precursor would constitute a rather small proportion of the endorphin-like immunoreactivity. The production of α-MSH involves a cleavage of ACTH after position 13, with an *N*-terminal enzymatic acetylation (cf. Gianoulakis *et al.*, 1979; Eipper *et al.*, 1976). Many α-MSH antisera are directed against the *N*-acetyl portion of that peptide. It appears more likely that an antiserum that responds to the acetylated group would be responding to that group only in its free or unattached form. There appears to be no literature supporting *N*-acetylation of ACTH within the precursor molecule. Finally, there are the studies of several groups (O'Donohue and Jacobowitz, 1979; Vaudry *et al.*, 1978;

Rudman *et al.*, 1974 and 1973) demonstrating that the α-MSH immunoreactivity and bioactivity detected in brain are associated with an α-MSH
sized peptide. Thus it would seem reasonable to conclude that both β-END
and α-MSH occur as free peptides and are not merely immunoreactivities
buried within the precursor molecule.

THE β-END/α-MSH SYSTEM: FUNCTION

The next question to arise is critical to the understanding of the nature of this
complex neuronal system. Are both of these substances active? In a wide
variety of test systems it has been demonstrated that β-END can produce
analgesia, tolerance, addiction and cross-tolerance (Hosobuchi *et al.*, 1979;
Catlin *et al.*, 1977; Wei *et al.*, 1977; Loh *et al.*, 1976; Tseng *et al.*, 1976a and
1976b; Wei and Loh, 1976). It competes at the opiate receptor against labelled
ligands and has been shown to produce endocrine, motor and electro-physio-
logical effects (Labrie *et al.*, 1979; Bloom *et al.*, 1978b and 1976; Dupont *et al.*,
1977; Jacquet and Marks, 1976). On the basis of these and other studies, it
seems clear that β-END is a very active neuropeptide. α-MSH has a very long
history, in which it has been shown to have significant effects on memory,
attention, motivation and learning (de Wied, 1977). Relatively less is known
about the specific neuronal system that it affects. It seems clear that β-END
acts as an opiate and produces most, if not all, of its effects, at the opiate
receptor; however, the receptor effects of α-MSH are unclear at this writing.
In light of the above description of α-MSH within β-END neurons, and a
second non-endorphin related set of α-MSH cells (Watson and Akil, 1979), it
is possible that some of the complexity of α-MSH, behavioural and pharmacological effects might well come from two sets of α-MSH neurons, axons and
receptor systems.

In approaching the question of whether β-END/α-MSH/16K are *stored*
together, the electron microscopic studies of Pelletier and co-workers (1979,
1978, 1977a and 1977b) are most relevant. In pituitary they have shown that
β-LPH and ACTH are stored within the same granules (1977b). As an
extension of that work to brain, Pelletier has seen (1979) that β-END, β-LPH
and 'ACTH'-like immunoreactivity are stored within the same vesicles of
arcuate neurons. It is possible that co-ordinate release of all 31K peptides
would occur, since it seems that the major pieces of the 31K pro-opiocortin are
stored within the same vesicles and granules of their parent cells.

The *release of* these peptides under various stimulating conditions has been
minimally studied. β-END seems to be released using electrical stimulation
and hormonal manipulations (Akil *et al.*, 1979b and 1978a). Specifically, in
stimulating thalamic region and withdrawing third ventricular fluids from
human pain patients, Akil and co-workers (1978a) have been able to see a
substantial rise in β-END immunoreactive levels. Hormonal release of brain

β-END using arginine vasotocin has also been observed (Akil *et al.*, 1979b). A decrease of brain β-END levels by 60% has been detected 20 minutes after 20 fmol of icv AVT. The question of release clearly needs more definite studies, with an emphasis on the question of whether β-END or α-MSH are released in a co-ordinate fashion or whether they have some separate release mechanisms.

Finally, the issue of separate neuronal *receptors* must be addressed. β-END is known to have action at the opiate receptors. In recent studies using [³H]β-END (Akil *et al.*, 1979a), its primary binding properties have been characterized. The binding of [³H]β-END is saturable and stereospecific in that only active opiate alkaloids are capable of displacing it; like other opiate agonists, β-END binding is inhibited by sodium. However, β-END also exhibits some unusual and interesting properties. It has a relatively slow dissociation rate, three times longer than that of enkephalin and ten times longer than that of naloxone. Furthermore, it exhibits a unique regional distribution, with similarities to and differences from opiate alkaloid binding.

α-MSH is known to have a wide range of biological actions and to contain a significant set of structure activity relationships for those actions in central nervous system (Eberle and Schwyzer, 1976). However, to date there is no evidence of binding of tritiated or iodinated α-MSH to brain synaptosomal preparations. In spite of these early negative reports on α-MSH binding, there is recent evidence to demonstrate that full [³H]ACTH$_{1-39}$ can bind to brain receptors (Akil *et al.*, unpublished). It is clear that ACTH/α-MSH binding is an extremely important logical and physiological link in establishing a dual transmitter system. In a more recent set of studies, ACTH appears to possess a significant capacity to inhibit [³H]β-END binding in brain membrane preparations in a dose-related fashion all across the concentration curve (Akil *et al.*, 1979a; Hökfelt *et al.*, 1977b). It therefore seems that there is substantial interaction of ACTH and related fragments at the opiate receptor.

In this brief overview, we have presented a summary of several lines of evidence which argue for the existence of two active peptides within the same neuronal system. These two substances are derived from a common precursor and are stored in the same vesicular system within the neuron of origin, as demonstrated by electron microscopy. There is preliminary evidence for release of β-END from brain and for its actions at an opiate receptor. Finally, studies are under way to evaluate the possibility of α-MSH receptors in brain. In sum, this pathway is a good candidate for a system which synthesizes and releases two active substances. In the case of 'one neuron, one transmitter', it is relatively straightforward to discuss problems of synthesis, receptors, regulation, feedback and the like. But these questions become considerably more complex in the case of a neuron involving two active substances, co-released, acting upon what may be two separate receptor systems. In the remaining space we shall discuss some of the problems and implications involved in understanding such systems.

FUTURE PROBLEMS AND IMPLICATIONS

Many of the concepts involving neuroregulation, receptor activity and release of substances intrinsically depend on the assumption of an almost one-to-one relationship between cellular activity and effective neurotransmission. Yet, in the case of a neuron that may release two active substances, possibly having two synthetic mechanisms, two receptors and two effects post-synaptically, the interactions become considerably more complex. The following are a series of questions and problems that require re-evaluation when one comes to study such a neuronal system.

(1) Biosynthesis and packaging

In the α-MSH and β-END system, biosynthesis and packaging may be relatively straightforward questions, since these two substances share a common precursor (Mains *et al.*, 1977; Roberts and Herbert, 1977), with a known synthetic route, common packaging (Pelletier *et al.*, 1977b) and therefore, quite possibly, common release. However, there are instances in the literature of common neuronal or cellular storage of active materials which most likely do not derive from a common precursor. For example, Hökfelt and co-workers have reported the presence of somatostatin in the norepinephrine-containing cells of the superior cervical ganglia (Hökfelt *et al.*, 1977b). They have also reported that some 5HT cells in the Raphe system contain Substance P (Hökfelt *et al.*, 1977c), and have visualized enkephalin within the adrenergic and noradrenergic cells of the adrenal medulla (Schultzberg *et al.*, 1978). These three neuronal pools are characterized by the coexistence of a peptide and a monoamine within the same cells. It is reasonable to assume that the monoamines come from enzymatic modification of existing amino acids, whereas somatostatin, enkephalin and Substance P are likely to be manufactured through the protein synthetic route. In these three cases, biosynthesis and packaging may well be a much more complex problem. Are norepinephrine and somatostatin stored within the same vesicles of the superior cervical ganglia? Or is it possible that norepinephrine and somatostatin and Substance P and 5HT are stored in separate vesicles within the parent neuron, with release of both of these substances being related to the specific release of particular vesicular type and size? There is new evidence suggesting that the enkephalin within the epinephrine/norepinephrine cells of the adrenal gland is stored in the same granules as these monoamines (Holz and Akil, unpublished observations). Recent studies of the release of enkephalin and catecholamine adrenal granules have shown that enkephalin and catecholamines can be co-purified along with the adrenal vesicles and that both are released in a parallel fashion. Thus, examples of monoamine-peptide systems and the β-END/α-MSH system suggest a wide variety of synthesis and packaging options for dual transmitter systems. In the case of a common synthetic route, it seems reasonable to assume that both peptides are stored within the same vesicle and therefore released simultaneously. However, in the case of different synthetic routes, it is possible that either the same vesicle or different vesicles could be used for storage of individual materials.

(2) Storage in multiple forms, metabolism and neuronal regulation

Evidence from studies of β-END suggest that it may be stored in multiple forms—some slightly shorter and some protected at the N-terminus. Smyth and Zakarian (1978) have described four forms of β-END, C fragment (β-END or β-LPH_{61-91}), C^1 fragment (β-LPH_{61-87}) and the N-acetylated forms of these two peptides. N-Acetylated forms are less active, and the proportion of the various forms differs from one brain region to the next. α-MSH may also be stored in multiple forms (O'Donohue and Jacobowitz, 1979; Vaudry et al., 1978; Rudman et al., 1974 and 1973). Is this multiplicity critical in determining the interactions between the two peptides and their final post-synaptic effects? Does the brain regulate this system by altering the ratio of active to inactive forms of one or both peptides?

A similar question can be raised with respect to breakdown of the peptides. Does a common enzyme control the metabolism of both α-MSH and β-END? Or, are their biological half-lives very different and independently regulated? In essence, does this system use typical feedback mechanisms to regulate its own level of activity, and, if so, does it code the status of one or both peptides, or their relative balance?

In adrenal, the regulation of enkephalins and its relationship to catechol-amine regulation promises to be a fascinating issue. While we know a good deal about catecholaminergic regulation, little is known about control of enkephalin. Does the system respond to both? Are enkephalins critical in modulating catecholamines, and vice versa? These questions point to the limits of our knowledge where regulation of multiplex systems is concerned.

(3) Receptors

In the case of the β-END/α-MSH system there appears to be good evidence for receptors for β-END (Akil et al., 1979a), whereas α-MSH receptors have yet to be demonstrated. There is some reason to suspect the existence of dual receptors for the monoamine-peptide systems mentioned above. There is general agreement that epinephrine, norepinephrine and 5HT have central and peripheral receptors. It is probable that enkephalin, somatostatin and Substance P also have receptors. However, the relationship between any of the above-mentioned receptor complexes and the release of two active substances has not been clearly delineated. For example, it is not known how the post-synaptic neuron responds to the presence of β-END and α-MSH in the synaptic cleft. If β-END and α-MSH are released simultaneously, they are likely to interact with the post-synaptic elements at approximately the same time. The nature of that interaction—for example, whether one acts as agonist and the other as antagonist—is not known. It seems equally possible that the state of the post-synaptic cell might determine whether α-MSH is more or less active in modulating the effects of β-END or vice versa. It is conceivable that the two peptide 'receptors' may have substantial interactions post-synaptically and may therefore be able to express a balanced action as a function of the biasing of that post-synaptic cell. Whether the post-synaptic interactions of the two substances are at one site or more, whether the sites are physically adjacent or disparate, whether the effects are mediated via the same or a different second messenger system, will determine our conceptualization of transmission and feedback regulation across that synapse.

(4) Pharmacology

Since the post-synaptic cell might interact with β-END and α-MSH simultaneously, the presence of only one of these substances in the synaptic cleft would be highly unusual. By analogy, the pharmacological administration of just one of these substances might also be physiologically atypical. This sort of distortion of the normal physiology may be part of the clue to the question of the nature of addiction and tolerance. For example, pharmacologically administered morphine and β-END have very similar actions on the opiate receptors. Yet *physiologically* released β-END might be co-released with α-MSH, resulting in their combined action post-synaptically. One major difference between the pharmacology of opiates and natural release of β-END might well be the presence of α-MSH. As a general principle, pharmacological experiments involving neurons with two active substances may need to take into account the normal physiology of these neurons and their propensity to release two substances in some specified ratio. Indeed, such pharmacological studies of ACTH–endorphin interactions have yielded some fascinating results (Wiegant et al., 1977).

Dual transmitter systems might also present other pharmacological problems, such as those associated with use of synthesis inhibitors, specific antagonists, etc. For example, in the 5HT/Substance P system, when monoamine synthesis inhibitors are used, only one component of the neuron's trans-synaptic modulation might be altered, whereas the other component (Substance P) might not be. In the β-END/α-MSH system, the use of a specific opiate antagonist (naloxone) might have quite different effects if an α-MSH antagonist were used in parallel with it.

CONCLUDING COMMENTS

The foregoing points were meant to emphasize the general pattern of problems that the field of neurosciences and neurochemistry in particular is likely to face over the next few years as it approaches the understanding of dual neurotransmitter systems. We are fortunate in that we have several active models currently and should be able to produce specific information about each of them prior to attempting to infer general principles. It is encouraging that we have been able to demonstrate these dual substance systems. Their existence may help explain some of the complexity of the pharmacological models associated with the respective neuronal pools and some of the problems in mimicking normal physiology using only a single pharmacological agent. By recognizing the increasingly complex elements of neurotransmission associated with these neurons, we may have a better opportunity to understand their normal modes of action.

Acknowledgements

This work was supported in part by the Mental Health Research Institute, University of Michigan and by National Institute of Drug Abuse Grant DA02265-01 and a grant from the Scottish Rite Schizophrenia Research Foundation. The authors gratefully acknowledge the assistance in the manuscript preparation of Ms Carol Criss.

References

Akil, H., Hewlett, W., Barchas, J. D. and Li, C. H. (1979a). Characterization of [³H]β-endorphin binding in rat brain. *Life Sci.* (In press)

Akil, H., Richardson, D. E., Barchas, J. D. and Li, C. H. (1978a). Appearance of β-endorphin-like immunoreactivity in human ventricular cerebrospinal fluid upon analgesic electrical stimulation. *Proc. Natl. Acad. Sci., USA*, **75**, 5170

Akil, H., Watson, S. J., Berger, P. A. and Barchas, J. D. (1978b). Endorphins, β-LPH and ACTH: biochemical, pharmacological and anatomical studies. In E. Costa and E. M. Trabucchi (eds.), *The Endorphins: Advances in Biochemical Psychopharmacology*, vol. 18, pp. 125–139. (New York: Raven Press)

Akil, H., Watson, S. J., Levy, R. and Barchas, J. D. (1979b). β-endorphin and other 31K fragments: pituitary and brain systems. In J. M. van Ree and L. Terenius (eds.), *Characteristics and Function of Opioids. Developments in Neuroscience*, vol. 4, pp. 123–134. (Amsterdam: Elsevier/North-Holland)

Bloch, B., Bugnon, C., Fellman, D. and Lenys, D. (1978). Immunocytochemical evidence that the same neurons in the human infundibular nucleus are stained with anti-endorphins and antisera of other related peptides. *Neurosci. Lett.*, **10**, 147

Bloom, F. E., Battenberg, E., Rossier, J., Ling, N. and Guillemin, R. (1978a). Neurons containing β-endorphin in rat brain exist separately from those containing enkephalin, immunocytochemical studies. *Proc. Natl. Acad. Sci., USA*, **75**, 1591

Bloom, F. E., Battenberg, E., Rossier, J., Ling, N., Leppaluoto, J., Vargo, T. M. and Guillemin, R. (1977). Endorphins are located in the intermediate and anterior lobes of the pituitary gland, not in the neurohypophysis. *Life Sci.*, **20**, 43

Bloom, F. E., Rossier, J., Battenberg, E. L. F., Bayon, A., French, E., Henricksen, S. J., Siggins, G. R., Segal, D., Browne, R., Ling, N. and Guillemin, R. (1978b). β-endorphin: cellular localization, electrophysiological and behavioral effects. In E. Costa and M. Trabucchi (eds.), *The Endorphins: Advances in Biochemical Psychopharmacology*, vol. 18, pp. 89–109. (New York: Raven Press)

Bloom, F. E., Segal, D., Ling, N. and Guillemin, R. (1976). Endorphins: profound behavioral effects in rats suggest new etiological factors in mental illness. *Science*, **194**, 630

Bradbury, A. F., Feldberg, W. F., Smyth, D. G. and Snell, C. (1976). Lipotropin C-fragment: an endogenous peptide with potent analgesic activity. In H. W. Kosterlitz (ed.), *Opiates and Endogenous Opioid Peptides*, pp. 9–17. (Amsterdam: Elsevier/North-Holland)

Catlin, D. H., Hui, K. K., Loh, H. H. and Li, C. H. (1977). Pharmacologic activity of β-endorphin in man. *Commun. Psychopharmacol.*, **1**, 493

Chretien, M., Benjannet, S., Dragon, N., Seidah, N. G. and Lis, M. (1976). Isolation of peptides with opiate activity from sheep and human pituitaries: relationship to β-lipotropin. *Biochem. Biophys. Res. Commun.*, **72**, 472

Cuello, A. C. and Paximos, G. (1978). Evidence for a long leu-enkephalin striopallidal pathway in rat brain. *Nature*, **271**, 178

Dupont, A., Cuson, L., Garon, M., Labrie, F. and Li, C. H. (1977). β-endorphin: stimulation of growth hormone release *in vivo*. *Proc. Natl. Acad. Sci., USA*, **74**, 358

Eberle, A. and Schwyzer, R. (1976). The message sequence of α-melanotropin: demonstration of two active sites. *Clin. Endocrinol.*, **5**, 41s

Eipper, B. A., Mains, R. E. and Guenzi, D. (1976). High molecular weight forms of adreno-corticotropic hormone are glycoproteins. *J. Biol. Chem.*, **251**, 4121

Elde, R., Hökfelt, T., Johansson, O. and Terenius, L. (1976). Immunohistochemical studies using antibodies to leucine-enkephalin: initial observations on the nervous system of the rat. *Neuroscience*, **1**, 349

Gianoulakis, C., Seidah, N. G. and Chretien. M. (1979). *In vitro* biosynthesis and chemical characterization of ACTH and ACTH fragments by the rat pars inter-media. Presented at the annual meeting of the *International Narcotics Research Conference*, June 11–15, N. Falmouth, Massachussetts

Goldstein, A. (1976). Opioid peptides (endorphins) in pituitary and brain. *Science*, **193**, 1081

Guillemin, R., Ling, N. and Burgus, R. (1976). Endorphins, peptides d'origine hypothalamique et neurohypophysaire d'activité morphinomimetique. Isolement et structure moleculaire d'alpha-endorphine. *C.R. Hebd. Seances Acad. Sci.*, Ser. D., **282**, 783

Hökfelt, T., Elde, R., Johansson, O., Terenius, L. and Stein, L. (1977a). The distribution of enkephalin-immunoreactive cell bodies in the rat central nervous system. *Neurosci. Lett.*, **5**, 25

Hökfelt, T., Elfvin, L. G., Elde, R., Schultzberg, M., Goldstein, M. and Luft, R. (1977b). Occurrence of somatostatin-like immunoreactivity in some peripheral sympathetic nor-adrenergic neurons. *Proc. Natl. Acad. Sci., USA*, **74**, 3587

Hökfelt, T., Ljungdahl, A., Terenius, L., Elde, R. and Nilsson, G. (1977c). Immunohistochemical evidence of substance P-like immunoreactivity in some 5-hydroxytryptamine-containing neurons in the central nervous system. *Neuroscience*, **3**, 517

Hosobuchi, Y., Adams, J. E. and Li, C. H. (1979). Intrathecal β-endorphin in humans. In E. Usdin and W. Bunney (eds.), *Endorphins in Mental Health Research*. (NewYork: MacMillan)

Hughes, J., Smith, T. W., Kosterlitz, H. W., Fothergill, L. A., Morgan, B. A. and Morris, H. R. (1975). Identification of two related pentapeptides from the brain with potent opiate agonist activity. *Nature*, **258**, 577

Jacquet, Y. F. and Marks, N. (1976). The C-fragment of β-lipotropin: an endogenous neuroleptic or antipsychotogen? *Science*, **194**, 632

Krieger, D. T., Liotta, A. and Brownstein, M. J. (1977). Presence of corticotropin in brain of normal and hypophysectomized rats. *Proc. Natl. Acad. Sci., USA*, **74**, 648

Labrie, F., Dupont, A., Cuson, L., Ferlund, L., Coy, D. H. and Li, C. H. (1979). Effects of endorphins and their analogues in neuroendocrine control. In E. Udsin and W. Bunney (eds), *Endorphins in Mental Health Research*. (New York: MacMillan)

Li, C. H. and Chung, D. (1976). Isolation and structure of an untriakontapeptide with opiate activity from camel pituitary glands. *Proc. Natl. Acad. Sci., USA*, **73**, 1145

Loh, H. H., Tseng, L. F., Wei, E. and Li, C. H. (1976). β-endorphin as a potent analgesic agent. *Proc. Natl. Acad. Sci., USA*, **73**, 2895

Mains, R. E., Eipper, B. A. and Ling, N. (1977). Common precursor to corticotropins and endorphins. *Proc. Natl. Acad. Sci., USA*, **74**, 3014

Moon, H. D., Li, C. H. and Jennings, B. M. (1973). Immunohistochemical and histochemical studies of pituitary β-lipotropin. *Anat. Rec.*, **175**, 524

Nilaver, G., Zimmerman, E. A., Defendini, R., Liotta, A., Krieger, D. A. and Brownstein, M. (1979). Adrenocorticotropin and β-lipotropin in hypothalamus. *J. Cell Biol.*, **81**, 50

O'Donohue, T. and Jacobowitz, D. (1979). Recent studies of α-melanotropinergic nerves in the brain. Presented to the *International Society of Psychoneuroendocrinology*, August 8–11, Salt Lake City

Pelletier, G. (1979). Ultrastructural localization of neuropeptides with the postembedment staining method. Presented at the annual meeting of the *Histochemical Society*, April 7–13, Keystone, Colorado

Pelletier, G., Desy, L., Lissitszky, J.-C., Labrie, F. and Li, C. H. (1978). Immunohistochemical localization of β-LPH in the human hypothalamus. *Life Sci.*, **22**, 1799

Pelletier, G. and Dube, D. (1977a). Electron microscopic immunohistochemical localization of α-MSH in the rat brain. *Am. J. Anat.*, **150**, 201

Pelletier, G., Leclerc, R., Labrie, F., Cote, J., Chretien, M. and Les, M. (1977b). Immunohisto-chemical localization of β-lipotropin hormone in the pituitary gland. *Endocrinology*, **100**, 770

Roberts, J. L. and Herbert, E. (1977). Characterization of a common precursor to corticotropin and β-lipotropin: identification of β-lipotropin peptides and their arrangement relative to corticotropin in the precursor synthesized in a cell-free system. *Proc. Natl. Acad. Sci., USA*, **74**, 5300

Rossier, J., Vargo, T. M., Minick, S., Ling, N., Bloom, F. E. and Guillemin, R. (1977). Regional dissociation of β-endorphin and enkephalin contents in rat brain and pituitary. *Proc. Natl. Acad. Sci., USA*, **74**, 5162

Rubinstein, M., Stein, S., Gerber, L. D. and Udenfriend, S. (1977). Isolation and characterization of the opioid peptides from rat pituitary: β-lipotropin. *Proc. Natl. Acad. Sci., USA*, **74**, 3052

Rudman, D., Del Rio, A. E., Hollins, B. M., Houser, D. H., Keeling, M. E., Sutin, J., Scott, J. W., Sears, R. A. and Rosenberg, M. Z. (1973). Melanotropic-lipolytic peptides in various regions of bovine, simian and human brains and in simian and human cerebrospinal fluids. *Endo-crinology*, **92**, 372

Rudman, D., Scott, J. W., Del Rio, A. E., Houser, D. H. and Sheen, S. (1974). Melanotropic activity in regions of rodent brain. *Am. J. Physiol.*, **226**, 682

Schultzberg, M., Lundberg, J. M., Hökfelt, T., Terenius, L., Brandt, J., Elde, R. P. and Goldstein, M. (1978). Enkephalin-like immunoreactivity in gland cells and nerve terminals of the adrenal medulla. *Neuroscience*, **3**, 1169

Simantov, R. and Snyder, S. H. (1976). Isolation and structure identification of a morphine-like peptide 'enkephalin' in bovine brain. *Life Sci.*, **18**, 781

Simantov, R., Kuhar, M. J., Uhl, G. R. and Snyder, S. H. (1977). Opioid peptide enkephalin: immunohistochemical mapping in rat central nervous system. *Proc. Natl. Acad. Sci., USA*, **74**, 2167

Smyth, D. G. and Zakarian, S. (1978). Endorphins: biological properties and distribution. In J. M. van Ree and L. Terenius (eds.), *Characteristics and Functions of Opioids*, pp. 293–296. (Amsterdam: Elsevier/North-Holland)

Sofroniew, M. V. (1979). Immunoreactive β-endorphin and ACTH in the same neurons of the hypothalamic arcuate nucleus in the rat. *Am. J. Anat.*, **154**, 283

Tseng, L. F., Loh, H. H. and Li, C. H. (1976a). β-endorphin as a potent analgesic by intravenous injection. *Nature*, **263**, 239

Tseng, L. F., Loh, H. H. and Li, C. H. (1976b). β-endorphin: cross-tolerance to and cross-physical dependence on morphine. *Proc. Natl. Acad. Sci., USA*, **73**, 4187

Uhl, G. R., Kuhar, M. J. and Snyder, S. H. (1978). Enkephalin containing pathway amygdaloid efferents in the stria terminalis. *Brain Res.*, **149**, 223

Vaudry, H., Tonon, M. C., Delarue, C., Vaillant, R. and Kraicer, J. (1978). Biological and radioimmunological evidence for melanocyte stimulating hormones (MSH) of extrapituitary origin in the rat brain. *Neuroendocrinology*, **27**, 9

Watson, S. J. and Akil, H. (1979). The presence of two α-MSH-positive cell groups in rat hypothalamus. *Eur. J. Pharmacol.* (In press)

Watson, S. J., Akil, H., Richard, C. W. and Barchas, J. D. (1978a). Evidence for two separate opiate peptide neuronal systems and the co-existence of β-lipotropin, β-endorphin, and ACTH immunoreactivities in the same hypothalamic neurons. *Nature*, **275**, 226

Watson, S. J., Akil, H., Sullivan, S. O. and Barchas, J. D. (1977a). Immunocytochemical localization of methionine-enkephalin: preliminary observations. *Life Sci.*, **25**, 733

Watson, S. J., Barchas, J. D. and Li, C. H. (1977b). β-lipotropin: localization of cells and axons in rat brain by immunocytochemistry. *Proc. Natl. Acad. Sci., USA*, **74**, 5155

Watson, S. J., Richard, C. W. and Barchas, J. D. (1978b). Adrenocorticotropin in rat brain: immunocytochemical localization in cells and axons. *Science*, **200**, 1180

Wei, E. and Loh, H. (1976). Physical dependence on opiate-like peptides. *Science*, **193**, 1262

Wei, E. T., Tseng, L. F., Loh, H. H. and Li, C. H. (1977). Comparison of the behavioral effects of β-endorphin and enkephalin analogs. *Life Sci.*, **21**, 321

de Wied, D. (1977). Behavioral effects of neuropeptides related to ACTH, MSH, β-LPH. *Ann. N.Y. Acad. Sci.*, **297**, 263

Wiegant, V. M., Gispen, W. H., Terenius, L. and de Wied, D. (1977). ACTH-like peptides and morphine: interaction at the level of the CNS. *Neuroendocrinology*, **2**, 63

Zimmerman, E. A., Liotta, A. and Krieger, D. T. (1978). β-lipotropin in brain: localization in hypothalamic neurons by immunoperoxidase technique. *Cell Tiss. Res.*, **186**, 393

Address for correspondence

Dr S. J. Watson, Mental Health Research Institute, University of Michigan, 205 Washtenaw Place, Ann Arbor, MI 48109, USA

1.8
Neurohypophysial hormones and their distribution in the brain

D. F. SWAAB

ABSTRACT

Arginine vasopressin is produced in the supraoptic nucleus (SON), paraventricular nucleus (PVN), and suprachiasmatic nucleus, and oxytocin in the SON and PVN. Neurosecretory fibres are found to terminate in neurohaemal organs and in extrahypothalamic area, while there is evidence of direct endings on the cerebral ventricles only in early brain development. In adulthood the neurohypophysial hormones in cerebrospinal fluid are thus considered to result rather from the removal of the hormones released in extrahypothalamic brain area than from direct terminations on the ventricular surface. The release of neurohypophysial hormones in extrahypothalamic area seems to take place via peptidergic synapses. Neurohypophysial hormones and exohypothalamic pathways are present early in fetal life, and are thought to be involved in brain development. Peptide transmitters may thus play an essential role both in brain maturation and in central processes in adult life.

INTRODUCTION

The two main subjects of this symposium, hormone production by the brain and the effects of these hormones on the central nervous system, can be traced back more than 40 years in the literature. Around the time that the Scharrers (1940) were advocating the possibility that nerve cells were capable of hormone production, Popa (1938) suggested that the pituitary may produce 'neurotropic principles' that were transported via the portal vessels and the cerebrospinal fluid to the brain. He supposed the existence of a 'neurotropine' which would be the mother-substance of all posterior-pituitary hormones, and talked of a 'cerebrostimuline' and a 'cerebrorelaxine'. Although we shall never know exactly which substances were responsible for the central effects described by Popa, neurohypophysial hormones were early candidates as centrally active substances. As early as 1932, Harvey Cushing demonstrated strong central, mainly parasympathetic, effects of pituitrin after injection of this extract into human brain ventricles. It was, however, the behavioural experiments of de Wied (1965) which really opened the experimental field on the effects of neurohypophysial hormones on the brain. De Wied showed that posterior lobectomy resulted in a more rapid extinction of a conditioned shuttle-box avoidance response, and that the administration of pitressin-tannate restored the extinction rate.

The present paper reviews the accumulating evidence that endogenous arginine vasopressin (AVP) and oxytocin (OXT) reveal their central actions in the adult rat brain via exohypothalamic fibres and peptide synapses, and that these hormones seem, moreover, to be involved in brain development. The limited related data on such systems in the human brain are also presented.

Observations in mammalian fetuses have suggested the existence of a third neurohypophysial hormone, arginine vasotocin (AVT). It has been said that this is present in adulthood in the pineal and the subcommissural organ (Pavel, 1978; Rosenbloom and Fisher, 1975), and, during fetal development, also in the mammalian neurohypophysis (Pavel, 1975). However, as the use of a specific and sensitive radioimmunoassay has not succeeded in confirming the presence of this hormone in mammalian brain (Dogterom *et al.*, 1979 and 1980), significant amounts of this hormone are not present in the mammalian brain, and it will not, therefore, be included in the present dissertation.

SITES OF PRODUCTION OF AVP AND OXT

The 'classical' and sometimes still propagated (Knigge *et al.*, 1978) view on the distribution of AVP and OXT in the brain was that the paraventricular nucleus (PVN) was predominantly or entirely responsible for OXT production, while the supraoptic nucleus (SON) synthesized mainly vasopressin. The development of immunocytochemical techniques and antibody purification procedures has enabled the specific localization of the sites of production, transport and release of the neurohypophysial hormones in the brain, and the data obtained by means of these techniques do not support the supposed functional differentiation of the SON and PVN.

In the rat the two hormones have been found in similar percentages in the SON and in the PVN (Figure 1). Within the SON and PVN, oxytocin cells have been found mainly in the rostral part of the nuclei, and vasopressin cells have been found mainly in the caudal part (Swaab *et al.*, 1975b).

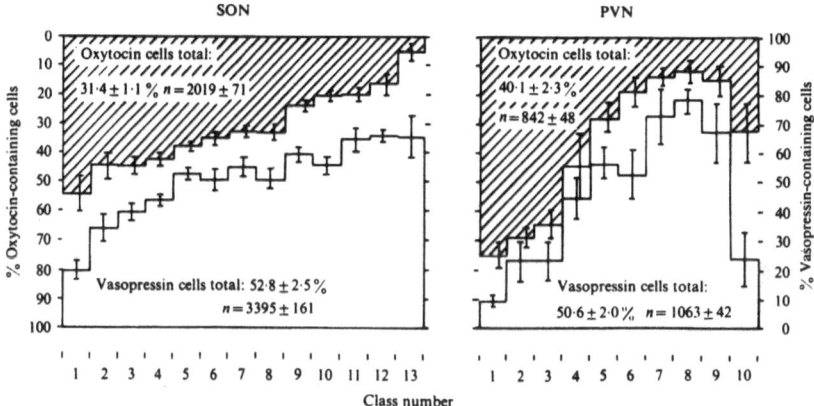

Figure 1 . Percentage of vasopressin- and oxytocin-containing cells in the supraoptic nucleus (SON) and paraventricular nucleus (PVN) from the rostral (left) to caudal (right) part, and the percentage and total number (*n*) of these cells per nucleus. The values given are means ± SEM (calculated from five mean values). The blank areas between the oxytocin and vasopressin cell areas in this figure represent the percentages of cells without hormones. Note that the SON contains about two-and-a-half times more oxytocin-containing cells than the PVN (Swaab *et al.*, 1975b; reproduced with permission)

In the SON, oxytocin cells have been found principally in the dorsal portion, while vasopressin cells have been found mainly in the ventral areas (van Leeuwen *et al.*, 1976; Vandesande and Dierickx, 1975). In the PVN the vasopressin neurons have been found to have a tendency to group in the centre of the nucleus, while the majority of the oxytocin cells have been found in the periphery (Vandesande and Dierickx, 1975). AVP and OXT are produced in different cells (Vandesande and Dierickx, 1979 and 1975; van Leeuwen and Swaab, 1977; Aspeslagh *et al.*, 1976; Swaab *et al.*, 1975b). An additional source of AVP and its related neurophysin appears to be the parvocellular suprachiasmatic nucleus (Swaab and Pool, 1975; Swaab *et al.*, 1975a; Vandesande *et al.*, 1975). These compounds are present in the suprachiasmatic nucleus in much smaller granules (94 nm) than in the SON (143 nm) (van Leeuwen *et al.*, 1978). Since Brattleboro rats homozygous for diabetes insipidus do not reveal such an AVP reaction in the suprachiasmatic nucleus (Swaab and Pool, 1975; Swaab *et al.*, 1975a), and extracts from the isolated nucleus of Wistar rats run parallel in our AVP radioimmunoassay, this nucleus most probably contains genuine AVP rather than a related compound. Apart from the accessory neurosecretory cell groups that are situated outside the SON and PVN (Palkovits *et al.*, 1974) and along the proximal parts of the exohypothalamic PVN tracts (Buijs *et al.*, 1978), these three nuclei—the SON, the PVN and the suprachiasmatic nucleus—are the only production sites of AVP and OXT in the brain.

In the human hypothalamus, separate AVP and OXT producing neurons have been found in the SON and PVN, while the suprachiasmatic nucleus only contains AVP. The total amount of AVP cells in the human hypothalamo-neurohypophysial system is, however, two-and-a-half times larger than the amount of OXT cells (Defendini and Zimmerman, 1978), while the AVP concentration is in some areas as much as ten times higher than that of OXT (George, 1978). In the SON, 80–90% of the cells contain AVP and some 10–20% OXT, while in the PVN the figures are 60–80% and 20–40% respectively (Defindini and Zimmerman, 1978; Dierickx and Vandesande, 1977).

TRANSPORT AND RELEASE OF NEUROHYPOPHYSIAL HORMONES

The SON, PVN and suprachiasmatic nucleus cells project fibres into a number of brain regions. Three types of neurohypophysial hormone-containing fibre terminations can be distinguished:

I. The classical sites of termination of the neurosecretory fibres are the neurohaemal regions. The fibres from the SON and PVN ending in the neurohypophysis (Sherlock *et al.*, 1975) are thought to be the main source of neurohypophysial hormones in the peripheral blood. In addition, vasopressin-containing fibres from the PVN terminate in the external zone of the median eminence (Vandesande *et al.*, 1977); it may be these fibres which are responsible for the high levels of neurohypophysial hormones found in portal blood (Zimmerman *et al.*, 1973). Electrophysiological observations suggest that these latter fibres are axon collaterals of those which run into the neurohypophysis (Blume *et al.*, 1978). The granular diameter in the external zone of the median eminence is, however, much smaller (90 nm) (Dube *et al.*, 1976) than that in the neurohypophysis, which would imply a selection mechanism for the small granula in the collaterals. Whether the suprachiasmatic nucleus contributes towards peripheral or portal AVP blood levels is not known. Although suprachiasmatic fibres run in the caudal direction (Buijs *et al.*, 1978; Swanson and Cowan, 1975; Makara *et al.*, 1972), they seem not to end in the external zone of the median eminence (Antunes *et al.*, 1977; Vandesande *et al.*, 1977). AVP-containing fibres from the suprachiasmatic nucleus seem to end in the organum vasculosum of the lamina terminalis (Buijs, 1978) and so may contribute to the cerebrospinal fluid (CSF) composition (Joseph and Knigge, 1978). However, since no correlation has been found between peripheral AVP levels and avoidance behaviour, the importance of this first class of neurohypophysial hormone-containing endings for central processes is seriously doubted (Dogterom, 1977), the more so since AVP and OXT do not readily penetrate the blood-brain barrier (Landgraf *et al.*, 1979).

II. In parallel with findings in lower animals, neurohypophysial hormone-containing fibres ending directly on the cerebral ventricles, and thus capable of hormone release directly into the CSF, have been thought to be present and functional in mammals (Rodriguez, 1976). However, no evidence of a frequent existence of such terminations in adulthood has been found. Despite much effort, Buijs (unpublished observations), using immunoelectron-microscopy, has been unable to demonstrate any neurohypophysial hormone-containing terminations on the ventricular surface, while Rodriguez (personal communication), using conventional electron-microscopy techniques to make serial electron-microscopy sections throughout the median eminence, suspected the presence of only a few such endings. Rodriguez, however, has not confirmed the endocrine content of these terminations by means of immunocytochemistry. In addition, hormones released into the CSF near to the

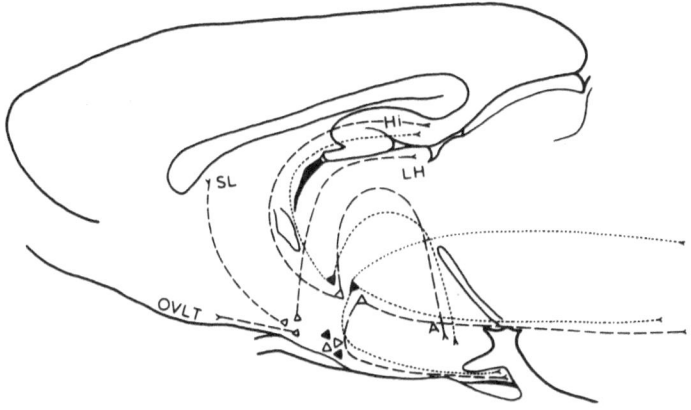

Figure 2 Intra- and exohypothalamic pathways originating in the suprachiasmatic nucleus (small triangles) and paraventricular nucleus (large triangles). The open triangles and broken lines indicate vasopressin-containing cell bodies and fibres respectively, and the closed triangles and dotted lines represent oxytocin-containing cell bodies and fibres. Fibres run from the suprachiasmatic nucleus to the organum vasculosum lamina terminalis (OVLT), the lateral septum (SL) and lateral habenula (LH). Paraventricular nucleus fibres run to the hippocampus (Hi), the amygdala (A), nuclei in the medulla oblongata, and into the spinal cord
(Diagram by R. M. Buijs)

infundibulum would have to be transported upstream in order to reach rostral target areas such as the lateral septum. Sterba suggested recently (personal communication) that the neuroendocrine 'endings' that were visualized on the ventricular surface might even be due to fixation artifacts. On the other hand, observations in the fetal brain of the rat have shown the presence of a number of such contacts during early brain development (Velis *et al.*, 1979). At present it thus seems most likely that in the adult rat the neurohypophysial hormones in the CSF come from the numerous fibres terminating in the brain (see below) and that they represent the elimination of centrally released peptides, rather than that they are using the CSF as the 'specific route' to their sites of action in the brain. In the fetal brain the CSF might be a transport medium for global central effects of neurohypophysial hormones, e.g. in brain development (see below).

III. The extensive networks of extrahypothalamic neurohypophysial hor-mone-containing fibres which are found in a number of brain areas (Figure 2) are currently thought to be the anatomical basis for the central effects described for these peptides. From the suprachiasmatic nucleus AVP-contain-ing fibres run to the lateral septum and the lateral habenular nucleus. The PVN sends AVP- and OXT-containing fibres to the hippocampus, the medial septum, the amygdala, nuclei in the medulla oblongata, and to the spinal cord. The more caudally one looks, the relatively more OXT fibres one finds (Buijs, 1978). These observations have been confirmed by radioimmunoassay in dissected brain areas (Dogterom and Buijs, 1980; Dogterom *et al.*, 1978). Only a few fibres have been found to run into the pineal stalk, the anterior part of the pineal, the subcommissural organ, and the attachment place of the choroid plexus (Buijs, 1978).

PEPTIDE SYNAPSES

These neurosecretory fibres seem to terminate on other neurons either as 'boutons' on the level of the dendritic tree or as punctate perineural structures on cell bodies (Buijs, 1978). The latter structures (Figure 3A) were first described in 1956 by Barry, who terminated his important work on the existence of extrahypothalamic fibres and possible 'neuroendocrine synapses' because he was convinced, already at that time, that this hypothesis could only be confirmed by combined studies, including electron-microscopy (personal communication). The recently developed technique of immunoelectron-microscopy has indeed revealed that both the structures mentioned above represent synapses which are morphologically indistinguishable from the conventional amine-containing synapses, except for the fact that the 'synaptic vesicles' contain neurohypophysial hormones (Figure 3B) (Buijs and Swaab, 1979; Dogterom and Buijs, 1980). The existence of 'true' synapses containing neurohypophysial hormones confirms Sterba's earlier expectations (Sterba, 1974). Release of neurohypophysial hormones from such peptidergic synapses is strongly suggested by the observations of Cooper *et al.* (1979). No infor-mation is yet available on the localization or characteristics of AVP or OXT receptors in the brain. The AVP 'receptors' reported to be present in the

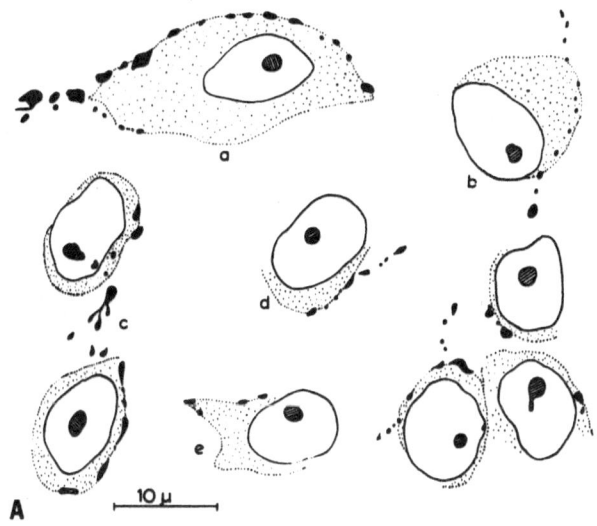

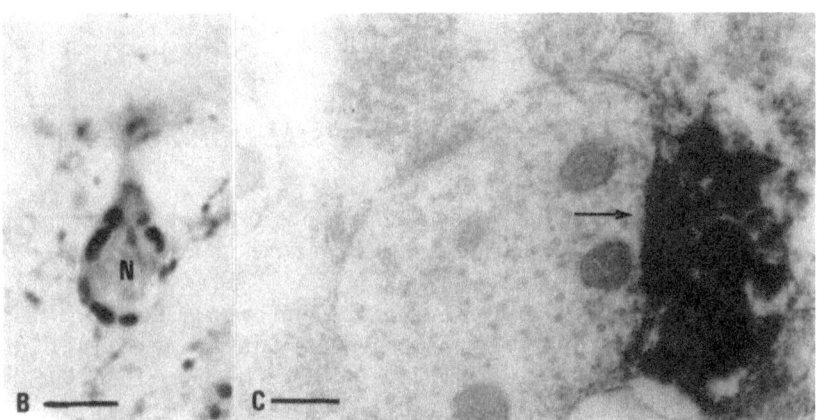

Figure 3 Peptidergic synapses in the central nervous system:

3A Camera lucida drawings of 'neurosecretory synapses' revealed by means of Gomori staining, by Barry (1956): 'Quelques types de synapses neurosécrétatoires. a et b: région du noyau périventriculaire postérieur et du noyau parafasciculaire chez *Rhinolophus ferrum equinum*. c: région du noyau de la strie semi-circulaire chez la souris blanche. d et f: région des noyaux amygdaliens basal et médian chez *Rhinolophus ferrum equinum*. e: région du noyau précommissural chez *Rhinolophus ferrum equinum*.' (Reproduced with permission)

3B Vasopressin positive reaction around a neuron (N) in the lateral septum, obtained by the unlabelled antibody enzyme technique. The bar represents 10 μm. Note the similarity with Figure 3A

3C Immunoelectron-microscopically demonstrated vasopressin positive terminal, which forms a synapse (arrow) with an unlabelled dendrite in the lateral septum. The bar represents 0.20 μm

(The photographs for Figure 3B and 3C were taken by R. M. Buijs)

intermediate lobe of the pituitary (Castel, 1978) are most probably the result of an artifactual staining of α-MSH (van Leeuwen et al., 1979).

Since hypothalamic hormone-producing neurons seem to effect hormone release not only in hypothalamic neurohaemal organs but also via synaptoid contacts in the extrahypothalamic area, the question arises as to whether the same cell is able to execute both functions. Support for this possibility comes from the bi- or multi-polar shape of hypothalamic hormone-producing cells (Buijs, 1978; Buijs et al., 1978) and from the finding that almost all cells of the supraoptic and paraventricular nuclei can be retrogradely stained by HPR from the neurohypophysis (Sherlock et al., 1975). However, electrophysio-logical studies have so far failed to confirm this possibility (Blume et al., 1978; Boer, unpublished observation). Recently, arguments have been made which support the alternative theory that whilst some cells project towards the neurohypophysis, others project towards the extrahypothalamic area. HRP injections into the neurohypophysis or the medulla are thought to label largely different populations of PVN cells (Armstrong et al., 1979; Hosoya and Matsushita, 1979; Ono et al., 1978; Schober, 1978). This opens the possibility of a differential release of neurohypophysial hormones into the peripheral bloodstream and into the brain.

THE PRESENCE OF NEUROHYPOPHYSIAL HORMONES DURING DEVELOPMENT

Yet unpublished radioimmunoassay data from our institute show that in rats AVP and OXT are present relatively early in development. At day 16 of pregnancy a content of approximately 100 pg of AVP and OXT per fetal brain has been found. While the AVP content in the fetal brain gradually increases during development, up to 3.6 ng on the first post-natal day, the course of the OXT content shows a U-shape, with its highest level (± 130 pg) at day 16, its lowest level (± 55 pg) at day 18 and a gradual increase (to ± 110 pg) up to the first post-natal day. These data suggest that considerable neuropeptide con-centrations may be present in the fetal brain even before day 16.

Current immunocytochemical studies show that the fetal SON contains neurohypophysial hormones from at least day 17 and the PVN from day 18, while neurohypophysial hormone-containing cells or fibres of the supra-chiasmatic nucleus appear only between 7 and 10 days post-partum (Velis et al., 1979). Exohypothalamic neurohypophysial hormone-containing fibres are present in the amygdala by day 18 and possibly earlier.

In the human fetal hypothalamus the earliest stainings of oxytocin and vasopressin neurons in the SON and PVN have been obtained in weeks 11–13 of gestation (Fellmann et al., 1979), and oxytocin and vasopressin were already present in the neurohypophysis in the youngest fetus (15 weeks) of our series (Visser and Swaab, 1979). Preliminary observations in the human nervous system reveal that exohypothalamic neurohypophysial hormone-containing fibres are present by mid-pregnancy (Buijs, unpublished observation).

ROLE OF NEUROHYPOPHYSIAL HORMONES IN THE ADULT BRAIN

The arguments in favour of AVP and OXT having a role in adaptive behaviour are dealt with by de Wied and by Bohus in the present volume, and other authors review the effects of these substances on the human central nervous system. It is suggested that in the rat the central effects of AVP are also of physiological importance, since the intraventricular injection of vasopressin antiserum has been found to inhibit memory consolidation (van Wimersma Greidanus *et al.*, 1975). Concerning the study of the physiological function of AVP in the brain, great expectations were raised by the finding of a complete absence of retention of a passive avoidance response in the homozygous Brattleboro rat, which is genetically lacking in AVP (de Wied *et al.*, 1975). However, homozygous animals showed only a partial performance deficit in a similar study by Bailey and Weiss (1979) and no deficit in a shuttlebox study by Celestian *et al.* (1975). In an extensive, as yet unpublished, study by van Oyen *et al.* on homozygous animals, no deficit was found at 60 days, while at 120 days the animals actually performed better than the heterozygous controls in the passive avoidance paradigm. Consequently, the Brattleboro rat does not seem to offer the simple and ideal model for endogenous AVP effects that we had all hoped. Interesting in this respect is the observation of van Oyen *et al.* that a slight but significant performance deficit was present in homozygous Brattleboro rats at 35 days of age, and the unpublished finding of Steinbusch that in the Brattleboro rat more serotoninergic endings are present in the suprachiasmatic nucleus, the lateral septum and the lateral habenula. If, in fact, during development the extra-hypothalamic AVP endings of the homozygous Brattleboro rat are replaced by other fibre systems the result is not just an AVP-less animal, but one which has a very different brain. Other central functions in which the neurosecretory fibres might be involved are drinking behaviour and the maintenance of water balance (Buijs, 1978), while the vasopressin-containing PVN fibres ending in the nucleus tractus solitaris might be involved in the regulation of blood pressure (Tanaka *et al.*, 1977), and those in the spinal cord might collect sensory information for the milk ejection reflex (Buijs, 1978).

It was felt that an alternative way of obtaining data on the physiological involvement of neurohypophysial hormones in central processes might be to measure the peptide content of isolated extrahypothalamic area during processes in which these hormones are involved. In order to show changes in the endogenous AVP and OXT content of brain structures during behaviour,

Dogterom and Buijs (1980) instituted a pilot study in which these hormones were measured in dissected areas during the passive avoidance paradigm 5 minutes after the learning trial. However, no changes were seen either in the AVP or in the OXT content in any of the structures studied. Of course, ideally such a study should be extended to longer intervals from the start of the learning trial, but here we are faced with the same type of problem that occurred before pituitary hormones could be determined in the peripheral blood and were measured in the pituitary itself. The hormone content in a brain area certainly reflects not only hormone release, but other variables as well, i.e. the rates of its production, transport and elimination. It is clear that more dynamic procedures of hormone release measurements have to be developed. So far we have not had success with push–pull procedures.

Our ignorance about the fundamental properties of the 'peptidergic synapse' is thus obvious. In view of this, neuronal systems with synapses that are more readily accessible for fundamental study than the.mammalian nervous system have to be looked for. Neurons of the pond snail (*Lymnaea stagnalis*) which seem to contain peptides which are similar or identical to AVP and OXT (Schot *et al.*, 1979) might be a suitable model system. It is also possible that the co-culture of neurosecretory cells (Gähwiler *et al.*, 1978) and an extrahypothalamic area where neurosecretory fibres usually terminate might form a useful model.

ROLE OF AVP AND OXT DURING DEVELOPMENT

Several possible functions of neurohypophysial hormones in fetal life are being studied at present. One role which has been suggested is in the maintenance of the amniotic fluid, but this is not sufficiently supported by the available data at present (Swaab *et al.*, 1978). Fetal OXT seems to be essential for speeding up the course of labour (Boer *et al.*, 1979). The early presence of neurohypophysial hormones in an extrahypothalamic area of the fetal brain suggests a possible involvement in developmental processes. Since the hereditary absence of AVP in the Brattleboro rat appears to result in seriously stunted post-natal brain development, persisting throughout life, AVP might be involved not only in adult brain function but also in brain development. A lower brain weight and total DNA content appears most pronounced in the cerebellum and medulla oblongata, and more detailed studies of this are currently in progress (Boer *et al.*, 1980 and 1978). Whether this is indeed a direct effect of AVP on brain development has still to be studied, but *in vivo* AVP has shown to be a potent mitogen for fibroblast and possibly also for chondrocytes and bone marrow cells (Rozengurt *et al.*, 1979).

Vasopressin and oxytocin are thus not only acting as neurohormones, but also play an essential role as neurotransmitters in brain maturation in the neonatal period and in a number of other central processes in adult life.

References

Antunes, J. L., Carmel, P. W. and Zimmerman, E. A. (1977). Projections from the paraventricular nucleus to the zona externa of the median eminence of the rhesus monkey: an immunohisto-chemical study. *Brain Res.*, **137**, 1

Armstrong, W. E., Hatton, G. I. and McNeill, T. H. (1979). Distribution of projection neurons in the rat paraventricular nucleus. Presented at the *Anatomy Meetings*, April and May, Miami, USA (Abstract)

Aspeslagh, M.-R., Vandesande, F. and Dierickx, K. (1976). Electron microscopic immunocyto-chemical demonstration of separate neurophysin–vasopressinergic and neurophysin–oxy-tocinergic nerve fibres in the neural lobe of the rat hypophysis. *Cell Tiss. Res.*, **171**, 31

Bailey, W. H. and Weiss, J. M. (1979). Evaluation of a 'memory deficit' in vasopressin-deficient rats. *Brain Res.*, **162**, 174

Barry, J. (1956). De l'existence probable de synapses interneuronales de type 'neurosécrétoire'. In J. Ariëns Kappers (ed.), *Progress in Neurobiology*, pp. 36–44. (Amsterdam: Elsevier)

Blume, H. W., Pittman, Q. J. and Renaud, L. P. (1978). Electrophysiological indications of a 'vasopressinergic' innervation of the median eminence. *Brain Res.*, **155**, 153

Boer, G. J., Swaab, D. F., Uylings, H. B. M., Boer, K., Buijs, R. M. and Velis, D. N. (1980). Neuropeptides in rat brain development. In P. McConnell *et al.* (eds.), *Adaptive Capabilities of the Nervous System. Progress in Brain Research*, vol. 54. (Amsterdam: Elsevier) (In press)

Boer, G. J., Uylings, H. B. M., van Rheenen-Verberg, C. M. F. and Fisser, B. (1978). Postnatal brain development in rats with hereditary diabetes insipidus (Brattleboro strain). In G. Dörner and M. Kawakami (eds.), *Hormones and Brain Development*, pp. 253–258. (Amsterdam: Elsevier/North-Holland)

Boer, K., Swaab, D. F. and Visser, M. (1979). The fetal brain and parturition. *Anim. Repr. Sci.*, **2**, 63

Buijs, R. M. (1978). Intra- and extra-hypothalamic vasopressin and oxytocin pathways in the rat. Pathways to the limbic system, medulla oblongata and spinal cord. *Cell Tiss. Res.*, **192**, 423

Buijs, R. M. and Swaab, D. F. (1979). Immunoelectronmicroscopical demonstration of vaso-pressin and oxytocin synapses in the rat limbic system. *Cell Tiss. Res.*, **204**, 355

Buijs, R. M., Swaab, D. F., Dogterom, J. and van Leeuwen, F. W. (1978). Intra- and extra-hypothalamic vasopressin and oxytocin pathways in the rat. *Cell Tiss. Res.*, **186**, 423

Castel, M. (1978). Immunocytochemical evidence for vasopressin receptors. *J. Histochem. Cytochem.*, **26**, 581

Celestian, J. F., Carey, R. J. and Miller, M. (1975). Unimpaired maintenance of a conditioned avoidance response in the rat with diabetes insipidus. *Physiol. Behav.*, **15**, 707

Cooper, K. E., Kasting, N. W., Lederis, K. and Veale, W. L. (1979). Evidence supporting a role for endogenous vasopressin in natural suppression of fever in the sheep. *J. Physiol.*, **295**, 33

Cushing, H. (1932). Posterior-pituitary hormone and parasympathetic apparatus. In *Papers Relating to the Pituitary Body, Hypothalamus and Parasympathetic Nervous System*, pp. 59–111. (Springfield: Charles C. Thomas)

Defendini, R. and Zimmerman, E. A. (1978). The magnocellular neurosecretory system of the mammalian hypothalamus. In S. Reichlin, R. J. Baldesarini and J. B. Martin (eds.), *The Hypothalamus*, pp. 137–152. (New York: Raven Press)

Dierickx, K. and Vandesande, F. (1977). Immunocytochemical localization of the vasopressin-ergic and the oxytocinergic neurons in the human hypothalamus. *Cell Tiss. Res.*, **184**, 15

Dogterom, J. (1977). The release and presence of vasopressin in plasma and cerebrospinal fluid as measured by radioimmunoassay; studies on vasopressin as a mediator of memory processes in the rat. Ph.D. thesis, State University of Utrecht

Dogterom, J. and Buijs, R. M. (1980). Vasopressin and oxytocin distribution in rat brain: radioimmunoassay and immunocytochemical studies. In Ajmone Marsan, C. and Traczyk, W. Z. (eds.), *Neuropeptides and Neural Transmission*, pp. 307–314. (New York: Raven Press)

Dogterom, J., Snijdewint, F. G. M. and Buijs, R. M. (1978). The distribution of vasopressin and oxytocin in the rat brain. *Neurosci. Lett.*, **9**, 341

Dogterom, J., Snijdewint, F. G. M., Pevet, P. and Buijs, R. M. (1979). On the presence of neuropeptides in the mammalian pineal gland and subcommissural organ. In J. Ariëns Kappers and P. Pevet (eds.), *The Pineal Gland of Vertebrates, including Man. Progress in Brain Research*, vol. 52, pp. 465–470. (Amsterdam: Elsevier)

Dogterom, J., Snijdewint, F. G. M., Pevet, P. and Swaab, D. F. (1980). Studies on the presence of vasopressin, oxytocin and vasotocin in the pineal gland, subcommissural organ and foetal pituitary gland: failure to demonstrate vasotocin in mammals. *J. Endocrinol.*, **84**, 115

Dube, D., Leclerc, R. and Pelletier, G. (1976). Electron microscopic immunohistochemical localization of vasopressin and neurophysin in the median eminence of normal and adrenalectomized rats. *Am. J. Anat.*, **147**, 103

Fellmann, D., Bloch, B., Bugnon, C. and Lenys, D. (1979). Étude immunocytologique de la maturation des axes neuroglandulaires hypothalamo-neurohypophysaires chez le foetus humain. *J. Physiol. (Paris)*, **75**, 37

Gähwiler, B. H., Sandoz, P. and Dreifuss, J. J. (1978). Neurones with synchronous bursting discharges in organ cultures of the hypothalamic supraoptic nucleus area. *Brain Res.*, **151**, 245

George, J. M. (1978). Immunoreactive vasopressin and oxytocin: concentration in individual human hypothalamic nuclei. *Science*, **200**, 342

Hosoya, Y. and Matsushita, M. (1979). Identification and distribution of the spinal and hypophysial projection neurons in the paraventricular nucleus of the rat. A light and electron microscopic study with the horseradish peroxidase method. *Exp. Brain Res.*, **35**, 315

Joseph, S. A. and Knigge, K. M. (1978). The endocrine hypothalamus: recent anatomical studies. In S. Reichlin, R. J. Baldessarini and J. B. Martin (eds.), *The Hypothalamus*, pp. 15–47. (New York: Raven Press)

Knigge, K. M., Joseph, S. A. and Hoffman, G. E. (1978). Organization of LRF- and SRIF-neurons in the endocrine hypothalamus. In S. Reichlin, R. J. Balessarini and J. B. Martin (eds.), *The Hypothalamus*, pp. 49–67. (New York: Raven Press)

Landgraf. R., Ermisch, A. and Hess, J. (1979). Indications for a brain uptake of labelled vasopressin and oxytocin and the problem of the blood-brain barrier. *Endokrinologie*, **73**, 77

van Leeuwen, F. W., de Raay, C., Swaab. D. F. and Fisser, B. (1979). The localization of oxytocin, vasopressin, somatostatin and luteinizing hormone in the rat neurohypophysis. *Cell Tiss. Res.*, **202**, 189

van Leeuwen, F. W. and Swaab, D. F. (1977). Specific immunoelectronmicroscopic localization of vasopressin and oxytocin in the neurohypophysis of the rat. *Cell Tiss. Res.*, **177**, 493

van Leeuwen, F. W., Swaab, D. F. and de Raay, C. (1978). Immunoelectronmicroscopic localization of vasopressin in the rat suprachiasmatic nucleus. *Cell Tiss. Res.*, **193**, 1

van Leeuwen, F. W., Swaab, D. F. and Romijn, H. J. (1976). Light and electron microscopic localization of oxytocin and vasopressin in rats. In G. Feldmann, P. Druet, J. Bignon and S. Avrameas (eds.), *Immunoenzymatic Techniques*, pp. 345–353. (Amsterdam: North-Holland)

Makara, G. B., Harris, M. C. and Spyer, K. M. (1972). Identification and distribution of tuberoinfundibular neurones. *Brain Res.*, **40**, 283

Ono, T., Nishino, H., Sasaka, K., Muramoto, K., Yano, I. and Simpson, A. (1978). Paraventricular nucleus connections to spinal cord and pituitary. *Neurosci. Lett.*, **10**, 141

Palkovits, M., Zaborszky, L. and Ambach, G. (1974). Accessory neurosecretory cell groups in the rat hypothalamus. *Acta Morphol. Acad. Sci. Hung.*, **22**, 21

Pavel, S. (1978). Arginine vasotocin as a pineal hormone. *J. Neural. Trans.*, **13** (suppl.), 135

Pavel, S. (1975). Vasotocin biocynthesis by neurohypophysial cells from human fetuses. Evidence for its ependymal origin. *Neuroendocrinology*, **19**, 150

Popa, G. T. (1938). Neurotropic principles in the sheep hypophysis including a 'cerebrostimuline'. *Academia Româna. Mem. Sect. Stiintif. Seria III. Tom. XIII. Mem. 6*

Rodriguez, E. M. (1976). The cerebrospinal fluid as a pathway in neuroendocrine integration. *J. Endocrinol.*, **71**, 407

Rosenbloom, A. A. and Fisher, D. A. (1975). Radioimmunoassayable AVT and AVP in adult mammalian brain tissue: comparison of normal and Brattleboro rats. *Neuroendocrinology*, **17**, 354

Rozengurt, E., Legg, A. and Pettican, P. (1979). Vasopressin stimulation of mouse 3T3 cell growth. *Proc. Natl. Acad. Sci.*, *USA*, **76**, 1284

Scharrer, E. and Scharrer, B. (1940). Secretory cells within the hypothalamus. In *The Hypothalamus and Central Levels of Autonomic Function*, vol. xx, pp. 170–194. (Publication of the ARNMD) (Baltimore: Williams & Wilkins)

Schober, F. (1978). Darstellung der neurosekretorischen hypothalamo-rhombenzephalen Verbindung bei der Ratte durch retrograden axonalen Transport von Meerrettich-Peroxidase. *Acta Biol. Med. Germ.*, **37**, 165

Schot, L. P. C., Boer, H. H. and Swaab, D. F. (1979). Peptidergic neurons in the pond snail, *Lymnaea stagnalis*. Presented at the *11th Summer School of Brain Research 'Adaptive Capabilities of the Nervous System'*, August 13–17, Amsterdam

Sherlock, D. A., Field, P. M. and Raisman, G. (1975). Retrograde transport of horseradish peroxidase in the magnocellular neurosecretory system of the rat. *Brain Res.*, **88**, 403

Sterba, G. (1974). Das oxytocinerge neurosekretorische System der Wirbeltiere, Beitrag zu einem erweiterten Konzept. *Zool. Jb. Physiol.*, **78**, 409

Swaab, D. F., Boer, G. J., Boer, K., Dogterom, J., van Leeuwen, F. W. and Visser, M. (1978). Fetal neuroendocrine mechanisms in development and parturition. In M. A. Corner, R. E. Baker, N. E. van de Poll, D. F. Swaab and H. B. M. Uylings (eds.), *Maturation of the Nervous System. Progress in Brain Research*, vol. 48, pp. 277–289. (Amsterdam: Elsevier)

Swaab, D. F. and Pool, C. W. (1975). Specificity of oxytocin and vasopressin immunofluorescence. *J. Endocrinol.*, **66**, 263

Swaab, D. F., Pool, C. W. and Nijveldt, F. (1975a). Immunofluorescence of vasopressin and oxytocin in the rat hypothalamo-neurohypophysial system. *J. Neural Trans.*, **36**, 195

Swaab, D. F., Nijveldt, F. and Pool, C. W. (1975b). Distribution of oxytocin and vasopressin in the rat supraoptic and paraventricular nucleus. *J. Endocrinol.*, **67**, 461

Swanson, L. W. and Cowan, W. M. (1975). The efferent connections of the suprachiasmatic nucleus of the hypothalamus. *J. Comp. Neurol.*, **160**, 1

Tanaka, M., de Kloet, E. R., de Wied, D. and Versteeg, D. H. G. (1977). Arginine[8]-vasopressin affects catecholamine metabolism in specific brain nuclei. *Life Sci.*, **20**, 1799

Vandesande, F. and Dierickx, K. (1979). The activated hypothalamic magnocellular neurosecretory system and the one neuron–one neurohypophysial hormone concept. *Cell Tiss. Res.*, **200**, 29

Vandesande, F. and Dierickx, K. (1975). Identification of the vasopressin-producing and of the oxytocin-producing neurons in the hypothalamic magnocellular neurosecretory system of the rat. *Cell Tiss. Res.*, **164**, 153

Vandesande, F., Dierickx, K. and de Mey, J. (1977). The origin of the vasopressinergic and oxytocinergic fibres of the external region of the median eminence of the rat hypophysis. *Cell Tiss. Res.*, **180**, 443

Vandesande, F., Dierickx, K. and de Mey, J. (1975). Identification of the vasopressin–neurophysin-producing neurons of the rat suprachiasmatic nuclei. *Cell Tiss. Res.*, **156**, 377

Velis, D. N., Buijs, R. M. and Swaab, D. F. (1979). Neurosecretory cells and their exohypothalamic fibers in rat brain development. Presented at the *11th International Summer School of Brain Research 'Adaptive Capabilities of the Nervous System'*, August 13–17, Amsterdam

Visser, M. and Swaab, D. F. (1979). Life span changes in the presence of α-melanocyte stimulating hormone containing cells in the human pituitary. *J. Dev. Physiol.*, **1**, 161

de Wied, D. (1965). The influence of the posterior and intermediate lobe of the pituitary and pituitary peptides on the maintenance of a conditioned avoidance response in rats. *Int. J. Pharmacol.*, **4**, 157 de Wied, D., Bohus, B. and van Wimersma Greidanus, T. B. (1975). Memory deficit in rats with hereditary diabetes insipidus. *Brain Res.*, **85**, 152

van Wimersma Greidanus, T. B., Dogterom, J. and de Wied, D. (1975). Intraventricular administration of anti-vasopressin serum inhibits memory consolidation in rats. *Life Sci.*, **16**, 637

Zimmerman, E. A., Carmel, P. W., Husain, M. K., Ferin, M., Tannenberg, M., Frantz, A. G. and Robinson, A. G. (1973). Vasopressin and neurophysin: high concentrations in monkey hypophysial portal blood. *Science*, **182**, 925

Address for correspondence

Professor D. F. Swaab, Nederlands Instituut voor Hersenonderzoek (Netherlands Institute for Brain Research), Ijdijk 28, 1095 KJ Amsterdam, The Netherlands

Section 2
Hormones
and behaviour

2.1
Peptides and adaptive behaviour

D. de WIED

ABSTRACT

During the last decade evidence has accumulated that pituitary and hypothalamic hormones are precursor molecules for biologically active fragments which affect a variety of brain functions. Examples of precursor hormones for neuropeptides which are involved in behavioural adaptation are adrenocorticotrophic hormone, melano-cyte-stimulating hormone, vasopressin, oxytocin and β-endorphin. The study of the influence of pituitary and hypothalamic hormones on the central nervous system has revealed the existence of peptide hormone fragments devoid of classical endocrine effects affecting motivational, attentional, learning and memory processes. In addition, these hormones generate fragments which modulate drug-seeking behaviour and the development of tolerance and physical dependence on opiates and alcohol, and neuropeptides which are involved in psychopathological processes. These findings suggest that psychopathological disturbances and impairment in mental performance may be caused by hormonal dysfunctions in the brain. Preliminary studies in man corroborate this view.

INTRODUCTION

Behavioural adaptation is essential for survival and is under the control of the central nervous system (CNS). Pituitary and hypothalamic hormones play an important role in this process by a direct action on the CNS. During the last decade evidence has accumulated that these hormones are precursor molecules for biologically active fragments which affect a variety of brain functions. These fragments, because of their neural action and their chemical structure, have been designated 'neuropeptides' (de Wied et al., 1974). The CNS effects of neuropeptides in general are independent of the peripheral classical endocrine effects of their precursor hormones. Examples of precursor hormones for neuropeptides which are involved in behavioural adaptation are adrenocorticotrophic hormone (ACTH), melanocyte-stimulating hormone (MSH), vasopressin, oxytocin and β-endorphin. The discovery of the CNS action of these hormones has initiated the development of psychoactive entities which may be used in the treatment of mental disease.

ACTH AND RELATED FRAGMENTS ON MOTIVATION, ATTENTION AND MEMORY

In the course of recent years it has become evident that ACTH, MSH and the smaller fragments of these hormones have a variety of behavioural effects. ACTH and related fragments affect conditioned behaviour motivated by fear, pain, food and sex (de Wied, 1979 and 1974). These effects have been interpreted as indicating that neuropeptides related to ACTH induce a temporary increase in motivation and selective attention (de Wied, 1976 and 1974; Kastin et al., 1975). Electrophysiological data support this notion. Following stimulation of the reticular formation, $ACTH_{4-10}$ induces a shift to higher frequencies in theta activity in hippocampus and thalamus in freely moving rats (Urban and de Wied, 1976). A similar frequency shift can be obtained by increasing the stimulus strength, indicating that $ACTH_{4-10}$ may facilitate transmission in midbrain limbic structures. This may temporarily augment arousal in selective limbic midbrain structures, which may lead to an increase in the motivational value of specific environment cues.

Evidence of the attentional effects of ACTH and related fragments has come from studies on cortical visual evoked responses after discharges related to theta activity. $ACTH_{4-10}$ suppresses the late visual evoked response components without affecting the amplitudes of the primary response or the latencies of any of the peaks in cortical area 17 of rats (Wolthuis and de Wied, 1976). This suggests that $ACTH_{4-10}$ has an activating effect on the vigilance regulating system, an effect which seems specific, since spontaneous motor behaviour as an index of a more generalized arousal is not affected by the peptide. Besides motivational and attentional effects, ACTH and related fragments affect memory processes (de Wied, 1979; Flood et al., 1976).

Clinical studies to date are in agreement with laboratory studies, suggesting motivational, attentional and memory effects of ACTH and related peptides. $ACTH_{4-10}$ restores the previously habituated orienting reaction in humans to a repetitive auditory stimulus (Endröczi et al., 1970). In healthy volunteers $ACTH_{4-10}$ has been shown to reduce performance deficits during serial reaction time tasks, retard the development of electroencephalographic signs of habituation, increase general arousal, improve the level of attention, and enhance attention and short-term visual memory (van Praag, 1980; van Riezen et al., 1977; Kastin et al., 1975). Since motivational, attentional and memory processes are generally reduced in the elderly, several studies have attempted to establish a more pronounced effect of $ACTH_{4-10}$ in this population. $ACTH_{4-10}$ has been found to improve cognitive function in the elderly, but the effect was small and only present in certain measures. $ACTH_{4-10}$ has been found to enhance attention in the mentally retarded. The same peptide has been found to facilitate retrieval from memory and to reduce depression and confusion in the elderly (Branconnier et al., 1979). On the other hand, Will et al. (1978) found no effect of a rather low dose of $ACTH_{4-10}$ in geriatric volunteers who complained of memory loss. Finally, in children with learning difficulties, Rapoport et al. (1976) found no effect on learning performance after a single intravenous injection of $ACTH_{4-10}$. Accordingly, the results to date with $ACTH_{4-10}$ in normal and in cognitive disturbed people confirm animal experiments, but are not very impressive. This may be due to the fact that, in general, only one dose has been used, though it must also be said that there has been only limited assessment of the effect of the mode of administration and of the amount and the potency of the peptide used.

The behavioural activity of ACTH fragments can be almost completely dissociated from inherent endocrine, metabolic and opiate-like activities by modification of the molecule. Substitution of Met[4] by methioninesulfoxide, D-Lys[8] by Arg, and Trp[9] by Phe yields a peptide which is behaviourally a thousand times more active than $ACTH_{4-10}$ (Table 1). It possesses, however, a thousand times less MSH activity, and its steroidogenic action is markedly reduced. It has no fat mobilizing action or opiate-like effects (Greven and de Wied, 1977). The increased behavioural potency is partly explained by protection against metabolic degradation (Witter et al., 1975). The peptide is orally

Table 1 Amino acid sequences of various ACTH fragments and analogues

	1	2	3	4	5	6	7	8	9	10	11	12	13	14	15	16	Potency ratio*
$ACTH_{4-10}$				H-Met-Glu-His-Phe-Arg-Trp-Gly-OH												1
$ACTH_{7-16}$							H-Phe-Arg-Trp-Gly-Lys-Pro-Val-Gly-Lys-Lys-NH₂									1
$ACTH_{4-9}$ analog				O↑				D									
				H-Met-Glu-His-Phe-Lys-Phe-OH												1000
$ACTH_{4-16}$ analog				O↑				D		D							
				H-Met-Glu-His-Phe-Lys-Phe-Gly-Lys-Pro-Val-Gly-Lys-Lys-NH₂												300 000

*Determined on extinction of pole-jumping avoidance behaviour (de Wied et al., 1975)

active in animals as well as in man. A number of clinical studies with this compound suggest that it acts, in principle, similarly to $ACTH_{4-10}$. Whether the results, particularly those following chronic administration, will be more pronounced than those of $ACTH_{4-10}$ has to await further investigation.

NEUROHYPOPHYSIAL HORMONES AND RELATED PEPTIDES ON MEMORY PROCESSES

Like ACTH and related fragments, vasopressin and related peptides stimulate acquisition of shuttle-box avoidance behaviour of hypophysectomized rats, normalize extinction of active avoidance behaviour in posterior lobectomized rats, and delay extinction of shuttle-box and pole-jumping avoidance behaviour in intact rats. In addition they facilitate retention of passive avoidance behaviour (de Wied, 1979 and 1969). In contrast to ACTH and related peptides, which have a short effect of several hours' duration, the influence of vasopressin is of a long-term nature lasting for days or even weeks and persisting beyond the actual presence of the injected material in the body. These findings have been taken to indicate that vasopressin and related peptides modulate memory processes. This is in agreement with findings showing that vasopressin and vasopressin analogues antagonize retrograde amnesia and protect against puromycin induced memory loss (van Wimersma Greidanus and Versteeg, 1979). Oxytocin has an effect on memory opposite to that of vasopressin and facilitates extinction of active and attenuation of passive avoidance behaviour (Schulz et al., 1976). These and other data suggest that oxytocin may be regarded as an amnesic peptide (Bohus et al., 1978b). The neurohypophysial peptides are physiologically involved in the modulation of memory processes, since diabetes insipidus rats, which lack the ability to synthesize vasopressin, have a serious memory deficit (Bohus et al., 1975). In addition, intracerebroventricularly administered specific vasopressin and oxytocin antisera, which temporarily neutralize the respective neurohypophysial hormones in the brain, have an effect which is opposite to that of the respective hormones (Bohus et al., 1978b; van Wimersma Greidanus et al., 1975).

Retention of passive avoidance behaviour provides a sensitive measure for the analysis of the nature of the vasopressin action. If injected immediately after the learning trial, vasopressin markedly facilitates passive avoidance behaviour. Postponing administration decreases the effect. However, injection 1 hour before the retention session, i.e. 23 hours after the learning trial, has the same facilitating effect on the retention of passive avoidance behaviour (Bohus et al., 1978a). This indicates that vasopressin is involved in consolidation as well as in retrieval processes.

Other studies have indicated that the effects of neurohypophysial hormones on consolidation and retrieval are located in different parts of the molecules (de Wied and Bohus, 1978): the covalent ring structures preferentially affect consolidation, while the linear parts seem to be involved in retrieval processes (Table 2). The differential action of the neurohypophysial hormones on memory processes might indicate that both consolidation and retrieval are separately located in the molecules and become apparent after biotransformation. Evidence is available for the existence of aminopeptidase activity and of C-terminal cleaving enzymes in hypothalamus and limbic structures. These enzymes may determine the generation of fractions which affect either consolidation or retrieval processes. Interestingly. there are regional differences in enzyme activity which degrades oxytocin. The highest activity is found in the medial basal hypothalamus while the activity in the region of the dorsal raphe nucleus and the nigrostriatal area is about twice as high as that found in the dorsal septal region (Burbach et al., unpublished observations). The sites of action of the neurohypophysial hormones are located in the midbrain limbic areas (van Wimersma Greidanus and de Wied, 1976), in particular in the projections of the dorsal noradrenergic bundle (Kovács et al., 1979).

Table 2   **Amino acid sequences of neurohypophysial hormones and fragments**

Arginine^8-vasopressin (AVP)	H-Cys-Tyr-Phe-Gln-Asn-Cys-Pro-Arg-Gly-NH$_2$
Desglycinamide^9-arginine^8-vasopressin (DGAVP)	H-Cys-Tyr-Phe-Gln-Asn-Cys-Pro-Arg-OH
Pressinamide (PA)	H-Cys-Tyr-Phe-Gln-Asn-Cys-NH$_2$
Prolyl-argyl-glycinamide (PAG)	H-Pro-Arg-Gly-NH$_2$
Oxytocin (OXT)	H-Cys-Tyr-Ile- Gln-Asn-Cys-Pro-Leu-Gly-NH$_2$
Tocinamide (TA)	H-Cys-Tyr-Ile- Gln-Asn-Cys-NH$_2$
Prolyl-leucyl-glycinamide (PLG)	H-Pro-Leu-Gly-NH$_2$

The evidence from laboratory findings that vasopressin is involved in memory processes has recently been supported by a number of human studies. Legros et al. (1978) were the first to show that vasopressin given by nasal spray for several days markedly improves attention, concentration and memory in the elderly. At the same time, Oliveros et al. (1978) found a dramatic recovery from amnesia in post-traumatic and alcohol amnesia. Other studies have since supported both findings. Moreover, a vasopressin analogue appears to be able to restore a passive avoidance learning defect, i.e. to stop automutilation in children with Lesch–Nyhan disease (Anderson et al., 1979). Lysine vasopressin (LVP) or deamino-d-arg-vasopressin (DDAVP) were used in these investigations. LVP has anti-diuretic and blood pressure increasing effects, while DDAVP possesses powerful anti-diuretic activities. Several years ago it was found that desglycinamide^9-lysine^8-vasopressin (DGLVP), isolated from hog pituitary material, is behaviourally nearly as effective as the parent molecule (de Wied *et al.*, 1972). This also holds for DGAVP. Such fragments are nearly devoid of classical endocrine effects, such as the effects on blood pressure, on water retention and on pituitary-adrenal activity. Thus, DGAVP or DGLVP may be much safer to use clinically in memory disturbances. In addition, the development of fragments which stimulate either consolidation or retrieval processes may yield more specific compounds for the treatment of mental disorders of cognitive origin.

The same may also hold for other CNS effects of the neurohypophysial hormones, such as drug-seeking behaviour. Intravenous self-administration in rats appears to be under the control of neurohypophysial hormones (van Ree *et al.*, 1978a). For example, DGAVP treatment reduces acquisition of heroin self-administration. As in memory processes, the covalent ring structure contains the essential elements for this effect. Conversely, the linear part of oxytocin, which may be involved in retrieval processes, stimulates acquisition of heroin self-administration. A preliminary study in heroin addicts points to a beneficial effect of DGAVP in detoxification with methadon (van Beek-Verbeek *et al.*, 1979).

ENDORPHINS AND ADAPTIVE BEHAVIOUR

Fragments of the pituitary hormone β-lipotrophin (β-LPH) have profound CNS effects. Peptides with the *N*-terminal amino acid residue tyrosine^{61} mimic the action of opiates in a variety of behavioural situations which are employed to assess opiate-like activity. The most potent peptide in this respect is β-endorphin (β-LPH$_{61-91}$); met-enkephalin (β-LPH$_{61-65}$), γ-endorphin (β-LPH$_{61-77}$) and α-endorphin (β-LPH$_{61-76}$) are less potent (Table 3), presumably due to their more rapid metabolic conversion. Apart from these opiate-like effects, β-endorphin and fragments also induce behavioural effects which are not mediated by opiate receptors. Thus, β-endorphin, α-endorphin

Table 3   Amino acid sequences of various β-endorphin (β-LPH$_{61-91}$) fragments

	1	2	3	4	5	6	7	8	9	10	11	12	13	14	15	16	17
γ-endorphin (β-LPH$_{61-77}$)	H-Tyr-Gly-Gly-Phe-Met-Thr-Ser-Glu-Lys-Ser-Gln-Thr-Pro-Leu-Val-Thr-Leu-OH
α-endorphin (β-LPH$_{61-76}$)	H-Tyr-Gly-Gly-Phe-Met-Thr-Ser-Glu-Lys-Ser-Gln-Thr-Pro-Leu-Val-Thr-OH
Met-enkephalin (β-LPH$_{61-65}$)	H-Tyr-Gly-Gly-Phe-Met-OH

	18	19	20	21	22	23	24	25	26	27	28	29	30	31
β-LPH$_{78-91}$	H-Phe-Lys-Asn-Ala-Ile-Val-Lys-Asn-Ala-His-Lys-Lys-Gly-Glu-OH

and met-enkephalin delay extinction of pole-jumping avoidance behaviour in rats. These behavioural effects cannot be antagonized by specific opiate antagonists. In addition, the removal of the N-terminal amino acid residue tyrosine, which eliminates the opiate-like activity of β-endorphin and related peptides, does not eliminate the influence on avoidance behaviour. Interestingly, γ-endorphin and des-tyrosine-γ-endorphin (DTγE) have an effect on extinction opposite to that of β- and α-endorphin. These neuropeptides facilitate extinction of pole-jumping avoidance behaviour (de Wied *et al.*, 1978a and 1978b). A similar opposite effect has been found in passive avoidance behaviour. Thus, whereas β- and α-endorphin facilitate passive avoidance behaviour, γ-endorphin and DTγE attenuate it.

Since the introduction of the neuroleptic drugs in 1952, acquisition and extinction of conditioned behaviour have been used as animal models to determine the activity of potential anti-psychotic drugs. Neuroleptics inhibit acquisition and facilitate extinction of conditioned behaviour. In view of the similar action of DTγE and neuroleptic drugs in facilitating extinction of pole-jumping avoidance behaviour and attenuating passive avoidance behaviour, it was postulated that this non-opiate-like neuropeptide might possess neuroleptic-like activities. It was therefore compared with the neuroleptic drug haloperidol in several assay systems. It is well known that neuroleptics decrease locomotor activity and cause sedation. DTγE did not affect gross behaviour in an open field as has been found following haloperidol. However, DTγE, like haloperidol, was found to cause a positive grasping response in various grip tests and to induce a slight immobility. Electrical self-stimulation via electrodes placed in the ventral segmental-medial substantia nigra area was reduced by DTγE and by haloperidol, but whilst the latter was active at threshold as well as at currents eliciting maximal performance, DTγE was active only at threshold currents. The same was found for electrical self-stimulation via electrodes placed in the nucleus accumbens area. Interestingly, α-endorphin, which delays extinction of active and facilitates passive avoidance behaviour, had the opposite effect on electrical self-stimulation elicited via electrodes in the ventral segmental-medial substantia nigra area at threshold currents. In this respect α-endorphin resembles amphetamine, which also stimulates electrical self-stimulation from this area at threshold as well as at currents inducing maximal performance (van Ree *et al.*, 1979). α-endorphin has other effects which are similar to those of amphetamine, but not its locomotor activation and stereotypy characteristics.

In view of these findings it was postulated that DTγE or a closely related peptide is an endogenous neuroleptic-like neuropeptide with a profile more specific than that of currently used neuroleptic drugs. However, the profile of DTγE does not allow it to be classified as a typical neuroleptic drug, since it does not displace [³H]haloperidol or [³H]spiperone from their stereospecific binding sites in membrane preparations of rat striatum, frontal cortex or nucleus accumbens area (van Ree *et al.*, 1978b). Thus DTγE is not, like the neuroleptic drugs, a post-synaptic dopamine antagonist. The hypothesis that DTγE is a neuroleptic-like neuropeptide has been supported by two clinical studies in chronic schizophrenic patients. In these, DTγE appeared to elicit marked anti-psychotic effects (Verhoeven et al., 1979). This, with our own laboratory findings, suggests that an inborn error in the generation or metabolism of DTγE might be an aetiological factor in schizophrenia. If this is correct one would assume that fragments of β-endorphin such as DTγE and DTαE are formed in the brain. In fact these and other β-endorphin fragments have been found to generate from β-endorphin in synaptosomal plasma membrane preparations of rat forebrain tissue (Burbach et al., 1980). The conversion of β-endorphin in this preparation depends on the pH, γ-endorphin and DTγE being formed preferentially at pH 6.7, while at pH 5.9 γ-endorphin, α-endorphin and DTαE are the main products. In addition, β-endorphin, γ-endorphin, DTγE, α-endorphin and DTαE are present in rat pituitary and brain and in human cerebrospinal fluid (Loeber et al., 1979a and 1979b).

CONCLUSION

The study of the influence of pituitary and hypothalamic hormones on the CNS suggests that psychopathological disturbances and impairment in mental performance may be caused by hormonal dysfunctions in the brain. These observations may provide new leads for the development of highly effective therapeutic agents with more specific actions and without the many side-effects of conventional psychoactive drugs. The studies reviewed here reveal the existence of peptide hormone fragments devoid of classical endocrine effects affecting motivational, attentional, learning and memory processes, molecules which modulate drug-seeking behaviour and the development of tolerance to and physical dependence on opiates, and neuropeptides which are involved in psychopathological processes.

Structure activity studies have already shown the possibilities for potentiating the CNS action of neuropeptides, for synthesizing antagonists or neuropeptides which act in an opposite way, and for the preparation of orally active compounds. The modification of $ACTH_{4-9}$ to a neuropeptide with a thousand-fold increase in behavioural activity and a concommittant decrease in inherent endocrine effects, has been followed by the construction of a modified $ACTH_{4-16}$ fragment which has a potency one million times that of the unmodified compound (Greven and de Wied, 1977).

The memory effects of vasopressin and oxytocin may be present in fragments of these hormones which preferentially affect memory consolidation or retrieval processes. It may be possible to potentiate the action of these entities and to develop highly active and specific principles for the treatment of cognitive disorders. Conversely, the amnesic effect of oxytocin may be of clinical importance for extinction of inadequate behaviour. The same may be said for drug-seeking behaviour, since preliminary observations suggest a beneficial effect of DGAVP in heroin detoxification.

The endorphins are not only a source of analgesic compounds; they also consist of non-opiate-like neuropeptides with neuroleptic-like and amphetamine-like effects. A balanced generation of α- and γ-type endorphins may be essential in brain homeostatic mechanisms. More knowledge of the generation of these fragments from β-endorphin may provide a better understanding of psychopathological processes.

These promising developments have come from animal studies which seem to have excellent predictive value. They may be followed by other exciting developments if we continue our efforts to build reliable animal models, which may contribute to the discovery of endogenous substances affecting brain function. The study of the biotransformation of hormones in brain tissue in relation to the CNS effects of the generated fragments and the determination of hormonal profiles, including those of the fragments of the respective hormones in brain, blood and CSF in animal and man, may further reveal new leads for the development of the psychoactive drugs of the future.

References

Anderson, L T., David. R., Bonnet, K. and Dancis, J. (1979). Passive avoidance learning in Lesch–Nyhan disease: effect of 1-desamino-8-arginine-vasopressin. *Life Sci.*, **24**, 905

van Beek-Verbeek. G., Fraenkel. M., Geerlings, P. J., van Ree. J. M. and de Wied, D. (1979). Des-glycinamide-arginine-vasopressin in methadon detoxification of heroin addicts. *Lancet*, **2**, 738

Bohus. B., Kovács. G. L. and de Wied, D. (1978a). Oxytocin, vasopressin and memory: opposite effects on consolidation and retrieval processes. *Brain Res.*, **157**, 414

Bohus. B., Urban. I., van Wimersma Greidanus, T. B. and de Wied. D. (1978b). Opposite effects of oxytocin and vasopressin on avoidance behavior and hippocampal theta rhythm in the rat. *Neuropharmacology*, **17**, 239

Bohus. B., van Wimersma Greidanus, T. B. and de Wied, D. (1975). Behavioral and endocrine responses of rats with hereditary hypothalamic diabetes insipidus (Brattleboro strain). *Physiol. Behav.*, **14**, 609

Branconnier. R. J., Cole. J. O. and Cardos. G. (1979). ACTH$_{4-10}$ in the amelioration of neuropsychological symptomatology associated with senile organic brain syndrome. *Psychopharmacology*, **61**, 161

Burbach, J. P. H., Loeber, J. G., Verhoef, J., Wiegart, V. M., de Kloet. E. R. and de Wied, D. (1980). Selective conversion of β-endorphin into peptides related to γ- and α-endorphin. *Nature*, **283**, 96

Endröczi, E., Lissák. K., Fekete. T. and de Wied, D. (1970). Effects of ACTH on EEG habituation in human subjects. In D. de Wied and J. A. W. M. Weijen (eds.), *Pituitary, Adrenal and the Brain. Progress in Brain Research*, vol. 32, pp. 254–262. (Amsterdam: Elsevier)

Flood, J. F., Jarvik, M. E., Bennett. E. L. and Orme. A. E. (1976). Effects of ACTH peptide fragments on memory formation. *Pharmacol. Biochem. Behav.*, **5** (suppl. 1), 41

Greven, H. M. and de Wied. D. (1977). Influence of peptides structurally related to ACTH and MSH on active avoidance behavior in rats. A structure-activity relationship study. In F. J. H.

Tilders, D. F. Swaab and T. B. van Wimersma Greidanus (eds.), *Melanocyte-stimulating Hormone: Control, Chemistry and Effects. Frontiers of Hormone Research*, vol. 4, pp. 140–152. (Basel: Karger)

Kastin, A. J., Sandman, C. A., Stratton, L. O., Schally, A. V. and Miller, L. H. (1975). Behavioral and electrographic changes in rat and man after MSH. In W. H. Gispen, T. B. van Wimersma Greidanus, B. Bohus and D. de Wied (eds.), *Hormones, Homeostasis and the Brain. Progress in Brain Research*, vol. 42, pp. 143–150. (Amsterdam: Elsevier)

Kovács, G. L., Bohus, B. and Versteeg, D. H. G. (1979). Facilitation of memory consolidation by vasopressin: mediation by terminals of the dorsal noradrenergic bundle? *Brain Res.* (In press)

Legros, J. J., Gilot, P., Seron, X., Claessens, J., Adam, A., Moeglen, J. M., Audibert, A. and Berchier, P. (1978). Influence of vasopressin on learning and memory. *Lancet*, 1, 41

Loeber, J. G., Verhoef, J., Burbach, J. P. H. and Witter, A. (1979a). Combination of high-pressure liquid chromatography and radioimmunoassay is a powerful tool for the specific and quantative determination of endorphins and related peptides. *Biochem. Biophys. Res. Commun.*, 86, 1288

Loeber, J., Verhoef, J., Burbach, J. P. H. and van Ree, J. M. (1979b). Endorphins and related peptides in human cerebrospinal fluid. *Acta endocr. (Kbh.)*, 91 (suppl. 225), 74

Oliveros, J. C., Jandali, M. K., Timsit-Berthier, M., Remy, R., Benghezal, A., Audibert, A. and Moeglen, J. M. (1978). Vasopressin in amnesia. *Lancet*, 1, 42

van Praag, H. M. (1980). Endorphins and schizophrenia. In D. de Wied and P. A. van Keep (eds.), *Hormones and the Brain*. (Lancaster: MTP Press)

Rapoport, J. L., Quinn, P. O., Copeland, A. P. and Burg, C. (1976). ACTH$_{4-10}$: cognitive and behavioral effects in hyperactive learning-disabled children. *Neuropsychobiology*, 2, 291

van Ree, J. M., Bohus, B., Versteeg, D. H. G. and de Wied, D. (1978a). Neurohypophyseal principles and memory processes. *Biochem. Pharmacol.*, 27, 1793

van Ree, J. M., Bohus, B. and de Wied, D. (1979). Similarity between behavioral effects of des-tyrosine-γ-endorphin and haloperidol and of α-endorphin and amphetamine. In E. Leong Way (ed.) *Endogenous and Exogenous Opiate Agonists and Antagonists*, pp. 459–462. (New York: Pergamon Press)

van Ree, J. M., Witter, A. and Leijsen, J. E. (1978b). Interaction of des-tyrosine-γ-endorphin (DTγE, β-LPH$_{62-77}$) with neuroleptic binding sites in various areas of rat brain. *Eur. J. Pharmacol.*, 52, 411

van Riezen, H., Rigter, H. and de Wied, D. (1977). Possible significance of ACTH fragments for human mental performance. *Behav. Biol.*, 20, 311

Schulz, H., Kovács, G. L. and Telegdy, G. (1976). The effect of vasopressin and oxytocin on avoidance behaviour in rats. In E. Endröczi (ed.), *Cellular and Molecular Bases of Neuro-endocrine Processes*, pp. 555–564. (Budapest: Akademiai Kiado)

Urban, I. and de Wied, D. (1976). Changes in excitability of the theta activity generating substrate by ACTH$_{4-10}$ in the rat. *Exp. Brain Res.*, 24, 325

Verhoeven, W. M. A., van Praag, H. M., van Ree, J. M. and de Wied, D. (1979). Improvement of schizophrenic patients treated with [Des-Tyr^1]-γ-endorphin (DTγE). *Arch. Gen. Psychiat.*, 36, 294

de Wied, D. (1979). Pituitary neuropeptides and behavior. In K. Fuxe, T. Hökfelt and R. Luft (eds.), *Central Regulation of the Endocrine System*, pp. 297–314. (New York: Plenum Press)

de Wied, D. (1976). Behavioral effects of intraventricularly administered vasopressin and vaso-pressin fragments. *Life Sci.*, 19, 685

de Wied, D. (1974). Pituitary-adrenal system hormones and behavior. In F. O. Schmitt and F. G. Worden (eds.), *The Neurosciences: Third Study Program*, pp. 653–666. (Cambridge: MIT Press)

de Wied, D. (1969). Effects of peptide hormones on behavior. In W. F. Ganong and L. Martini (eds.), *Frontiers in Neuroendocrinology*, pp. 97–140. (New York: Oxford University Press)

de Wied, D. and Bohus, B. (1978). The modulation of memory processes by vasotocin, the evolutionarily oldest neurosecretory principle. In M. A. Corner, R. E. Baker, N. E. van de Pol, D. F. Swaab and H. B. M. Uylings (eds.), *Maturation of the Nervous System. Progress in Brain Research*, vol. 48, pp. 327–334. (Amsterdam: Elsevier)

de Wied, D., Bohus, B., van Ree, J. M. and Urban, I. (1978a). Behavioral and electrophysiological effects of peptides related to lipotropin (β-LPH). *J. Pharmacol. Exp. Ther.*, **204**, 570

de Wied, D., Greven, H. M., Lande, S. and Witter, A. (1972). Dissociation of the behavioral and endocrine effects of lysine vasopressin by tryptic digestion. *Br. J. Pharmacol.*, **45**, 118

de Wied, D., Kovács, G. L., Bohus, B., van Ree, J. M. and Greven, H. M. (1978b). Neuroleptic activity of the neuropeptide β-LPH$_{62-77}$ ([Des-Tyr^1]γ-endorphin; DTγE). *Eur. J. Pharmacol.*, **49**, 427

de Wied, D., van Wimersma Greidanus, T. B. and Bohus, B. (1974). Pituitary peptides and behavior: influence on motivational, learning and memory processes. *Neuropsychopharmacology*. Excerpta Medica International Congress Series, no. 359, pp. 653–658. (Amsterdam: Excerpta Medica)

de Wied, D., Witter, A. and Greven, H. M. (1975). Behaviorally active ACTH analogues. *Biochem. Pharmacol.*, **24**, 1463

Will, J. C., Abuzzahab, F. S. Sr and Zimmerman, R. L. (1978). The effects of ACTH$_{4-10}$ versus placebo on the memory of symptomatic geriatric volunteers. *Psychopharmacol. Bull.*, **14**, 25

van Wimersma Greidanus, T. B., Dogterom, J. and de Wied, D. (1975). Intraventricular administration of anti-vasopressin serum inhibits memory consolidation in rats. *Life Sci.*, **16**, 637

van Wimersma Greidanus, T. B. and Versteeg, D. H. G. (1979). Neurohypophyseal hormones: their role in endocrine function and behavioral homeostasis. In C. B. Nemeroff and A. J. Dunn (eds.), *Behavioral Neuroendocrinology*. (New York: Spectrum)

van Wimersma Greidanus, T. B. and de Wied, D. (1976). Dorsal hippocampus: a site of action of neuropeptides on avoidance behavior. *Pharmacol. Biochem. Behav.*, **5** (suppl. 1), 29

Witter, A., Greven, H. M. and de Wied, D. (1975). Correlation between structure, behavioral activity and rate of biotransformation of some ACTH$_{4-9}$ analogs. *J. Pharmacol. Exp. Ther.*, **193**, 853

Wolthuis, O. L. and de Wied, D. (1976). The effect of ACTH analogues on motor behavior and visual evoked responses in rats. *Pharmacol. Biochem. Behav.*, **4**, 273

Address for correspondence

Professor D. de Wied, Rudolf Magnus Instituut voor Farmacologie, Medische Faculteit, Rijksuniversiteit Utrecht, Vondellaan 6, 3521 GD Utrecht, The Netherlands.

2.2
Structure and behavioural activity of peptides related to corticotrophin and lipotrophin

H. M. GREVEN and D. de WIED

ABSTRACT

Behavioural activities of peptides related to corticotrophin and lipo-trophin were studied in active and passive avoidance tests in rats. When searching for an active core in the ACTH-molecule which would be responsible for activity in the pole-jumping test, we found that essential information for this type of activity was not confined to the minimal fragment 4–7, but was also present in the sequences 7–10, Ac-(11–13)-NH_2 and 25–39, indicating a redundancy of information. Through the introduction of certain modifications in the sequence $ACTH_{4-10}$, selectivity of action could be improved and the potency increased a thousandfold. Another increase in potency by a factor of at least 1000 could be obtained by C-terminal elongation with a modified $ACTH_{1f-16}$ sequence. The finding that [Met⁵]enkephalin was equally as active as $ACTH_{4-10}$ in the pole-jumping test was used as an additional argument for the suggestion that the latter peptide assumes an α-helix conformation at the receptor site. When fragments of β-endorphin were tested for their capacity to inhibit extinction of a conditioned avoidance response in the pole-jumping test, the sequence 62–76 appeared to be the most active one, whereas in the series of peptides related to γ-endorphin which accelerate extinction, the fragment 66–77 appeared to be the shortest one to give a significant response. The possible function of peptides related to corticotrophin and lipotrophin in situations of stress or in psychotic disorders is discussed.

INTRODUCTION

There is growing evidence (Mains *et al.*, 1977) that under conditions of stress the secretion by the pituitary of both adrenocorticotrophin- and lipotrophin-like peptides is stimulated through the production of a common precursor, namely pro-opiocortin (Rubinstein *et al.*, 1978). Peptides derived from pro-opiocortin function not only as hormones for peripheral targets, but also by affecting neural processes in the brain, probably after transportation by reverse flow to the brain via the pituitary portal vessels, or by way of the cerebrospinal fluid (Krieger and Liotta, 1979).

These peptides may be conceived of as an emergency supply in addition to stores of similar peptides produced locally in the brain (Krieger and Liotta, 1979). Apparently they affect the level of arousal, alertness and attention, the processing of sensory input, and, less directly, consolidation and retrieval of memory, all aspects thought to be essential for coping with situations of stress and for adaptation to changing external conditions.

It appears that a remarkable wealth of information is stored in different part-sequences of pro-opiocortin. These fragments may be released by selective enzymatic cleavage in the pituitary (e.g. the anterior or intermediate lobe) (Lowry and Scott, 1975), during transportation to the target in the brain, or near the receptor site (Burbach *et al.*, 1979).

In this paper we show that the messages contained in these fragments partially overlap each other, indicating redundant information and underlining the importance of their function; some, however, are mutually antagonistic, serving to maintain a delicate equilibrium between opposing actions.

Disturbance of this balance, in our opinion, may eventually lead to psychotic disorders (de Wied, 1978). Such disorders may be treated by supplementation to correct a deficiency of a particular peptide fragment (Verhoeven *et al.*, 1979).

METHODS

In this communication we report on results of structure-activity studies aimed at unravelling the behavioural information contained in peptides derived from adrenocorticotrophin (ACTH) and lipotrophin (LPH). For behavioural activity we used data primarily obtained in the pole-jumping test on the extinction of a conditioned, active, avoidance response in intact rats, as described in detail in a previous publication (Greven and de Wied, 1973). In our opinion this assay has the following advantages:

(1) The results are representative of adaptive behavioural activity.

(2) The test can distinguish between acceleration and retardation of extinction, thus giving a clear indication of the type of activity.

(3) The numerical avoidance scores give reliable potency relationships. When data obtained over a period of more than 15 years were recently used in a quantitative Free–Wilson-type of structure-activity analysis (Kelder and Greven, 1979), a coherent picture emerged with a calculated standard error of about 3, i.e. of the same magnitude as the accuracy of the assay method, demonstrating a remarkable consistency for the test results over a long period of time.

Additional information on the type of behavioural activity was obtained from one-trial passive avoidance studies in rats (Greven and de Wied, 1973). In this test the peptide may be administered at three different points in time, i.e. before or after the acquisition trial or before the retention test. Results obtained after the first route of application are associated with effects on learning, whereas data from post-acquisition or pre-retention dosing are interpreted as effects on memory, the former on consolidation, the latter on retrieval.

PEPTIDES RELATED TO ACTH

In earlier reports we have described the results of our search for an active core in the ACTH molecule which is responsible for the behavioural activity in our active and passive avoidance tests (Greven and de Wied, 1977 and 1973). We found that essential information of this type of behavioural activity was not confined to a single centre, but was present in a number of different loci. In addition to the minimal fragment 4–7, the sequences 7–10, Ac-(11–13)-NH_2 and 25–39 appeared to be complete agonists, though with a lower potency in the pole-jumping test. These results are summarized in Figure 1. The relative potencies are corrected for molecular weight and expressed with $ACTH_{4-10}$ as a reference. It was concluded that in this respect there appeared to be a redundancy of information stored in the ACTH molecule, accentuating the importance of this message.

This is the more remarkable since we know that in the process of biosynthesis, ACTH and LPH are contained in a common precursor, pro-opiocortin. It now appears that the sequence $ACTH_{4-10}$ is repeated, not only in the β-MSH fragment of LPH, but also twice more, though slightly modified, in the N-terminal part of pro-opiocortin, according to the structure proposed by Nakanishi et al. (1979).

Although the different parts of the ACTH molecule show similar activity in the pole-jumping test, their information content is not identical, as can be seen when they are tested for other CNS activities, e.g. they differ in affinity for an opiate receptor (Terenius *et al.*, 1975) and in their ability to induce a grooming response (Gispen *et al.*, 1975).

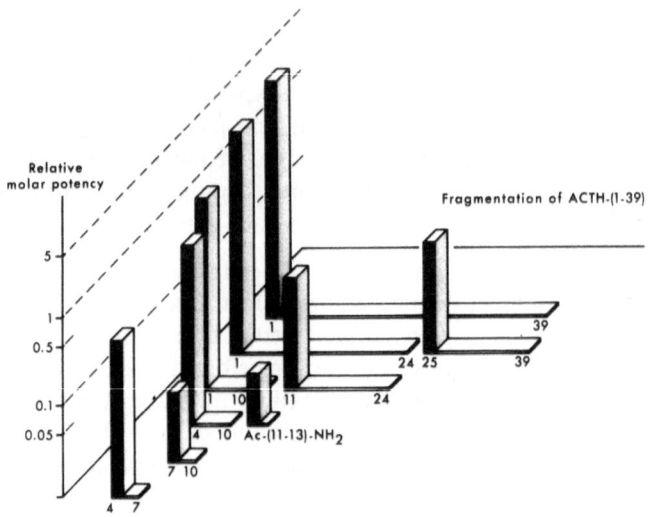

Figure 1   Relative molar potencies of ACTH fragments assayed in the pole-jumping test, and expressed with $ACTH_{4-10}$ as a reference. The peptides, dissolved in saline, are injected subcutaneously

Through the introduction of some modifications in the sequence $ACTH_{4-10}$ it appeared possible to further improve the selectivity of action. Substitution, for instance, of a D-lysine residue for arginine in position 8, combined with two minor modifications at the *C*- and *N*-terminus, resulted in an analogue named Org 2766, i.e. H-Met(O_2)-Glu-His-Phe-D-Lys-Phe-OH, which showed a thousandfold increase of potency in the pole-jumping test (Greven and de Wied, 1973), but which had lost all activity both in the grooming test (Gispen *et al.*, 1975) and in the opiate receptor assay.

On the other hand, exchange of the phenylalanine residue in position 7 by its optical antipode gave the analogue, coded Org OI 64, i.e. H-Met-Glu-His-D-Phe-Arg-Trp-Gly-OH, which showed at least the same affinity for the opiate receptor (Terenius *et al.*, 1975), increased activity in the grooming test (Gispen *et al.*, 1975), but a completely different type of activity in the pole-jumping test. Instead of a delay in extinction, this analogue induced an acceleration in extinction, not as a competitive antagonist, but via a new mechanism of action (Wiegant *et al.*, 1978; Greven and de Wied, 1973). These data are summarized in a Venn-diagram in Figure 2.

In the course of many years we have synthesized a large number of analogues, first of the fragment $ACTH_{4-10}$ and later of the sequence $ACTH_{4-16}$. Recently, working with J. Kelder, we have performed a Free–Wilson-type of structure-activity analysis (Kelder and Greven, 1979), and found that our data satisfied the conditions for such an approach. This implies that we may conceive of the behavioural potency in the pole-jumping test as being composed of individual group contributions which are constant, mutually independent and additive.

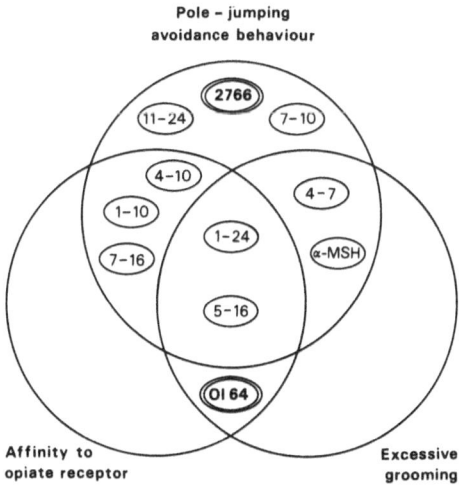

Figure 2 Venn-diagram showing the distribution of a number of ACTH fragments and analogues over three partially overlapping circles. Each circle encloses a collection of ACTH fragments or analogues active in a particular test on CNS activity

The group contributions of a number of modifications are listed in a level diagram in Figure 3, and are expressed relative to the contributions of the original amino acid residues present in the natural sequence of ACTH. It can be seen, first, that the residues of glutamic acid and histidine in the positions 4 and 5 can be exchanged for that of the relatively simple alanine without loss of behavioural activity, and second, that elongation of the analogue Org 2766 with the sequence [D-Lys^{11}]ACTH$_{10-16}$-NH$_2$ further increases its potency by at least a factor 1000. Concurrent introduction of both these modifications resulted in the analogue Org 5042, i.e. [Met(O$_2$)^4,Ala^{5,6},D-Lys^{8,11},Phe^9]-ACTH$_{4-10}$-NH$_2$, which appeared to be a million times as active as our reference peptide ACTH$_{4-10}$, i.e. Org OI 63.

In Figure 4 the log dose-response lines are given of Org OI 63 and of the two analogues Org 2766 and Org 5042 upon three modes of application: oral, subcutaneous and intracerebroventricular. A remarkable feature is the

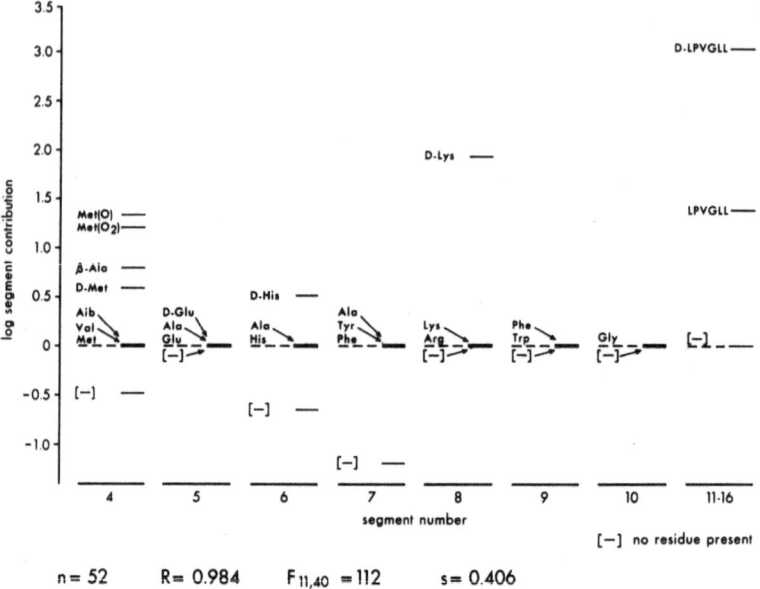

Figure 3   Level diagram of the segment or group contributions to the behavioural potency in the pole-jumping test relative to the contributions of the amino acid residues of $ACTH_{4-10}$

finding that the potency ratios, irrespective of the route of administration, remain fairly constant.

Although we have shown in a study undertaken in conjunction with A. Witter that the high potency of analogue Org 2766 could, in part, be ascribed to an increase in half-life (Witter *et al.*, 1975), the constancy of the potency ratios after different routes of application indicates that metabolic degradation during transportation, either from the gastrointestinal tract or from the peripheral site of injection to the brain, is of the same order of magnitude for all three compounds. The possibility remains that enzymatic inactivation near the receptor site is quite different. Another factor which may contribute to the high potencies of the analogues may be an increased affinity for the receptor site. This suggestion is supported by the finding that the introduction of a D-arginine* instead of a D-lysine residue in position 8 is accompanied by only one-tenth of the potentiation produced by the latter substitution, whereas the same metabolic stabilization may be expected. We therefore suppose that the flexible 8-D-lysine side chain can function as an efficient electrostatic anchor at the receptor site, whereas the more bulky and rigid arginine side chain cannot.

---

*The analogue [D-Arg⁸]$ACTH_{4-10}$ is three times as active as the reference peptide $ACTH_{4-10}$ in the pole-jumping test (unpublished results)

Results of our Free–Wilson analysis also gave a suggestion for a stereo-chemical conformation of the sequence $ACTH_{4-10}$ at the receptor site, i.e. that the residues of methionine in position 4 and arginine in position 8 would be in close proximity, indicating a loop or helix-like structure. This conclusion was based on the observation that the result of concurrent substitution of a D-amino acid residue in the positions 4 and 8 was not additive, but mutually annihilating, suggesting spatial interaction. This was one of the very few instances where data did not satisfy the conditions for a Free–Wilson analysis. Other arguments for a helical conformation at the receptor site have come from circular dichroism studies on N-terminal ACTH fragments by Fermand-jian et al., and from the application of Chou and Fasman's method for the prediction of protein conformation to this sequence (Greven and de Wied, 1977). We now have additional evidence which supports this hypothesis. We not only found [Met⁵]enkephalin to be equally as active as $ACTH_{4-10}$ in the pole-jumping test, but we also observed that the introduction of methionine-sulfoxide into enkephalin resulted in a potentiation similar to that found for

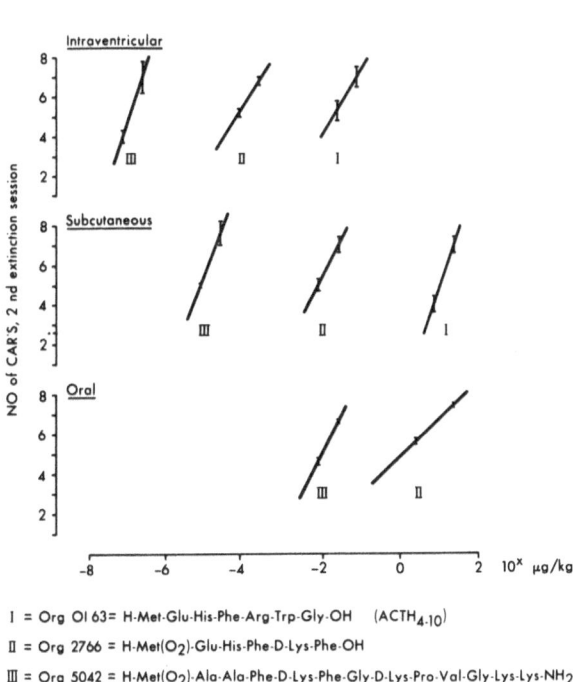

I = Org OI 63= H·Met·Glu·His·Phe·Arg·Trp·Gly·OH   (ACTH₄.₁₀)

II = Org 2766 = H·Met(O₂)·Glu·His·Phe·D·Lys·Phe·OH

III = Org 5042 = H·Met(O₂)·Ala·Ala·Phe·D·Lys·Phe·Gly·D·Lys·Pro·Val·Gly·Lys·Lys·NH₂

Figure 4   Log dose–response lines of Org OI 63 and the two analogues Org 2766 and Org 5042 in the pole-jumping test upon three modes of administration: intracerebroventricular, sub-cutaneous and oral. The number of conditioned avoidances scored during the second extinction session serves as the response for the dose of peptide given. The peptides are dissolved in saline

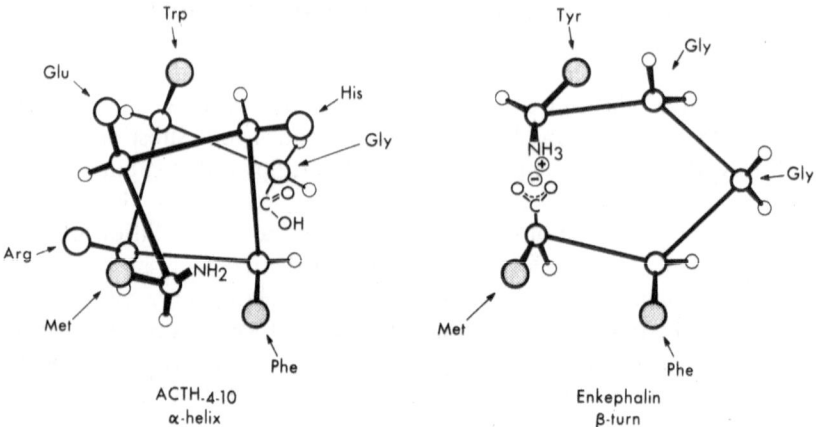

Figure 5 Schematic representation of ACTH$_{4-10}$ in an α-helix conformation and [Met^5]-enkephalin in a β-turn conformation, showing the close proximity of the residues of phenylalanine and methionine

analogues in the ACTH series. This suggests a common feature for both classes of compounds, which, in our opinion, is that the methionine and phenylalanine residues are intra-chain neighbours in enkephalin and extra-chain neighbours in ACTH, provided the latter assumes an α-helix, as shown in Figure 5.

PEPTIDES RELATED TO LPH

When we tested two fragments of β-LPH, namely α- and γ-endorphin, i.e. β-LPH$_{61-76}$ and β-LPH$_{61-77}$ respectively, which only differ in one C-terminal leucine residue, we made the striking observation that the two peptides affected extinction in the pole-jumping test in an opposite way (de Wied *et al.*, 1978b). Whereas α-endorphin, like the ACTH-like peptides, delayed extinction, γ-endorphin induced an acceleration in extinction resembling the effect of the analogue [D-Phe^7]ACTH$_{4-10}$. We shall use the latter as a reference compound for this type of activity, though the mechanism of action may be quite different. We then synthesized and tested a series of peptides with different chain lengths and found the sequence β-LPH$_{66-77}$ to be the shortest peptide, which, upon subcutaneous administration, induced an acceleration in extinction (Figure 6). This not only means that the N-terminal tyrosine residue, essential for opiate-like activity, can be left out, but also that the whole enkephalin sequence 61–65, which may be considered to bear important, latent, information for inhibition of extinction, can be removed. This gives the shorter peptide β-LPH$_{66-77}$ a potential advantage over des-1-tyrosine-γ-endorphin, i.e. Org GK 78, which was shown to be clinically

effective in the treatment of a small number of patients with psychotic disorders (Verhoeven *et al.*, 1979 and 1978). This preference may be due to the
fact that metabolic degradation by a carboxypeptidase, removing the *C*-ter-
minal leucine from Org GK 78, can generate peptides related to α-endorphin
with considerable potency of the opposite type of activity. Similar peptides
derived from β-LPH$_{66-77}$ are much less active; the potency of β-LPH$_{66-76}$, for
instance, in delaying extinction is only one-eightieth that of β-LPH$_{62-76}$.

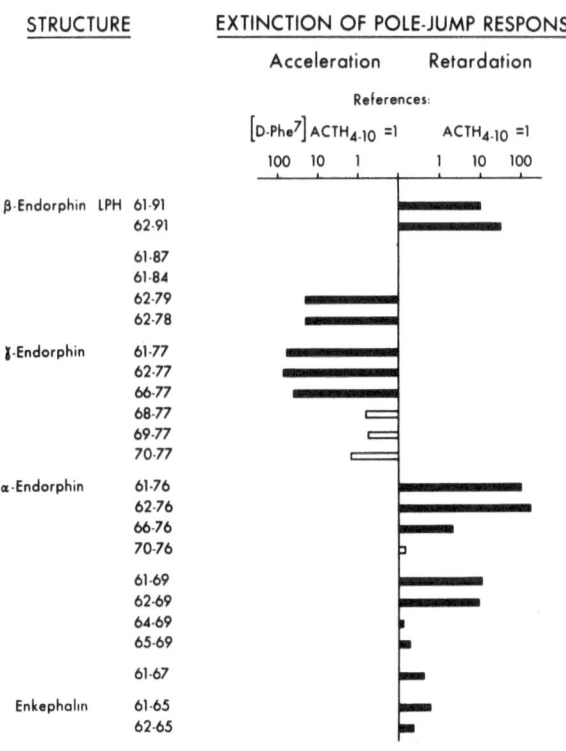

Figure 6 Relative molar potencies of progressively shortened β-LPH fragments assayed in the
pole-jumping test on extinction of an active avoidance response in rats. The peptides, dissolved in
saline, were injected subcutaneously. Open bars: no maximal response could be obtained

Although peptides related to α-endorphin resemble ACTH$_{4-10}$ in their
capacity to induce a delay in extinction in the pole-jumping test, they can be
differentiated from ACTH$_{4-10}$ when tested in the passive avoidance test. We
found that whereas ACTH-related peptides were only active when given
shortly before the retention test, the α-endorphin-like peptides were active
both upon post-trial and pre-retention application, indicating an effect both
on consolidation and on retrieval of memory. It can be seen in Figure 7 that
behavioural information for a passive avoidance response is apparently

present in a latent form in β-endorphin, but becomes expressed after removal of the *N*-terminal tyrosine residue or part of the *C*-terminus (de Wied *et al.*, 1978b; Kovács and de Wied, unpublished results).

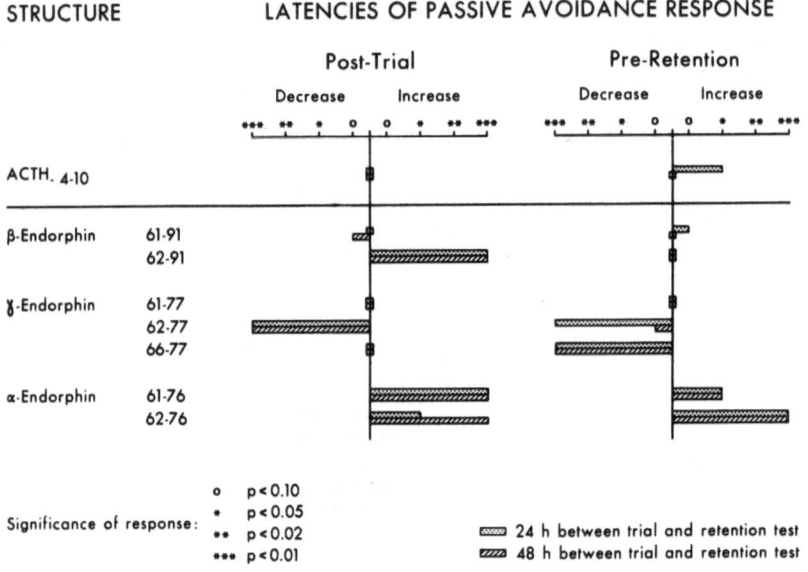

Figure 7   Significance of response latencies in a one-trial passive avoidance test of peptides related to α-, β- and γ-endorphin compared with $ACTH_{4-10}$. The peptides, at a fixed dose of 1.5 µg per rat for the endorphin-like peptides and 15 µg per rat for $ACTH_{4-10}$ were dissolved in saline and injected subcutaneously either post-trial or pre-retention

DISCUSSION

We have shown that peptides derived from ACTH and LPH affect conditioned avoidance behaviour in the pole-jumping test, mostly by inducing a delay in extinction. Only a special family of peptides, related to γ-endorphin, causes an acceleration of extinction. We have also indicated that some ACTH-like peptides show *in vitro* affinity for an opiate receptor and induce *in vivo* a grooming response upon intracerebroventricular administration, an effect thought to be mediated via an opiate receptor, because it can be antagonized by naltrexone (Gispen and Wiegant, 1976); this is opposite to the effects seen in the pole-jumping test, which cannot be modified by naltrexone (de Wied *et al.*, 1978a).

In more general terms, it appears that the effects of peptides derived from pro-opiocortin are, in part, parallel and seem to overlap, but, on the other hand, are sometimes mutually opposing. The latter holds for sequences of

ACTH, antagonizing the effect of morphine, and thus, in all probability, of β-endorphin (Jacquet, 1978; Wiegant *et al.*, 1977; Zimmermann and Krivoy, 1973), as well as for sequences related to α- and γ-endorphin. But what all these peptides have in common is that they are released in response to conditions of stress, which means, with a teleological argument, that they serve to induce a co-ordinated and well-balanced reaction to the new situation.

In our opinion, a common feature of peptides related to ACTH and LPH may be that they affect the processing of sensory information from the level of input (for instance, MSH on retinal function (Dubois, 1979), endorphins on the transmission of the pain stimulus), via phases of gate or filter control, where the relevance of the information is checked (Oades, 1979), to the state of conscious perception. In this respect ACTH- and α-endorphin-related peptides apparently share a stimulating activity, resulting in an increase of awareness. This increased level of awareness may induce the subject to pay more attention to the cues for conditioned behaviour (Sandman *et al.*, 1977), and, by the same mechanism, may cause an improvement in memory retrieval.

CONCLUSION

A complex picture emerges from the interactions of ACTH- and LPH-related peptides with their receptors. Their effects appear, in part, synergistic and mutually supporting, in part, however, mutually opposing. In our opinion they both serve to induce a co-ordinated and balanced response to cope with changing or stressful conditions. Disturbance of this balance may eventually lead to psychotic disorders. Insight into the nature of such disturbances may open new approaches towards their therapeutic treatment.

References

Burbach, J. P. H., Loeber, J. G., Verhoef, J., de Kloet, E. R. and de Wied, D. (1979). Biotransformation of endorphins by a synaptosomal plasma membrane preparation of rat brain and by human serum. *Biochem. Biophys. Res. Commun.*, **86**, 1296

Dubois, M. (1979). Immunocytologie de la rétine: mise en évidence d'antigènes apparentes aux sécrétions polypeptidiques du complexe hypothalamo-hypophysaire. Presented at the *10 ème Colloque de la Société Française de Neuroendocrinologie Expérimentale, Faculté de Médicine Lyon-Sud*, September 6–7, Oullins, France

Gispen, W. H. and Wiegant, V. M. (1976). Opiate antagonists suppress ACTH$_{1-24}$-induced excessive grooming in the rat. *Neurosci. Lett.*, **2**, 159

Gispen, W. H., Wiegant, V. M., Greven, H. M. and de Wied, D. (1975). The induction of excessive grooming in the rat by intraventricular application of peptides derived from ACTH: structure-activity studies. *Life Sci.*, **17**, 645

Greven, H. M. and de Wied, D. (1977). Influence of peptides structurally related to ACTH and MSH on active avoidance behaviour in rats. A structure-activity relationship study. In F. J. H. Tilders, D. F. Swaab and T. B. van Wimersma Greidanus (eds.), *Melanocyte Stimulating*

Hormone: Control, Chemistry and Effects. Frontiers of Hormone Research, vol. 4, pp. 140–152. (Basel: Karger)

Greven, H. M. and de Wied, D. (1973). The influence of peptides derived from corticotropin (ACTH) on performance. Structure-activity studies. In E. Zimmermann, W. H. Gispen, B. H. Marks and D. de Wied (eds.), *Drug Effects on Neuroendocrine Regulation. Progress in Brain Research*, vol. 39, pp. 429–441. (Amsterdam: Elsevier)

Jacquet, Y. F. (1978). Opiate effects after adrenocorticotropin or β-endorphin injection in the periaqueductal gray matter of rats. *Science*, **201**, 1032

Kelder, J. and Greven, H. M. (1979). A quantitative study on the relationship between structure and behavioural activity of peptides related to ACTH. *Recl. Trav. Chim. Pays-Bas*, **98**, 168

Krieger, D. T. and Liotta, A. S. (1979). Pituitary hormones in brain: where, how, and why? *Science*, **205**, 366

Lowry, P. J. and Scott, A. P. (1975). The evolution of vertebrate corticotrophin and melanocyte stimulating hormone. *Gen. Comp. Endocrinol.*, **26**, 16

Mains, R. E., Eipper, B. A. and Ling, N. (1977). Common precursor to corticotropins and endorphins. *Proc. Natl. Acad. Sci., USA*, **74**, 3014

Nakanishi, S., Inoue, A., Kita, T., Nakamura, M., Chang, A. C. Y., Cohen, S. N. and Numa, S. (1979). Nucleotide sequence of cloned cDNA for bovine corticotropin-β-lipotropin precursor. *Nature*, **278**, 423

Oades, R. D. (1979). Search and attention: interactions of the hippocampal–septal axis, adrenocortical and gonadal hormones. *Neurosci. Biobehav. Rev.*, **3**, 31

Rubinstein, M., Stein, S. and Udenfriend, S. (1978). Characterization of pro-opiocortin, a precursor to opioid peptides and corticotropin. *Proc. Natl. Acad. Sci., USA*, **75**, 669

Sandman, C. A., George, J., McCanne, T. R., Nolan, J. D., Kaswan, J. and Kastin, A. J. (1977). MSH/ACTH$_{4-10}$ influences behavioral and physiological measures of attention. *J. Clin. Endocrinol. Metab.*, **44**, 884

Terenius, L., Gispen, W. H. and de Wied, D. (1975). ACTH-like peptides and opiate receptors in the brain: structure-activity studies. *Eur. J. Pharmacol.*, **33**, 395

Verhoeven, W. M. A., van Praag, H. M., Botter, P. A., Sunier, A., van Ree, J. M. and de Wied, D. (1978). [Des-Tyr^1]-γ-endorphin in schizophrenia. *Lancet*, **1**, 1046

Verhoeven, W. M. A., van Praag, H. M., van Ree, J. M. and de Wied, D. (1979). Improvement of schizophrenic patients treated with [Des-Tyr^1]-γ-endorphin (DTγE). *Arch. Gen. Psychiat.*, **36**, 294

de Wied, D. (1978). Psychopathology as a neuropeptide dysfunction. In J. M. van Ree and L. Terenius (eds.), *Characteristics and Function of Opioids. Developments in Neuroscience*, vol. 4, pp. 113–122. (Amsterdam: Elsevier/North-Holland)

de Wied, D., Bohus, B., van Ree, J. M. and Urban, I. (1978a). Behavioral and electrophysiological effects of peptides related to lipotropin (β-LPH). *J. Pharmacol. Exp. Ther.*, **204**, 570

de Wied, D., Kovács, G. L., Bohus, B., van Ree, J. M. and Greven, H. M. (1978b). Neuroleptic activity of the neuropeptide β-LPH$_{62-77}$ ([Des-Tyr^1]γ-endorphin; DTγE). *Eur. J. Pharmacol.*, **49**, 427

Wiegant, V. M., Colbern, D., van Wimersma Greidanus, T. B. and Gispen, W. H. (1978). Differential behavioral effects of ACTH$_{4-10}$ and [D-Phe^7]ACTH$_{4-10}$. *Brain Res. Bull.*, **3**, 167

Wiegant, V. M., Gispen, W. H., Terenius, L. and de Wied, D. (1977). ACTH-like peptides and morphine: interaction at the level of the CNS. *Psychoneuroendocrinology*, **2**, 63

Witter, A., Greven, H. M. and de Wied, D. (1975). Correlation between structure, behavioral activity and rate of biotransformation of some ACTH$_{4-9}$ analogs. *J. Pharmacol. Exp. Ther.*, **193**, 853

Zimmermann, E. and Krivoy, W. (1973). Antagonism between morphine and the polypeptides ACTH, ACTH$_{1-24}$ and β-MSH in the nervous system. In E. Zimmermann, W. H. Gispen, B. H. Marks and D. de Wied (eds.), *Drug Effects on Neuroendocrine Regulation. Progress in Brain Research*, vol. 39, pp. 383–392. (Amsterdam: Elsevier)

Address for correspondence

Dr H. M. Greven, Organon International BV, Scientific Development Group, Research Laboratory for Peptide Chemistry, PO Box 20, 5340 BH Oss, The Netherlands

2.3
Effects of neuropeptides on adaptive autonomic processes

B. BOHUS

ABSTRACT

Neuropeptides related to adrenocorticotrophic hormone (ACTH), vasopressin and oxytocin influence centrally regulated cardiovascular responses. In recent studies $ACTH_{4-10}$ and lysine^8-vasopressin (LVP) were seen to delay the extinction of a classically conditioned cardiac response in the rat. Cardiac response during an emotional behaviour was affected, but differentially, by $ACTH_{4-10}$ and by des-glycinamide^9-lysine^8-vasopressin (DGLVP). DGLVP intensified the bradycardia which accompanied passive avoidance behaviour, while $ACTH_{4-10}$ caused tachycardia. The behavioural effect of the two neuropeptides was, however, indistinguishable. In accordance with current psychophysiological views, it is suggested that $ACTH_{4-10}$ signals intense stress to brain centres which regulate cardiovascular reactions. This signalization may result in a facilitated arousal state which increases the probability of the appropriate behavioural coping. DGLVP, on the other hand, may affect both generalized and specific emotional (fear) responses. This effect of the peptide may be related to an influence on attentional and/or expectancy processes. Observations in rats with hereditary hypothalamic diabetes insipidus indicate that in the genetic absence of vasopressin, behavioural coping is impaired: a specific cardiac response failed to occur but the generalized cardiac reaction was preserved. The likelihood that the autonomic effects of neuropeptides occur as a result of a direct action on cardiovascular control mechanisms rather than as a consequence of their behavioural actions is indicated by an examination of the effects of neuropeptides on centrally evoked pressor responses. Intra-cerebroventricularly administered arginine[8]-vasopressin and frag-ments of this peptide have been seen to attenuate blood pressure increase evoked by the electrical stimulation of the mesencephalic reticular formation.

The outlined observations indicate neuropeptide influences on adaptive autonomic processes, and suggest that neuropeptide dys-functions may be involved in psychosomatic disorders.

INTRODUCTION

The adaptation of the organism to environmental conditions requires a chain or behavioural, autonomic, endocrine and metabolic responses in order to preserve homeostasis. The integration of these adaptive functions is assured by complex brain mechanisms. The study of the mechanisms by which the organism adapts to physical and chemical stressors has long been of interest. It is only recently, however, that research has been undertaken into the mechanisms which assure homeostasis when the organism is affected by adverse psychological stimuli. Such stimuli induce changes in emotionality resulting in fear, anxiety, disappointment and frustration. These psycho-logical stimuli are among the strongest to activate the release of pituitary hormones such as ACTH, α-MSH and vasopressin (Sandman *et al.*, 1973; Thompson and de Wied, 1973; Mason, 1968). A prominent development of the last decade was the recognition that the brain is a target organ for pituitary- and/or brain-borne peptides related to ACTH, β-LPH, vasopressin and oxytocin, and that the effects of these neuropeptides on brain mechanisms influence behavioural adaptation (Bohus, 1979; de Wied, 1977).

Alterations in autonomic functions, primarily of the cardiovascular system, in response to psychic (emotional) stimuli are among the most prominent bodily reactions of animal and man. Interactions between behavioural and cardiovascular adaptive processes are widely recognized (Henry, 1976). The malfunctioning of these integrative adaptive mechanisms can lead to psycho-somatic disorders.

Our interest in autonomic changes related to emotional behaviour started from the wish to understand the exact role and the mechanism of action of peptide hormones in centrally controlled adaptive processes. In addition, the eventual pathological consequence of increased neuropeptide production or of its absence on cardiovascular function seemed worth exploring. This paper reviews our work to date, which indicates that neuropeptides related to

ACTH and vasopressin profoundly affect centrally controlled autonomic processes. Some of our observations further suggest that neuropeptides may be helpful in correcting psychosomatic disorders.

NEUROPEPTIDE INFLUENCES ON CARDIOVASCULAR RESPONSES ACCOMPANYING EMOTIONAL BEHAVIOUR

Neuropeptides and heart rate changes during classical fear conditioning

One of the most prominent behavioural effects of neuropeptides, as observed in the rat, is that on the maintenance of acquired behavioural responses. Resistance to extinction of conditioned avoidance responses is increased after the administration of ACTH-related peptides, such as $ACTH_{4-10}$, of vasopressin and of fragments of this peptide (Bohus, 1979; de Wied, 1977). Since Pavlov's classic studies, it has been well known that, similarly to behavioural responses, cardiovascular changes to noxious stimuli can be conditioned. It was therefore of interest to us to investigate whether neuropeptides affect the autonomic component of classically conditioned emotionality. In our experiments free-moving rats were presented with a conditioned stimulus (CS) which was randomly followed by an unavoidable electric foot-shock. An acquisition period was followed by extinction training during which no punishment followed the CS. The electrocardiogram of the rats was recorded by means of wire leads from transcutaneous electrodes, and the heart rate, as determined from R-R intervals, served as the index of autonomic activity. Changes in the heart rate during the presentation of CS indicated the development and retention of a conditioned cardiac response (Bohus, 1975). A decrease in heart rate during CS indicated a conditioned cardiac response. Extinction training resulted in a gradual disappearance of this cardiac response. Administration of $ACTH_{4-10}$ or of lysine[8]-vasopressin (LVP) before each extinction session led to a delay in the extinction of the conditioned cardiac reaction. This means that behaviourally active neuropeptides modulate not only conditioned behaviour but also adaptive cardiac responses.

Measurement of the base-line heart rate of the classically conditioned rats provided additional information on the nature of the effect of neuropeptides on brain mechanisms. The heart rate of the control rats during the extinction period was not substantially changed from that prior to the extinction. That of the rats receiving $ACTH_{4-10}$, however, was markedly higher during the extinction period, whilst that of the rats treated with LVP was substantially lower. Administration of these two peptides failed to affect the heart rate of pseudo-conditioned rats (non-contingent presentation of CS and foot-shock), of rats which received non-signalled foot-shock and of non-conditioned rats. This observation indicated that the influence of the peptides on heart rate is specifically related to conditioning-dependent emotional responses. The differential changes in heart rate following $ACTH_{4-10}$ and LVP treatment may have indicated different central activity states, but both activity states promoted the maintenance of the conditioned cardiac response.

It was felt that the tachycardia which developed after $ACTH_{4-10}$ treatment may have reflected intensified conditioning-related arousal, and that the bradycardia in LVP-treated rats may have been the consequence of a facilitated specific response to the fear-provoking environment.

Neuropeptides and cardiac responses accompanying passive avoidance behaviour

The assumption that different central activity states are induced by $ACTH_{4-10}$ and by LVP gained support from subsequent behavioural studies. Despite the similarity of the effects of these two peptides on avoidance extinction behaviour, i.e. increased resistance to extinction, the duration of their effects is different. The influence of $ACTH_{4-10}$ is of a short-term nature and is observed only during treatment, whereas LVP induces long-term changes in conditioned behaviour, and its effect on the developed behavioural response is not affected by the cessation of treatment (Bohus et al., 1973).

In order to obtain more evidence to support the hypothesis that the two substances have different central activity states it was decided to institute an experimental project, again using rats, in which the cardiac responses could be studied at the same time as the behavioural ones. For this purpose a one-trial learning passive paradigm seemed the most suitable. In this experiment, which takes advantage of the highly predictable behaviour of the rat, the effect of psychological stimulus (conditioned fear) is not confounded by the stress of punishment (foot-shock), since passive avoidance behaviour and cardiac responses are studied 24 h after the learning trial during which the punishment is applied. This experiment uses the innate preference of the rat for darkness over light. From an elevated lit platform the rat quickly, within a few seconds, chooses to enter a dark compartment. After four pre-training trials the rat receives a single electric foot-shock immediately after entering the dark compartment. Learning experience, as tested 24 h later, is manifest by the rat avoiding re-entering the dark compartment (Ader et al., 1972). In this experiment the electrocardiogram of the rat was recorded from transcutaneous electrodes with the aid of radiotelemetry (Bohus, 1974a). Passive avoidance behaviour was found to depend upon the intensity of the foot-shock during the learning trial: the stronger the aversive stimulus, the more time the animal took to re-enter the preferred dark compartment. This emotional behaviour was accompanied by tonic and phasic changes in cardiac rhythm. Tonic changes were represented by a decrease in heart rate (HR) during avoidance behaviour relative to pre-learning values. The degree of this bradycardia also depended on the intensity of the aversive stimulus: the more pronounced bradycardia occurring after the higher intensity shocks. Phasic changes in HR, in the form of an abrupt decrease in HR and arrhythmia, occurred when the animal approached or partially entered the dark compartment. Unlike the tonic changes, the degree of phasic alterations did not correlate with the intensity of punishment. Based on a detailed analysis of the HR responses and behaviour, it was concluded that the tonic response may reflect generalized emotionality changes, while the phasic changes in HR during passive avoidance behaviour are probably the correlates of a more specific discriminative function and reflect the conditioned fear response (Bohus, 1977).

Both $ACTH_{4-10}$ and desglycinamide^9-lysine^8-vasopressin (DGLVP), a vasopressin fragment practically devoid of classical endocrine activities (de Wied *et al.*, 1972), facilitated passive avoidance behaviour. The cardiac responses accompanying passive avoidance behaviour of the peptide-treated rats were, however, different. Tonic HR response in rats receiving $ACTH_{4-10}$ appeared to be tachycardia. Enhanced passive avoidance behaviour in rats treated with DGLVP was accompanied by a decrease in HR. The degree of bradycardia was substantially greater in the peptide-treated rats than in controls which received the same punishment during the learning trial. Phasic changes in HR were, however, qualitatively the same in the peptide-treated rats. As in the controls, abrupt bradycardia occurred when these rats approached the dark compartment. The degree of the HR decreases was more pronounced in rats treated with DGLVP than in controls or in those which received $ACTH_{4-10}$ (Bohus, 1977).

These observations substantiated our assumption that the behavioural effect of the two peptides is the consequence of different central mechanisms. The increased HR of $ACTH_{4-10}$-treated rats is most probably due to an increased sympathetic influence on HR, which is normally minimal during this type of emotional behaviour. This suggestion is based on the fact that neonatal chemical sympathectomy prevents the appearance of tachycardia during passive avoidance in rats which have received $ACTH_{4-10}$ (Bohus *et al.*, 1976). Current psycho-physiological opinion maintains that HR does not provide a simple, uni-dimensional measure of brain processes, such as motivational or affective states. However, a decrease of HR, which is mediated through the vagus nerve in a mildly stressful behavioural paradigm, is related to attentional and expectancy processes, while sympathetic influences are evoked by more intense stress in which the organism is actively engaged in the preparation or execution of activities which will cope with the stress (Pribram and McGuiness, 1975; Obrist *et al.*, 1970). If one accepts this view, the tachycardia in the rats which received $ACTH_{4-10}$ may have occurred because the peptide signalled intense stress to the appropriate brain centres. This signalization may result in a facilitated arousal state which increases the probability of the appropriate behavioural coping. The fact that $ACTH_{4-10}$ facilitates arousal in the limbic–midbrain system has been shown by electrophysiological observations in the rat (Urban and de Wied, 1976). Interestingly, recent human observations have led to a similar conclusion. Brunia and van Boxtel found that $ACTH_{4-10}$ increased the heart rate and the magnitude of tendon reflexes in young healthy volunteers during a binary choice reaction test (Brunia and van Boxtel, 1978). They suggested that $ACTH_{4-10}$ intensified the arousal effect of the task. Branconnier et al. (1979) reported that $ACTH_{4-10}$ ameliorated the symptoms of senile organic brain syndrome due to an increase in non-specific arousal.

The more marked tonic and phasic bradycardiac changes in HR in rats treated with DGLVP, relative to controls, suggest that this neuropeptide intensifies both the generalized emotional reaction and the specific conditioned fear response. Vasopressin and related neuropeptides, similarly to $ACTH_{4-10}$, may increase arousal within the limbic–midbrain system, as has been indicated by electrophysiological experiments (Urban and de Wied, 1978). The difference in the quality of the tonic HR response of $ACTH_{4-10}$-treated rats and of those treated with DGLVP during passive avoidance, however, indicates that the behavioural effect of DGLVP is induced by mechanisms other than an increased arousal. The intensified tonic and phasic HR response may mean that this peptide modulates brain processes which are already specific for the given situation.

Neuropeptide deficiency and cardiac responses during passive avoidance behaviour

The above observations indicated that the same form of behavioural expression of emotion need not necessarily be accompanied by a uniform autonomic response. It was suggested that the same behavioural expression may occur under different central activity states. Our subsequent experiments, however, brought forward an alternative possibility: behavioural and autonomic changes may be under parallel but separate control of the same environmental stimulus events which evoke alterations in emotionality. Evidence favouring this alternative hypothesis and suggesting the importance of neuropeptides in both behavioural and autonomic responses was obtained from observations in rats with hereditary hypothalamic diabetes insipidus (Bohus, 1977). Rats homozygous for this disease lack the ability to synthesize vasopressin. This vasopressin deficiency is associated with a severe impairment of adaptive behaviour, particularly of memory function (Bohus et al., 1975; de Wied et al., 1975). Administration of vasopressin or of DGLVP normalizes the behaviour of the diabetes insipidus rat (de Wied et al., 1975). Impairment of passive avoidance behaviour in diabetes insipidus rats relative to that of their heterozygous litter-mates is not associated with a deficit of tonic HR response. Phasic changes in HR are, however, absent in these rats. Administration of vasopressin or DGLVP normalizes behaviour and leads to the re-occurrence of phasic HR responses. These observations indicate that in the absence of vasopressin the emotional experience is preserved but that the rat is not able to cope adequately with his behaviour to environmental stimuli. Such dissociation between behavioural and autonomic reactions may be of importance in the aetiology of psychosomatic disorders. It remains to be seen if neuropeptides play a role in these processes.

NEUROHYPOPHYSIAL PEPTIDES AND CENTRALLY EVOKED PRESSOR RESPONSES

Vasopressin inhibits the pressor response evoked by brain stimulation: a central site of action

The influence of neuropeptides on cardiac responses during classical conditioning and passive avoidance behaviour clearly indicates that the modulatory effects are not restricted to behavioural adaptation. The possibility of dissociation of behavioural and autonomic responses as found in the diabetes insipidus rats, however, led us to question whether the cardiac effect of the peptides is not the result of an action on the integrated control of the cardiovascular system rather than a consequence of their behavioural action. In order to investigate this matter we adopted another experimental approach: an examination of the effects of neuropeptides on centrally evoked pressor responses. The hypothalamus and brain stem areas are intimately involved in the central control of the cardiovascular system and in the organization of cardiovascular responses during defence reactions. By electrical stimulation of these areas one may simulate the activation of the system: an increase in blood pressure (pressor response) and a decrease in heart rate is induced. Our first findings with vasopressin on the centrally evoked pressor responses were rather surprising. Intravenous administration of LVP, although causing a temporary increase in basal blood pressure, resulted in a significant reduction of the pressor response evoked by posterior hypothalamic stimulation and increased the threshold to evoke pressor response from the mesencephalic reticular formation (Bohus, 1974b). It took 60 min, however, for the maximal inhibitory effect to develop. This long latency period was indicative that the inhibition could not be due to the vasopressor property of the peptide and presupposed a central site of action. This assumption was further supported by the finding that the administration of DGLVP resulted in a similar inhibition of the centrally evoked pressor response. DGLVP does not possess pressor activity, but it is highly active behaviourally (de Wied *et al.*, 1972).

The ultimate evidence that vasopressin and DGLVP act centrally in inhibiting the pressor response was obtained following intracerebroventricular administration of the peptides (Versteeg, 1979a). It was found that arginine[8]-vasopressin (AVP) injected into a lateral ventricle attenuated the pressor response evoked by the stimulation of the mesencephalic reticular formation of urethane-anaesthetized rats. The attenuation was dose-dependent in a range of 3 to 25 ng. A dose of 25 ng AVP was effective after 20 min and caused a diminution of about 40%. Intracerebroventricular administration of DGLVP had a similar effect on the pressor response.

Although these findings were at first rather unexpected, recently acquired knowledge makes sense of the hypothesis that centrally available vasopressin is a modulator of cardiovascular regulation. It is generally acknowledged that noradrenaline is an inhibitory transmitter in central cardiovascular regulation (de Jong *et al.*, 1975). It has also been shown that centrally administered vasopressin increases the turnover rate of noradrenaline in limbic–midbrain areas and in the lower brain stem (Tanaka *et al.*, 1977). Pronounced effects have been found in areas such as the nucleus tractus solitarii and reticularis lateralis, which play an important role in cardiovascular regulation. Furthermore, it has been demonstrated that the dorsal noradrenergic bundle system is involved in certain behavioural effects of vasopressin (Kovács *et al.*, 1979). Accordingly, it is felt that an inhibitory effect of vasopressin on the centrally evoked pressor responses may be mediated through the activation of central noradrenergic inhibitory mechanisms. The physiological significance of the inhibitory effect of vasopressin, however, is not yet clear. It is of interest that vasopressinergic neurons, which arise from the neurosecretory nuclei of the hypothalamus, terminate in limbic, mesencephalic and lower brain stem areas which have been implicated in cardiovascular control (Buijs *et al.*, 1978; Sofroniew and Weindl, 1978). Modulation of behavioural and cardiovascular responses by vasopressin may occur in the same sites. Local micro-injection of AVP in the dentate gyri of the hippocampi facilitates adaptive processes such as memory consolidation (Kovács *et al.*, 1979). Destruction of the dentate area by electrolytic lesions prevents the inhibitory effect of AVP on the centrally evoked pressor responses, while local micro-injection of the peptide in this area results in a mimicking of intraventricular administration (Versteeg *et al.*, 1979b).

Inhibition of a centrally evoked pressor response by vasopressin: structure-activity relations

Behavioural studies have suggested that neurohypophysial hormones may serve as mother-molecules for behaviourally active fragments (de Wied, 1977). It has been found that AVP contains two active sites in attenuating centrally evoked pressor response. One is located in the pressinoic ring structure and the other in the C-terminal linear portion of the molecule. Both pressinamide and Pro-Arg-Gly-NH$_2$ (PAG) attenuate the pressor response when administered intracerebroventricularly. Interestingly, the structurally related oxytocin has a similar activity. The ring structure of oxytocin (tocinamide) remains inactive, but the C-terminal fragment Pro-Leu-Gly-NH$_2$ (PLG) is even more active than AVP or PAG on a weight basis (Versteeg *et al.*, 1979a). It is not unlikely that PLG, which also has an MSH-release-inhibiting activity and can be formed in the brain, and neurohypophysis (Walter *et al.*, 1973) represents another modulatory system independent of the vasopressin-ergic one.

CONCLUDING REMARKS

The experiments reviewed here clearly indicate that neuropeptides related to ACTH, vasopressin and oxytocin influence adaptive cardiovascular responses. The effects of the peptides on autonomic processes may be related to their modulatory role in behavioural adaptation. Neurohypophysial peptides may also modulate the activity of integrative cardiovascular regulatory centres. Our findings have helped to explain the mechanisms of action of neuro-peptides through which the behavioural effects are exerted, and have suggested that central peptidergic systems may play a modulatory role in the inhibitory control of the cardiovascular system. Centrally evoked pressor response may be considered a model of neurogenic hypertension. Disturb-ances in central catecholamine metabolism may be important in the genesis of hypertension (Yamori *et al.*, 1970). Vasopressin and its fragments modulate the activity of central noradrenergic neurons. It would therefore be interesting to explore whether dysfunction of the neuropeptide system contributes to the development of neurogenic hypertension, and whether neuropeptide treat-ment can restore the activity of the catecholaminergic system, thereby pre-venting the genesis of centrally induced hypertension.

References

Ader, R., Weijnen, J. A. W. M. and Moleman, P. (1972). Retention of a passive avoidance response as a function of the intensity and duration of electric shock. *Psychon. Sci.*, **26**, 125

Branconnier, R. J., Colemi, J. O. and Gardos, G. (1979). ACTH$_{4-10}$ in the amelioration of neuropsychological symptomatology associated with senile organic brain syndrome. *Psycho-pharmacology*, **61**, 161

Bohus, B. (1979). Effects of ACTH-like neuropeptides on animal behavior and man. *Pharma-cology*, **18**, 113

Bohus, B. (1977). Pituitary neuropeptides, emotional behavior and cardiac responses. In W. de Jong, A. P. Provoost and A. P. Shapiro (eds.), *Hypertension and Brain Mechanisms. Progress in Brain Research*, vol. 47, pp. 277–288. (Amsterdam: Elsevier)

Bohus, B. (1975). Pituitary peptides and adaptive autonomic responses. In W. H. Gispen, T. B. van Wimersma Greidanus, B. Bohus and D. de Wied (eds.), *Hormones, Homeostasis and the Brain. Progress in Brain Research*, vol. 42, pp. 275–283. (Amsterdam: Elsevier)

Bohus, B. (1974a). Telemetered heart rate responses of the rat during free and learned behavior. *Biotelemetry*, **1**, 193

Bohus, B. (1974b). The influence of pituitary peptides on brain centers controlling autonomic responses. In D. F. Swaab and J. P. Schadé (eds.), *Integrative Hypothalamic Activity. Progress in Brain Research*, vol. 41, pp. 175–183. (Amsterdam: Elsevier)

Bohus, B., Gispen, W. H. and de Wied, D. (1973). Effect of lysine vasopressin and ACTH$_{4-10}$ on conditioned avoidance behavior of the rat. *Neuroendocrinology*, **11**, 137

Bohus, B., de Jong, W., Provoost, A. P. and de Wied, D. (1976). Emotionales Verhalten und Reaktionen des Kreislaufs und Endokriniums bei Ratten. In A. W. von Eiff (ed.), *Seelische und Körperliches Störungen Durch Stress*, pp. 140–157. (Stuttgart: Gustav Fisher)

Bohus, B., van Wimersma Greidanus, T. B. and de Wied, D. (1975). Behavioral and endocrine responses of rats with hereditary hypothalamic diabetes insipidus (Brattleboro strain). *Physiol. Behav.*, **14**, 609

Brunia, C. H. M. and van Boxtel, A. (1978). MSH/ACTH$_{4-10}$ and task-induced increase in tendon reflexes and heart rate. *Pharmacol. Biochem. Behav.*, **9**, 615

Buijs, R. M., Swaab, D. F., Dogterom, J. and van Leeuwen, F. W. (1978). Intra- and extra-hypothalamic vasopressin and oxytocin pathways in the rat. *Cell Tiss. Res.*, **186**, 423

Henry, J. P. (1976). Mechanisms of psychosomatic disease in animals. *Adv. Vet. Sci.*, **20**, 115

de Jong, W., Zandberg, P. and Bohus, B. (1975). Central inhibitory noradrenergic control. In W. H. Gispen, T. B. van Wimersma Greidanus, B. Bohus and D. de Wied (eds.), *Hormones, Homeostasis and the Brain. Progress in Brain Research*, vol. 42, pp. 285–298. (Amsterdam: Elsevier)

Kovács, G. L., Bohus, B. and Versteeg, D. H. G. (1979). The effects of vasopressin on memory processes: the role of noradrenergic neurotransmission. *Neuroscience*, **4**, 1529

Mason, J. W. (1968). A review of psychoneuroendocrine research on the pituitary-adrenal cortical system. *Psychosom. Med.*, **30**, 576

Obrist, P. A., Webb, R. A., Sutterer, J. R. and Howard, J. L. (1970). The cardiac–somatic relationship: some reformulations. *Psychophysiology*, **6**, 569

Pribram, K. H. and McGuiness, D. (1975). Arousal, activation and effort in the control of attention. *Psychol. Rev.*, **82**, 116

Sandman, C. A., Kastin, A. J., Schally, A. V., Kendall, J. W. and Miller, L. H. (1973). Neuroendocrine responses to physical and psychological stress. *J. Comp. Physiol. Psychol.*, **84**, 386

Sofroniew, M. W. and Weindl, A. (1978). Projections from the parvocellular vasopressin- and neurophysin-containing neurons of the suprachiasmatic nucleus. *Am. J. Anat.*, **153**, 391

Tanaka, M., de Kloet, E. R., de Wied, D. and Versteeg, D. H. G. (1977). Arginine[8]-vasopressin affects catecholamine metabolism in specific brain nuclei. *Life Sci.*, **20**, 1799

Thompson, E. A. and de Wied, D. (1973). The relationship between the antidiuretic activity of rat eye plexus blood and passive avoidance behaviour. *Physiol. Behav.*, **11**, 377

Urban, I. and de Wied, D. (1978). Neuropeptides: effects on paradoxical sleep and theta rhythm in rats. *Pharmacol. Biochem. Behav.*, **8**, 51

Urban, I. and de Wied, D. (1976). Changes in excitability in the theta activity generating substrate by ACTH$_{4-10}$ in the rat. *Exp. Brain Res.*, **24**, 325

Versteeg, C. A. M., Bohus, B. and de Jong, W. (1979a). Inhibitory effects of neuropeptides on centrally evoked pressor responses. In W. Lovenberg (ed.), *Prophylactic Approach to Hypertensive Diseases*, pp. 329–335. (New York: Raven Press)

Versteeg, C. A. M., Bohus, B. and de Jong, W. (1979b). Involvement of the hippocampus in the attenuation of a centrally evoked pressor response by neuropeptides. *Procs. of the 20th Dutch Federation Meeting, Groningen*, abs. 437

Walter, R., Griffiths, E. C. and Hooper, K. C. (1973). Production of MSH-release-inhibiting hormone by a particulate preparation of hypothalami: mechanisms of oxytocin-inactivation. *Brain Res.*, **60**, 449

de Wied, D. (1977). Peptides and behavior. *Life Sci.*, **20**, 195

de Wied, D., Bohus, B. and van Wimersma Greidanus, T. B. (1975). Memory deficit in rats with hereditary diabetes insipidus. *Brain Res.*, **85**, 152

de Wied, D., Greven, H. M., Lande, S. and Witter, A. (1972). Dissociation of the behavioural and endocrine effects of lysine vasopressin by tryptic digestion. *Br. J. Pharmacol.*, **45**, 118

Yamori, Y., Lovenberg, W. and Sjoerdsma, A. (1970). Norepinephrine metabolism in brainstem of spontaneously hypertensive rats. *Science*, **170**, 544

Address for correspondence

Dr B. Bohus, Rudolf Magnus Instituut voor Farmacologie, Medische Faculteit, Rijksuniversiteit Utrecht, Vondellaan 6, 3521 GD Utrecht, The Netherlands

2.4
Endorphins
and schizophrenia

H. M. VAN PRAAG and W. M. A. VERHOEVEN

ABSTRACT

Clinical endorphin research in schizophrenia has so far fanned out in the following directions: (a) studies of endorphin concentration in body fluids, and (b) studies of the effects in schizophrenic patients of opiate (endorphin) antagonists, and of endorphins and endorphin derivatives. The main results are reviewed in this paper. The conclusions drawn are:

(1) Body fluid research has so far yielded no conclusive evidence of disrupted endorphin metabolism in schizophrenia. Technology for the measurement of small quantities of endorphins is, however, still deficient.

(2) The opiate antagonist issue is controversial. One of the major problems is that the studies undertaken differ considerably from each other in patient selection, dose and route of administration, making comparisons difficult. Furthermore, only single dose studies have been reported; the results of repeated administrations may be different.

(3) To date only β-endorphin, DTγE (a fragment of γ-endorphin) and FK33-824 (a synthetic met-enkephalin derivative) have been studied therapeutically. Of these, DTγE is the most interesting in scientific terms, firstly because, pharmacologically, it seems to be related to the 'true' neuroleptics, and secondly because its lacks morphinomimetic properties. The

141

therapeutic potential of this substance, if confirmed, would therefore not be related to morphine-like activity but to a 'genuine' opiate-receptor-independent anti-psychotic action.

INTRODUCTION

The discovery of endorphins resulted from the following observations:

(a) The mammalian central nervous system was found to contain receptors which had a high affinity for morphine and related compounds but which were insensitive to any of the known neurotransmitters (Pert and Snyder, 1973; Simon *et al.*, 1973; Terenius, 1973).

(b) Pain can be alleviated in test animals by electrical stimulation of certain brain areas. The stimulation-induced analgesia can be antagonized with an opiate antagonist such as naloxone (Akil *et al.*, 1976; Mayer *et al.*, 1971).

These observations suggested the existence of an endogenous ligand for these so-called opiate receptors. Within a remarkably short space of time, two such compounds were isolated in the brain and identified (Hughes, 1975; Terenius and Wahlström, 1975). They were pentapeptides named enkephalins: methionine-enkephalin (met-enkephalin) and leucine-enkephalin (leu-enkephalin).

After the discovery of the enkephalins, the search for other peptides with opiate-like effects was further intensified when the amino-acid sequence of met-enkephalin proved to be present in the 91-amino-acid pituitary hormone β-lipotropin (β-LPH). There then followed the discovery of β-endorphin (β-LPH$_{61-91}$) (Li and Chung, 1976), which consists of the terminal 31 amino acids of β-LPH, γ-endorphin (β-LPH$_{61-76}$) and α-endorphin (β-LPH$_{61-77}$) (Figure 1),

All endorphins and enkephalins except leu-enkephalin, therefore, are β-LPH fragments. The endorphins—the larger β-LPH fragments—are chiefly found in the pituitary gland, like β-LPH itself. The enkephalins, on the other hand, are found almost exclusively in the brain. Neurons and pituitary cells containing β-endorphin also contain β-LPH and ACTH. The brain contains neurons with β-endorphin as well as with enkephalin. There are sound reasons for assuming that in these cells β-endorphin and enkephalin play a role in impulse transmissions or modulation (Snyder and Childers, 1979). In the present paper 'endorphins' will be used collectively for endorphins in the strict sense and for enkephalins.

Endorphins attracted psychiatric attention from the start for the following reasons:

(1) High endorphin concentrations are found in brain areas involved in

pain conduction, motor activity and, probably, regulation of mood and affects (Snyder and Childers, 1979).

(2) Opiates have a distinct effect on pain threshold, mood and level of psychological integration. A similar effect could be expected of the 'endogenous morphines'.

(3) Patients whose medial thalamus was electrically stimulated to alleviate chronic pain were found to have increased enkephalin-like activity in the cerebrospinal fluid (CSF) (Akil *et al.*, 1978a).

(4) Stress increases the release of ACTH as well as of β-endorphin by the pituitary gland (Watson *et al.*, 1979; Guillemin *et al.*, 1977).

(5) β-endorphin exerts an unmistakable influence on animal behaviour. In large doses it gives rise to a catatonia-like condition with motor retardation (Snyder, 1978; Bloom *et al.*, 1976; Jacquet and Marks, 1976).

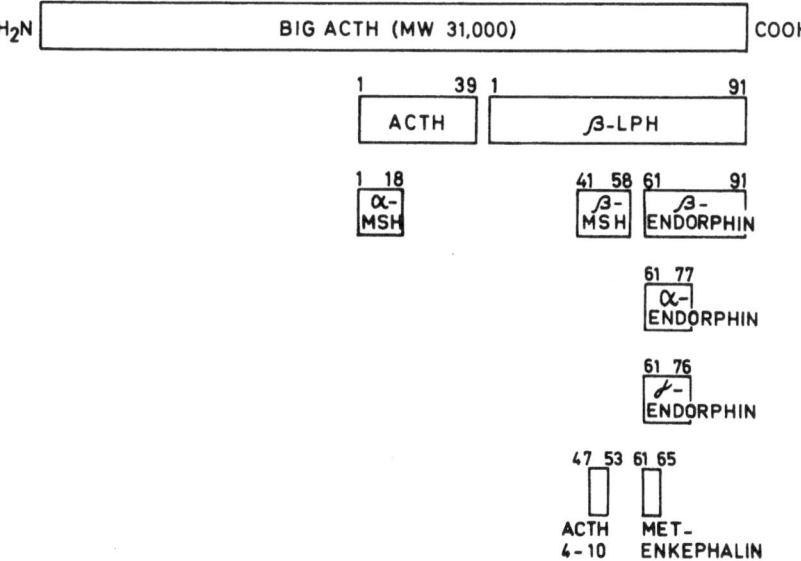

Figure 1 Precursor relationships of corticotrophins and pituitary endotrophins. The 31 000 molecular weight peptide 'big ACTH' contains the ACTH and β-lipotropin (β-LPH) molecules, which appear to be located next to each other. Within the ACTH molecule lies the sequence of α-MSH, while the sequences of β-MSH and of β-endorphin are contained within the structure of β-LPH. The sequence of the fourth to tenth amino acids of ACTH is contained within the β-LPH sequence, so that this portion of the ACTH molecule is contained twice within the big ACTH precursor. The sequence of γ-endorphin, α-endorphin and met-enkephalin is contained within that of β-endorphin. Supposedly, α- and γ-endorphin are formed from β-endorphin. There is no evidence that β-endorphin is the precursor of met-enkephalin in the brain. (From Snyder and Childers, 1979)

Clinical endorphin research to date has consisted of studies of endorphin concentrations in body fluids, principally of CSF and dialysate after haemodialysis, and into the effects of opiate (endorphin) antagonists and of endorphins and endorphin derivatives in psychiatric patients. The following is a brief survey of these activities.

ENDORPHIN RESEARCH IN PSYCHIATRIC PATIENTS

Endorphins in human cerebrospinal fluid

In 1975, Terenius and Wahlström isolated two 'endorphin fractions' (opiate-like material) from human CSF, neither of which is identical to any of the endorphins as we now know them. The concentrations of these fractions were determined in 13 patients with schizophrenic and in seven with manic-depressive psychoses (Lindström et al., 1978; Terenius et al., 1977 and 1976). An increased fraction I and II endorphin concentration was found in several, not in all, schizophrenic patients. This was normalized by neuroleptic medication, which resulted in a reduction of psychotic symptoms. In all manic patients an increased fraction I endorphin fraction was found during the manic phase. A correlation between fraction II endorphin and clinical symptoms was not demonstrable.

The β-endorphin concentration in the CSF was found to be markedly increased in patients with acute schizophrenic psychoses, whereas in chronic psychotic patients it was normal or slightly decreased (Domschke et al., 1979). Loeber et al. (1979) demonstrated the presence of α- and γ-endorphin in human CSF. Whether the concentrations of these two endorphins can show changes in psychiatric patients has yet to be established.

Opiate antagonists

Opiate antagonists block opiate receptors and have therefore been used in efforts to establish the (patho)physiological significance of endorphins, at least that of their effects which are produced via opiate receptors. The two pure opiate antagonists, naloxone and naltrexone, have been used in human studies. (Naltrexone has a slightly prolonged effect and, unlike naloxone, can be administered orally in normal subjects.) Naltrexone has been found to have a dysphoric effect (Mendelson et al., 1979). In psychiatric patients these compounds have been studied mostly in schizophrenic and manic syndromes. The results of relevant studies are shown in Table 1.

In three out of eight controlled clinical trials, those of Akil et al. (1978a), Watson et al. (1978) and Emrich et al. (1977), a favourable effect of naloxone was demonstrated, i.e. a transient reduction, and sometimes disappearance, of acoustic hallucinations. Some 30% of the patients so far treated with naloxone have responded to this medication. There are sound reasons to believe that the

Table 1 Effects of naloxone and naltrexone in schizophrenic and manic syndromes

Study	Diagnosis	N	Neuroleptic medication	Design	Dosage naloxone*	Result	Duration	Attenuation of symptoms
Emrich et al., 1977	Schizophrenia	20	−: 2 / +: 18	Double-blind cross-over	4 mg i.v.	+12	2–7h	Auditory hallucinations
Watson et al., 1978	Schizophrenia	11	−: 6 / +: 5	Double-blind cross-over: 9 / Single-blind: 2	10 mg i.v.	+6	3–6 h: 4 / 48 h: 2	Auditory hallucinations
Akil et al., 1978a	Schizophrenia	8	−: 4 / +: 4	Double-blind cross-over	10 mg i.v.	+8	1¼–1½h	Auditory hallucinations
Gunne et al., 1977	Schizophrenia	6	+: 6	Single-blind	0.4 mg i.v.	+4	1–6h	Auditory hallucinations
Kurland et al., 1977	Schizophrenia	12	+: 12	Double-blind	0.4–1.2 mg i.v.	−		
Mielke and Gallant, 1977	Schizophrenia	5	−: 5	Open	Naltrexone 250 mg 9 days	−		
Gitlin and Rosenblatt, 1978	Schizophrenia	3	−: 1 / +: 2	Single-blind	Naltrexone 50–100 mg 14 days	−		
Davis et al., 1977	Schizophrenia	14	−: 9 / +: 5	Double-blind	0.4–10 mg i.v.	−		
Volavka et al., 1977	Schizophrenia	7	+: 7	Double-blind	0.4 mg i.v.	−		
Janowsky et al., 1977	Schizophrenia	8	+: 8	Double-blind cross-over	1.2 mg i.v.	−		
Hertz et al., 1978	Schizophrenia	20	−: 20	Double-blind cross-over	4 mg i.v.	−		
Janowsky et al., 1978	Manic syndrome	12	−: 3 / +: 9	Double-blind cross-over	20 mg i.v. (infusion)	+12	½–1½h	Manic symptoms
Judd et al., 1978	Manic syndrome	12	−: 12	Double-blind cross-over	20 mg i.v. (infusion)	+4	½–2 h	Manic symptoms
Verhoeven et al., 1979b	Schizophrenia 5 / Manic syndrome 5		+: 10	Double-blind	20 mg s.c.	−		
TOTAL	Schizophrenia 119 / Manic syndrome 29					+30 / +16	2–7h / ½–2 h	Auditory hallucinations / Manic symptoms

* So far only single administration studies have been carried out

therapeutic effect of neuroleptics depends on their ability to block dopamine receptors (van Praag, 1980b and 1977). However, as naloxone, unlike neuroleptics, has no effect on serum prolactin (Lal *et al.*, 1979), the dopamine receptors in the tubero-infundibular system are not blocked. The antipsychotic properties of naloxone must, therefore, be produced via another mechanism.

The two controlled clinical studies of Janowsky *et al.* (1978) and Judd *et al.* (1978) revealed a transient reduction of manic symptoms in 16 out of a total of 24 patients. One controlled study, that of Verhoeven *et al.* (1979b), produced negative results.

It is tentatively concluded from these data that there could exist a subgroup of psychotic patients, or some psychotic symptoms, which are susceptible to opiate antagonists. However, further definition of this range of indications is not yet possible.

Dialysate studies

In 1977, Wagemaker and Cade described a favourable effect of long-term haemodialysis in chronic schizophrenic patients. Several centres are now conducting studies in which dialysis and sham-dialysis are being compared. A conclusion on the therapeutic validity of this method in schizophrenic patients would be premature at the present time, however.

Also in 1977, Palmour *et al.* isolated a hitherto unknown peptide from the dialysate of dialysed schizophrenic patients. This was believed to be β-endorphin in which the methionine in the five-position has been replaced by leucine (βH-leu^5-endorphin). It was a sensational discovery, implying the possibility of a correlation between disorders of endorphin metabolism and schizophrenic psychoses. However, Lewis *et al.* have recently reported (1979) that they have been unable to isolate a peptide of this structure from the haemodialysate of two schizophrenic patients.

THERAPEUTIC APPLICATIONS OF ENDORPHINS AND ENDORPHIN DERIVATIVES

β-Endorphin

In an open study, without a clearly defined protocol, a total dose of 9 mg β-endorphin was injected intravenously over 4 days in five patients with schizophrenic psychoses and in two with depressions, one unipolar and the other bipolar (Kline *et al.*, 1977). Within a few minutes of the injection an activating, anxiolytic and anti-depressant effect was seen, which persisted for 2–3 h. There then followed a period of drowsiness, and about 12 h after the injection a therapeutic effect was observed, characterized by a reduction of the psychotic or depressive symptoms, which lasted 1–10 days. Berger *et al.*, however, in a carefully controlled study, have been unable to confirm these findings (personal communication). This group found that only one item, hallucinations, improved after β-endorphin administration, and that although this improvement was statistically significant, therapeutically it was insignificant.

Des-tyrosine-γ-endorphin (DTγE)

Most endorphins, certainly β-endorphin, α-endorphin, met-enkephalin and leu-enkephalin, have the following properties:

(1) They are morphinomimetics. Elimination of the terminal tyrosine molecule in position six leads to loss of the morphinomimetic characteristics.

(2) They are able to delay the extinction of conditioned behaviour (e.g. conditioned active and passive avoidance behaviour). This effect is independent of the opiate receptors, for it persists after the blocking of these receptors by means of naloxone.

One endorphin deviates from this general pattern: γ-endorphin (de Wied *et al.*, 1978). This endorphin does have morphinomimetic properties, but it facilitates extinction instead of retention of new information. In this respect it behaves like the traditional neuroleptics of, say, the phenothiazine and butyrophenone series. If the terminal tyrosine molecule is split off (thus producing DTγE), the molecule loses its morphinomimetic characteristics and its facilitating effect on the extinction of conditioned behaviour is intensified.

Apart from its suppressive effect on conditioned behaviour, DTγE has other properties in common with traditional neuroleptics, e.g. a positive grip test. In some ways its profile differs from that of traditional neuroleptics: it has no effect on gross behaviour in an open field, nor does it antagonize the effects of apomorphine and amphetamine, compounds with a dopamine-potentiating capacity. In biochemical terms, too, there is a similarity between DTγE and neuroleptics. Both types of compound increase the dopamine turnover in certain brain areas. With the neuroleptics, this effect is probably secondary to the blockade of post-synaptic dopamine receptors. Exactly how DTγE increases the dopamine turnover remains to be established (Versteeg *et al.*, 1979).

In view of the similarities between DTγE and the traditional neuroleptics we decided to study this peptide in patients with schizophrenic psychoses. To date one open and one controlled study have been undertaken, involving a total of 14 patients with recurrent schizophrenic and schizo-affective psychoses (Verhoeven *et al.*, 1979b and 1978). Twelve of these patients had been hospitalized for at least 6 months when the study began and were still psychotic despite medication with neuroleptics. The remaining two were treated with DTγE immediately upon admission to hospital for acute schizo-phrenic psychoses. In the past these two patients had repeatedly been hospital-ized for acute psychotic episodes; at the time of the study they were not being treated with neuroleptics.

In the first study, six of the long-term patients were given a single intra-muscular dose of 1 mg DTγE per day for 7 days. Treatment with neuroleptics had been discontinued 1 week before the DTγE injections were started. All six patients showed marked exacerbation of psychotic symptoms upon dis-continuation of neuroleptics. From day 4 of DTγE medication, three patients showed a reduction of psychotic symptoms and were entirely free of them from day 6 of DTγE treatment until the third week after its discontinuation. Two then showed a recurrence of psychotic symptoms; the follow-up of the third patient had to be discontinued when she was transferred to another hospital. The remaining three patients showed a reduction of psychotic symptoms on days 3 and 4 of medication, but from day 5 on became psychotic again with severe agitation and aggressiveness. DTγE was then discontinued and neuroleptic medication reinstituted.

In the second study, a double-blind, placebo-controlled, cross-over design, six long-term patients received 1 mg DTγE per day by intramuscular injection for 8 days, but in these patients the neuroleptic treatment was continued. A progressive reduction of psychotic symptoms was observed in all six patients from the first day of DTγE medication (Figure 2). Four patients became psychotic again 4–10 days after discontinuation of treatment, but their symptoms seemed less severe than prior to DTγE medication. The other two patients remain free from psychotic symptoms.

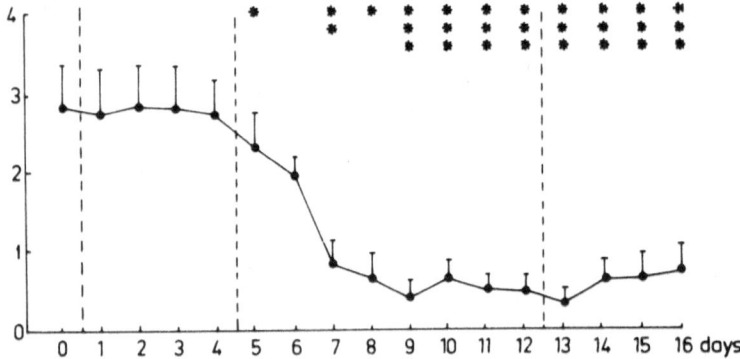

Figure 2 Summary of data relating to the item delusions and hallucinations obtained in a controlled (des-tyr[1])-γ-endorphin study. Days 1 to 4 are those preceding (des-tyr[1])-γ-endorphin treatment (days 5 to 12) and days 13 to 16 are those on which placebo was administered. Mean scores of six patients are plotted against days of treatment. Vertical bars indicate SEM. Student's paired t test was used to compare individual values on a given day with those obtained on day 4. *indicates $p < 0.05$, **$p < 0.01$, ***$p < 0.005$. (From Verhoeven et al., 1979b)

The same double-blind cross-over design was used for the two acutely psychotic drug-free patients treated with DTγE immediately after hospitalization. Both showed reduction of psychotic symptoms from day 3 of medication, and from day 6 onwards were free of psychotic symptoms for some months.

All 14 patients treated with DTγE showed an improved emotional responsiveness, and no extrapyramidal, cardiovascular or gastrointestinal side-effects were observed.

Like γ-endorphin, DTγE has recently been found in human CSF (Loeber *et al.*, 1979). It therefore seems plausible that this compound is normally formed in the brain, probably from γ-endorphin, which, like α-endorphin, is probably a split product of β-endorphin (Figure 3).

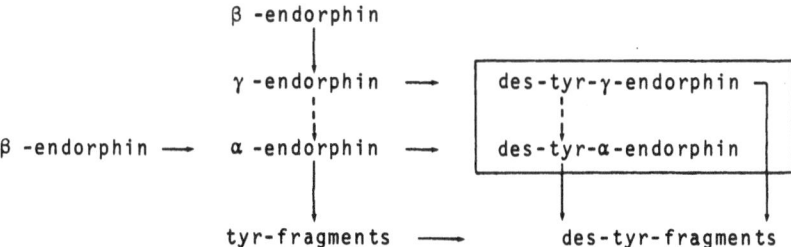

Figure 3 Schematic representation of the fragmentation of β-endorphin. (From de Wied, 1978)

It is conceivable that DTγE was effective in the studies described above because the patients involved were suffering from a DTγE deficiency (de Wied, 1978), a deficiency which could, in principle, develop in two ways: as a result of a deficient formation of DTγE from β-endorphin, or because of its accelerated conversion to α-endorphin. This hypothesis is being investigated in our current endorphin research. If arguments are found to support it, it would mean that a disturbed endorphin metabolism plays a role in the pathogenesis of (some types of) schizophrenic psychoses, and, further, that treatment with DTγE could be regarded as a form of substitution therapy (de Wied, 1978).

A similar development, i.e. treatment of a psychiatric syndrome with exogenous substances in which the brain is probably deficient, has already occurred in the field of depression, where the serotonin precursor 5-hydroxytryptophan has been successfully used in the treatment and prevention of certain types of vital depression (van Praag, 1980a).

In three patients in the first DTγE study mentioned above, initial improvement was followed by marked psychotic exacerbation with intensive agitation and aggressiveness. In principle there are two possible explanations for this: firstly, the exacerbation may have resulted from the discontinuation of neuroleptic therapy; secondly, it may have been due to the DTγE medication itself. In the context of the latter possibility, it could be that the exogenous DTγE is unusually quickly converted to DTαE and that DTαE is responsible for the exacerbation. This seems a reasonable hypothesis because de Wied (personal communication) has demonstrated that, at least in animals, DTαE has amphetamine-like properties, and central stimulants are known to be able to induce psychoses or exacerbate existing psychoses. The fact that this complication did not develop in the second experiment could have been due to the fact that in this study neuroleptic maintenance therapy was continued during the DTγE study. Verification of the hypothesis has to be postponed until reliable methods are evolved to determine DTγE and its split products in body fluids.

FK33-824: a synthetic met-enkephalin

FK33-824 is a met-enkephalin derivative with the following amino-acid sequence: Tyr-D-Ala-Gly-Mephe-Met(0)-ol. The amino-acid sequence of met-enkephalin is: Tyr-Gly-Gly-Phe-Meth. FK33-824 differs from met-enkephalin in (a) the replacement of glycine by d-alanine, (b) the N-methylation of phenylalanine, and (c) the alteration of methionine by the oxidization of its sulphur to sulphoxide and the conversion of the carboxyl to a carbinol.

Jørgensen *et al.* (1979) used FK33-824 in nine patients with chronic psychoses: eight chronic schizophrenics and one patient with alcohol hallucinosis. The patients had been hospitalized for 7–15 years. Their medication was continued, but in addition they received, in a single-blind design, intramuscular injections of 1, 2 and 3 mg FK33-824 on three consecutive days. An unmistakable therapeutic effect was observed in six patients. Four of them showed a striking effect against hallucinations ('voices') and an increased sense of well-being: they 'felt better than they had for years'. In two patients there was no effect on the hallucinations, but these patients became more open and spontaneous, more freely speaking than usual, and euphoric. The effect persisted for 4–7 days after the last injection. A rebound effect was observed (as it was after DTγE) in three patients. Initial improvement in these patients was followed by exacerbation, which in turn was followed by improvement. The DTγE patients who showed exacerbation were given neuroleptics to control it, and consequently it was not established whether their rebound effect was transient.

These findings were confirmed by Nedopil and Rüther (1979) who demonstrated, in an open study, a beneficial effect of FK33-824 in five out of six patients suffering from acute and chronic schizophrenia. The drug was given in doses of 0.5 and 1.0 mg per i.v. infusion on two consecutive days. In contrast to the former study, the patients in this study were drug-free.

Unlike DTγE, FK33-824 has retained its terminal tyrosine molecule and so possesses morphinomimetic properties. It is therefore uncertain whether its therapeutic effect is based on these properties or on a 'genuine' opiate-receptor-independent anti-psychotic action.

CONCLUSIONS

Since 1975 the identification of the endorphins, which can perhaps be regarded as neurotransmitters or neuromodulators, has given the field of psychoneuroendocrinology a new dimension. Animal experiments have shown that, in addition to a morphinomimetic effect, endorphins exert other influences on behaviour which may or may not be mediated by opiate receptors.

Therapeutic effects have so far been obtained with β-endorphin, DTγE (a split product of γ-endorphin) and FK33-824 (a synthetic-met-enkephalin derivative). However, the clinical data available are far too limited at the present time to permit any definitive conclusions to be drawn. So far, observations on DTγE have been the most interesting in scientific terms. DTγE is an endogenous peptide in the brain, with properties which are also found in the pharmacological action profile of 'true' neuroleptics. It is therefore conceivable that DTγE, or a compound closely related to it, is an endogenous 'anti-psychotic' and that a DTγE deficiency based on disturbed endorphin metabolism contributes to the pathogenesis of (certain types of) schizophrenia. The heuristic value of this theory is quite substantial, for it generates a number of hypotheses that could be clinically tested, always provided that reliable methods can be evolved to separate and measure endorphins in body fluids.

References

Akil, H., Mayer, D. J. and Liebeskind, J. C. (1976). Antagonism of stimulation-produced analgesia by naloxone, a narcotic antagonist. *Science*, **191**, 961

Akil, H., Richardson, D. E., Hughes, J. and Barchas, J. D. (1978a). Enkephalin-like material elevated in ventricular cerebrospinal fluid of pain patients after analgesic focal stimulation. *Science*, **201**, 463

Akil, H., Watson, S. J., Berger, P. A. and Barchas, J. D. (1978b). Endorphins, β-LPH and ACTH: biochemical, pharmacological and anatomical studies. In E. Costa and M. Trabucci (eds.), *Advances in Biochemical Psychopharmacology*, pp. 125–137. (New York: Raven Press)

Bloom, F., Segal, D., Ling, N. and Guillemin, R. (1976). Endorphins: profound behavioral effects in rats suggest new etiological factors in mental illness. *Science*, **194**, 630

Davis, G. C., Bunney, W. E., Jr, DeFraites, E. G., Kleinman, J. E., van Kammen, D. P., Post, R. M. and Wyatt, R. J. (1977). Intravenous naloxone administration in schizophrenia and affective illness. *Science*, **197**, 74

Domschke, W., Dickschas, A. and Mitznegg, P. (1979). CSF β-endorphine in schizophrenia. *Lancet*, **1**, 1029

Emrich, H. M., Cording, C., Pirée, S., Kölling, A., von Zerssen, D. and Hertz, A. (1977). Indication of an anti-psychotic action of the opiate antagonist naloxone. *Pharmakopsychiat.*, **10**, 265

Gitlin, M. and Rosenblatt, M. (1978). Possible withdrawal from endogenous opiates in schizophrenics. *Am. J. Psychiat.*, **135**, 377

Guillemin, R., Vargo, T., Rossier, J., Minick, I., Ling, N., Rivier, C., Vale, W. and Bloom, F. (1977). β-endorphin and adrenocorticotropin are secreted by the pituitary gland. *Science*, **197**, 1367

Gunne, L. M., Lindström, L. and Terenius, L. (1977). Naxolone-induced reversal of schizophrenic hallucinations. *J. Neural. Trans.*, **40**, 13

Hertz, A., Bläsig, J. M., Emrich, H. M., Cording, C., Pirée, S., Kölling, A. and von Zerssen, D. (1978). In E. Costa and M. Trabucchi (eds.), *Advances in Biochemical Psychopharmacology*. (New York: Raven Press)

Hughes, J. (1975). Isolation of an endogenous compound from the brain with pharmacological properties similar to morphine. *Brain Res.*, **88**, 295

Jacquet, Y. F. and Marks, N. (1976). The C-fragment of β-lipotropin: an endogenous neuroleptic of anti-psychotogen. *Science*, **194**, 632

Janowsky, D. S., Judd, L. L., Huey, L., Roitman, N., Parker, D. and Segal, D. (1978). Naloxone effects on manic symptoms and growth hormone levels. *Lancet*, **2**, 320

Janowsky, D. S., Segal, D. S., Bloom, F., Abrams, A. and Guillemin, R. (1977). Lack of effect of naxolone on schizophrenic symptoms. *Am. J. Psychiat.*, **134**, 926

Jørgensen, A., Fog, R. and Veilis, B. (1979). Synthetic enkephalin analogue in treatment of schizophrenia. *Lancet*, **1**, 935

Judd, L. L., Janowsky, D. S., Segal, D. S., Leighton, P. D. and Huey, L. (1978). Nalaxone related attenuation of manic symptoms in certain bipolar depressives. In J. M. van Ree and L. Terenius (eds.), *Characteristics and Function of Opioids. Developments in Neuroscience*, vol. 4, pp. 173–175. (Amsterdam: Elsevier/North-Holland)

Kline, N. S., Li, C. H., Lehmann, H. E., Lajtha, A., Laski, E. and Cooper, T. (1977). β-endorphin-induced changes in schizophrenic and depressed patients. *Arch. Gen. Psychiat.*, **34**, 1111

Kurland, A. A., McCabe, O. L., Hanlon, T. E. and Sullivan, D. (1977). The treatment of perceptual disturbances in schizophrenia with naloxone hydrochloride. *Am. J. Psychiat.*, **134**, 1408

Lal, S., Nair, N. P. V., Cervantes, P., Pulman, J. and Snyder, H. (1979). Effects of naloxone or levallorphan on serum prolactin concentrations and apomorphine induced growth hormone secretion. *Acta Psychiat. Scand.*, **59**, 173

Lewis, R. V., Gerber, L. D., Stein, S., Stephen, R. L., Grosser, B. I., Velick, S. F. and Udenfriend, S. (1979). On βH-leu⁵-endorphin and schizophrenia. *Arch. Gen. Psychiat.*, **36**, 237

Li, C. H. and Chung, D. (1976). Isolation and structure of an untriakontapeptide with opiate activity from camel pituitary glands. *Proc. Natl. Acad. Sci., USA*, **73**, 1145

Lindström, L. H., Widerlöv, E., Gunne, L. M., Wahlström, A. and Terenius, L. (1978). Endorphins in human cerebrospinal fluid: clinical correlations to some psychotic states. *Acta Psychiat. Scand.*, **57**, 153

Loeber, J., Verhoef, J., Burbach, J. P. H. and van Ree, J. M. (1979). Endorphins and related peptides in human cerebrospinal fluid. *Acta Endocrinol. (Kbh.)*, **91**, suppl. 225, 74

Mayer, D. J., Wolfe, T. L., Akil, H., Cardner, B. and Liebeskind, J. C. (1971). Analgesia from electrical stimulation in the brain-stem of the rat. *Science*, **174**, 1351

Mendelson, J. H., Ellingboe, J., Keuhule, J. C. and Mello, N. K. (1979). Effects of naltrexone on mood and neuroendocrine function in normal adult males. *Psychoneuroendocrinology*, **3**, 231

Mielke, D. H. and Gallant, D. M. (1977). An oral opiate antagonist in chronic schizophrenia: a pilot study. *Am. J. Psychiat.*, **134**, 1430

Nedopil, N. and Rüther, E. (1979). Effects of the synthetic analogue of methionine enkephalin FK33-824 on psychotic symptoms. *Pharmakopsychiat.*, **12**, 277

Palmour, R. M., Ervin, F. R. and Wagemaker, H. (1977). Characterization of a peptide derived from the serum of psychiatric patients. *Abstr. Soc. Neurosci.*, **7**, 32

Pert, C. B. and Snyder, S. H. (1973). Opiate receptor: demonstration in nervous tissue. *Science*, **179**, 1011

van Praag, H. M. (1980a). Central monoamine metabolism in depressions. I. Serotonin and related compounds. *Compr. Psychiat.*, **21**, 30

van Praag, H. M. (1980b). Observations within and beyond the boundaries of catecholamine research in psychosis. *Int. J. Neurol.* (In press) van Praag, H. M. (1977). The significance of dopamine for the mode of action of neuroleptics and the pathogenesis of schizophrenia. *Br. J. Psychiat.*, **130**, 463

Simon, E., Hiller, J. M. and Edelman, I. (1973). Stereospecific binding of the potent narcotic analgesic [³H]etorphine to rat brain homegenate. *Proc. Natl. Acad. Sci., USA*, **70**, 1947

Snyder, S. H. (1978). The opiate receptor and morphine-like peptides in the brain. *Am. J. Psychiat.*, **135**, 645

Snyder, S. H. and Childers, S. R. (1979). Opiate receptors and opioid peptides. *Ann. Rev. Neurosci.*, **2**, 35

Terenius, L. (1973). Characteristics of the receptor for narcotic analgesics in synaptic plasma membrane fraction from rat brain. *Acta Pharmacol. (Kbh.)*, **33**, 377

Terenius, L. and Wahlström, A. (1975). Search for an endogenous ligand for the opiate receptor. *Acta Physiol. Scand.*, **94**, 74

Terenius, L., Wahlström, A. and Agren, H. (1977). Naloxone (Narcan ᴵᴵ) treatment in depression: clinical observations and effects on CSF endorphins and monoamine metabolites. *Psychopharmacol.*, **54**, 31

Terenius, L., Wahlström, A., Lindström, L. and Widerlöv, E. (1976). Increased CSF levels of endorphins in chronic psychosis. *Neurosci. Lett.*, **3**, 157

Verhoeven, W. M. A., de Jong, J. T. V. M. and van Praag, H. M. (1979a). The effects of naloxone on psychotic symptoms. *Proc. 20th Dutch Fed. Meeting*, p. 435

Verhoeven, W. M. A., van Praag, H. M., Botter, P. A., Sunier, A., van Ree, J. M. and de Wied, D. (1978). (Des-tyr¹)-γ-endorphin in schizophrenia. *Lancet*, **1**, 1046

Verhoeven, W. M. A., van Praag, H. M., van Ree, J. M. and de Wied, D. (1979b). Improvement of schizophrenic patients by treatment with (des-tyr¹)-γ-endorphin (DTγE). *Arch. Gen. Psychiat.*, **36**, 294

Versteeg, D. H. G., de Kloet, E. R. and de Wied, D. (1979). Effects of α-endorphin, β-endorphin and (des-tyr¹)-γ-endorphin on α-MPT-induced catecholamine disappearance in discrete regions of the rat brain. *Brain Res.* (In press)

Volavka, J., Mallya, A., Baig, S. and Perez-Cruet, J. (1977). Naloxone in chronic schizophrenia. *Science*, **196**, 1227

Wagemaker, H. and Cade, R. (1977). The use of hemodialysis in chronic schizophrenia. *Am. J. Psychiat.*, **134**, 684

Watson, S. J., Akil, H., Berger, P. A. and Barchas, J. D. (1979). Some observations on the opiate peptides and schizophrenia. *Arch. Gen. Psychiat.*, **36**, 35

Watson, S. J., Berger, P. A., Akil, H., Mills, M. J. and Barchas, J. D. (1978). Effects of naloxone on schizophrenia: reduction in hallucinations in a subpopulation of subjects. *Science*, **201**, 73

de Wied, D. (1978). Psychopathology as a neuropeptide dysfunction. In J. M. van Ree and L. Terenius (eds.), *Characteristics and Function of Opioids. Developments in Neuroscience*, vol. 4, pp. 113–123. (Amsterdam: Elsevier/North-Holland)

Address for correspondence

Professor H. M. van Praag, Universiteitskliniek voor Psychiatrie, Academisch Ziekenhuis Utrecht, Catharijnesingel 101, 3500 CG Utrecht, The Netherlands

2.5
Effects of MIF-I and TRH on the brain

R. H. EHRENSING and A. J. KASTIN

ABSTRACT

MIF-I (prolyl-leucyl-glycinamide) and TRH (pyroglutamyl-histidyl-proline amide) have direct central nervous system effects in animals. In a series of double-blind, placebo and imipramine controlled studies in humans, MIF-I has shown promise as a rapidly acting antidepressant in a dose of approximately 1 mg/kg but not in doses of 0.1, 2 and 10 mg/kg. MIF-I stimulates motor activity in monkeys with a similar curvilinear dose response curve. MIF-I is also reported to lower ACTH and may act in depression by decreasing activity of the hypothalamic–pituitary–adrenal axis known to be increased in depression. Because MIF-I potentiates the effects of dopa, it has been tried as a treatment in Parkinson's disease with generally favourable results that suggest a curvilinear dose response curve. MIF-I has also been found to increase the sensitivity of animals to naloxone, to block the development of physical dependency on morphine and to reduce the effect of morphine on animals. Despite its early promise, TRH has not been found to be a clinically effective antidepressant in humans. However, the blunted TSH response to TRH in mental depression has diagnostic and prognostic value. The persistence of a blunted TSH response to TRH indicates a strong likelihood of early relapse, while the recovery of a normal TSH response is a good prognostic indication for continued recovery without maintenance therapy. Future indicated research with MIF-I and TRH is discussed.

INTRODUCTION

MIF-I (prolyl-leucyl-glycinamide) and TRH (pyroglutamyl-histidyl-proline amide) have a special chronological position in any consideration of the brain as an endocrine target. These two peptides were the first hypothalamic hormones demonstrated to have direct central nervous system (CNS) effects not mediated by the pituitary (Plotnikoff *et al.*, 1973, 1972a, 1972b and 1971), phenomena from which we derived our hypothesis of 'extra endocrine' effects of peptide hormones (Kastin *et al.*, 1974). This hypothesis was advanced at a time when the reality of the hypothalamic peptides was finally being accepted, several years before the discovery of the enkephalins and the endorphins excited the imagination and further demonstrated a direct effect of peptides on the CNS. Furthermore, MIF-I and TRH were the first hypothalamic peptides used in clinical trials for direct CNS effects in non-endocrine disease processes (Ehrensing and Kastin, 1974; Kastin and Barbeau, 1972; Kastin *et al.*, 1972; Prange *et al.*, 1972).

MIF-I

Depression

Since MIF-I was active in the dopa potentiation test (Plotnikoff *et al.*, 1971), and reversed the sedative effects of deserpidine when given orally to mice and monkeys (Plotnikoff *et al.*, 1973), both tests considered by some to be animal models for depression, clinical trials with MIF-I in mental depression were undertaken. In the first study (Ehrensing and Kastin, 1974), women with unipolar endogenous depression, all of whom in retrospect would have met the criteria for major depressive illness (Spitzer *et al.*, 1978), received either 60 mg MIF-I, 150 mg MIF-I or placebo in a single oral morning dose for 6 days in a double-blind design after a 3-day single-blind placebo lead in. Four of five patients receiving the 60 mg dose of MIF-I improved markedly and met the criteria established for substantial improvement. However, two of four patients receiving placebo and two of five patients receiving 150 mg MIF-I a day also demonstrated marked improvement. On one rating scale, the Line Self Rating, the improvement with the 60 mg dose of MIF-I was significantly superior to that seen with placebo and the MIF-I 150 mg dose. The effectiveness of MIF-I at a given dosage in alleviating mental depression was not, of course, clearly established in this small, pilot investigation. It was from this study, however, that we proposed our hypothesis that MIF-I might have a biphasic or curvilinear (inverted U) dose response curve, which hypothesis was then used to cast light on some of the clinical results with the high doses of MIF-I in Parkinson's disease and tardive dyskinesia to be discussed later.

In a subsequent study we compared the effects of 75 mg/d and 750 mg/d MIF-I and of placebo in patients with both unipolar and bipolar major depressive illnesses (Ehrensing and Kastin, 1978). In this double-blind 5-day study, the lower dose of MIF-I showed clearer superiority with five of eight patients meeting the criteria for substantial improvement, while only one of ten in the 750 mg/d MIF-I dose group and one of five of the placebo group showed such improvement. The lower dose of MIF-I was associated with significantly greater improvement than both the higher dose and placebo on all the rating scales employed. In this study it did not seem to make any difference whether the low dose of MIF-I was administered in three divided doses or in a single morning dose. The improvement in most patients was sustained for at least several weeks and in some patients indefinitely. In both studies improvement began approximately 36 to 48 hours after the first dose of MIF-I. Mood, self-esteem and concentration all improved to a greater extent than did disturbances in sleep.

Other investigations support these clinical observations of different effects of low and high doses of MIF-I. Itil (1976) demonstrated an EEG profile similar to that seen with the tricyclic antidepressants in human beings given low oral doses of MIF-I and a pattern similar to the psycho-stimulants with higher doses. Crowley and Hydinger (1976) demonstrated a significant increase in motor activity in monkeys given MIF-I parenterally, with the maximum effect occurring at the dose of 0.1 mg/kg on a curvilinear dose response curve. In a new animal model for depression which measures the struggle or 'hopelessness' of a rat in an impossible swimming situation, a model in which the tricyclic antidepressants are active, we found that MIF-I was similarly active at a dose of 0.1 mg/kg and showed no significant effect at higher or lower doses (Kastin et al., 1978b).

In our most recent study we explored the effect of the 0.1 mg/kg dose range of MIF-I which was found to be most effective in stimulating the motor activity of primates. Ten patients received either 10 mg MIF-I or 75 mg imipramine at 8 p.m. for seven consecutive days in a double-blind, in-patient study of patients having unipolar major depressive illnesses. This dose of imipramine was chosen to decrease the chance of side-effects, which would unblind the rater, and to approximate clinical practice where a full therapeutic dose of a tricyclic antidepressant is not usually administered during the first few days of treatment. In this study there were no significant differences on any of the rating scales between the improvement seen with MIF-I 10 mg/d and that seen with imipramine 75 mg/d. One of five patients receiving MIF-I and two of five patients receiving imipramine met the pre-established criteria for substantial improvement. These results strongly suggest that an oral dose of 10 mg MIF-I, a dose in the range of 0.1 mg/kg, is not adequate. It may be that an oral dose of 1 mg/kg is degraded in the gastrointestinal tract and/or poorly absorbed and is equivalent to the parenteral dose of 0.1 mg/kg which is the most active dose in some of the animal models. Another possibility is that the time of administration may be crucial. Primates given this dose (0.1 mg/kg) MIF-I parenterally showed increased motor activity for 12 hours.

Therefore, the administration of MIF-I at the usual time for tricyclic anti-depressants, at night before sleep, might be expected to increase sleep disturb-ances and the dysphoric effects of insomnia. Only one of the patients receiving MIF-I showed improvement in her sleep disturbance. Hopefully these questions will be answered by a similar study with MIF-I 10 mg administered in the morning.

MIF-I has been reported to significantly lower serum ACTH levels in patients with Addison's disease (Voigt *et al.*, 1977). The high incidence of depression described in Cushing's disease, a primary hypothalamic condition with stimulation of the basophilic cells of the pituitary and resulting increase in ACTH levels and, secondarily, cortisol levels, has been reviewed by Carroll and Mendels (1976), who compared it to Cushing's syndrome, involving primary adrenal hyperactivity with increased cortisol levels resulting in sup-pression of ACTH which has a lower incidence of depression. Many depressed patients have high serum cortisol levels and are resistant to dexamethasone suppression (Carroll and Mendels, 1976). It could be that MIF-I intervenes in the endocrine sequelae of mental depression by lowering ACTH and reducing the hyperactivity of the hypothalamic–pituitary–adrenal axis. The timing of the dose of MIF-I might then be crucial in normalizing a disrupted diurnal cortisol rhythm. Serum cortisols measured in patients finishing our second study of MIF-I in depression, collected 3 days after the study concluded, did not show any significant difference between those patients who had received MIF-I and those who had received placebo, but, as expected, decrease in serum cortisol correlated with improvement (Spearman Rank Order, $p < 0.01$).

Parkinsonism

The first clinical trials with MIF-I were conducted in Parkinson's disease (Kastin and Barbeau, 1972). The original hypothesis that preceded this clinical trial was an endocrine hypothesis, the inhibition of MSH release by MIF, outlined by Kastin in 1967, but modified to a non-endocrine, non-pituitary mediated hypothesis when it was demonstrated that MIF-I poten-tiated the effect of dopa in hypophysectomized animals (Plotnikoff *et al.*, 1971) as well as reduced the tremor induced by oxotremorine, also in hypo-physectomized animals (Plotnikoff *et al.*, 1972a). The initial study by Kastin and Barbeau (1972) with MIF-I in Parkinsonism employed an oral dose of 30 to 50 mg/d. Mild improvement in rigidity, tremor, akinesia and dopa-induced dyskinesias occurred with these lower doses. In a subsequent study, oral doses as high as 1 g/d were employed with a lessening of improvement in the Parkinson's disease as the dose increased. A much more favourable response was seen with MIF-I given intravenously in a dose of 200 mg in conjunction with L-dopa therapy (Barbeau, 1975). Subsequent investigations with MIF-I by others have, for the most part, confirmed the beneficial effect of MIF-I in Parkinson's disease, with particular improvement in akinesia and rigidity as well as mood (Gerstenbrand *et al.*, 1979; Fischer *et al.*, 1974). One study has been termed 'essentially negative', even though improvement seemed to be observed on most measurements (Caraceni *et al.*, 1979).

The mechanism of action of MIF-I in Parkinsonism is not clear. MIF-I has increased striatal dopamine synthesis in some studies (e.g. Friedman *et al.*, 1973) but not in others (Kostrzewa *et al.*, 1975; Plotnikoff *et al.*, 1974). MIF-I has been demonstrated to potentiate the effect of apomorphine on rotational behaviour in rats lesioned unilaterally by 6-OHDA, presumably by increasing the sensitivity of post-synaptic receptors (Kostrzewa *et al.*, 1978). In other models MIF-I has sometimes (Plotnikoff and Kastin, 1974) and sometimes not (Cox *et al.*, 1976) potentiated apomorphine, but this may be dose related. Evoked potential studies in cats also suggest a post-synaptic site of action of MIF-I (Kastin *et al.*, 1975). It may be that MIF-I stabilizes the post-synaptic dopamine receptor or acts on its own receptor.

A substance that ameliorates Parkinsonism, a hypoactive dopamine tract disorder, would be expected to worsen tardive dyskinesia thought secondary to hypersensitive or increased post-synaptic dopamine receptors. However, improvement in the tardive dyskinesia of one patient was observed while the patient received MIF-I for depression in a research study (Ehrensing and Kastin, 1974). In a subsequent un-blinded study of 13 patients with tardive dyskinesia there was a suggestion that MIF-I in low doses improved their condition, while with higher doses their condition worsened (Ehrensing *et al.*, 1977). Our final conclusion that a placebo response was a more likely explanation for the improvement seen in this study is supported by the failure of MIF-I to show a beneficial effect in animal models of tardive dyskinesia (Davis *et al.*, 1980).

Morphine interaction

Van Ree and de Wied have reported (1976) that MIF-I and its possible pro-hormone oxytocin both facilitate the development of morphine dependence. In their study, rats were pre-treated with MIF-I and morphine on day one and then on day two were given morphine and naloxone and tested for analgesia. Rats pre-treated with MIF-I showed a significant decrease in analgesia on day two compared to those pre-treated with saline and morphine, implying that these rats had become more sensitive to the effects of naloxone, a sign of the development of morphine dependence. They found similar results with MIF-I increasing the development of tolerance to the analgesic effects of the C-fragment of lipotropin (van Ree *et al.*, 1976). Walter *et al.* (1979), on the other hand, found MIF-I in a dose of 0.02–2 mg/kg to be a most potent peptide in blocking physical dependence on morphine in mice as measured by the withdrawal syndrome induced by naloxone. They suggested the clinical possibility that MIF-I could be used to prevent narcotic addiction. Others have reported that chronic pre-treatment with MIF-I blocks morphine-induced catalepsy in mice (Chiu and Mishra, 1979). In the vas deferens assay, MIF-I shows no opiate activity by itself (Kastin et al., 1978a). Recently, Dunn and Ciofalo (unpublished personal communication) have found that MIF-I has no analgesic properties when given alone in the mouse hot-plate test and rat yeast paw-pressure test, but is able to significantly reduce the analgesic effects of morphine when given as an oral pre-treatment.

TRH

Depression

TRH was not as active as MIF-I in the dopa potentiation test (Plotnikoff et al., 1972b), but it was available for clinical testing before MIF-I which led to its being tested first in mental depression. Although the initial reports concerning TRH in mental depression were encouraging for a short-acting beneficial effect (Kastin et al., 1972; Prange et al., 1972), subsequent studies have, in the main, failed to substantiate any real clinical effectiveness of TRH in depression, as we have reviewed elsewhere (Ehrensing and Kastin, 1977). Improvement in depression with TRH is relatively uncommon, and when it does occur it is more in the order of an idiosyncratic side-effect. A study of TRH administered in addition to a tricyclic antidepressant failed to demonstrate any substantial benefit of combining TRH with conventional antidepressants (Coppen et al., 1975). Very high doses of oral TRH have been shown to have a dysphoric effect (Kiely et al., 1976).

One group consistently continues to report an ameliorating effect of TRH in mental depression. In a recent study they reported a significant decrease in depression and 'nervousness' lasting several days from a single injection of TRH (500 µg) intravenously administered to five women with unipolar depression (Loosen and Prange, 1979). In a second similar group, administered 25 µg T_3 and 100 µg T_4 as a pre-treatment to TRH, this improvement in depression and nervousness was not observed. They have also reported a brief but significant decrease in the secondary depression of alcoholic men in withdrawal (Loosen et al., 1979). But even this group does not view TRH as an effective clinical treatment for depression (Loosen et al., 1979).

The blunted TSH response to TRH in depression was originally described by us (Kastin et al., 1972) and by Prange et al. (1972), and has been a consistent finding in approximately 25% to 50% of depressed patients (Ehrensing and Kastin, 1977). In one investigation we observed three depressed patients who responded to saline and had a normal TSH response to TRH (Ehrensing et al., 1974). We speculated that the TSH response to TRH might be of some diagnostic value in mental depression. Kirkegaard et al. (1978) have differentiated neurotic depression from unipolar depression and mixed manic depression, both of which have a significantly lower TSH response to TRH. Some investigators have found a significantly higher TSH response to TRH in bipolar-depressed patients compared to that in unipolar-depressed patients (Gold *et al.*, 1977), but others have not (Kirkegaard *et al.*, 1978; Takahashi *et al.*, 1973). Kirkegaard and Smith have further explored the prognostic value of this blunted response and observed that the persistence of a diminished TSH response to TRH in patients who have recovered from depression indicates a strong prognosis for an early relapse within a few months; but that recovery of a normal TSH response to TRH is a good prognostic indication for continued recovery without maintenance therapy (Kirkegaard and Smith, 1978).

The basis of this blunted TSH response to TRH in often the most depressed patients remains obscure. We observed high serum cortisols, known to blunt the TSH response, tending to correlate with a blunted response in depression (Ehrensing and Kastin, 1977), and Loosen *et al.* were able to show a significant correlation between the two (1978). However, we both observed exceptions to this correlation. The sometimes observed increased GH response to TRH in depression (Brambilla *et al.*, 1978; Maeda *et al.*, 1978) tends to rule out elevated somatostatin levels as the cause of the blunted response (Hall *et al.*, 1973). Gold *et al.* observed a significant correlation between CSF levels of 5-HIAA and blunted TSH response and raised the possibility of serotonin hyperactivity as an aetiology (Gold *et al.*, 1977). Others have argued for a dopamine aetiology (Loosen *et al.*, 1979).

Miscellaneous conditions

In some animals TRH reduces the sleeping time and hypothermia induced by alcohol and barbiturates (Breese *et al.*, 1974; Prange *et al.*, 1974). It may also exert some type of 'organizing' effect on the brain when injected during the first week of life in infant rats as manifested by later increased open field activity, fewer signs of emotionality and increased maze running ability in these rats as adults (Stratton *et al.*, 1976).

An initial report of a therapeutic effect of TRH in schizophrenia (Wilson *et al.*, 1973) was followed by negative reports (Bigelow *et al.*, 1975; Davis et al., 1975). Recently, a significant, although clinically slight, improvement, i.e. activation of apathetic and withdrawn patients with chronic schizophrenia with oral TRH, was reported (Inanga *et al.*, 1978).

FUTURE RESEARCH WITH MIF-I AND TRH

MIF-I is so devoid of known side-effects and toxicity in the human being that even if it could be demonstrated to be equal in clinical efficacy to other compounds, it would be desirable for its safety characteristics alone. In depression, we are proceeding with research to more clearly establish the dose response curve of MIF-I, its best time of administration, and its effect on

ACTH and serum cortisol. It also should be determined if MIF-I on a maintenance basis will be effective in mental depression, or if there would develop a cumulative dose effect which would bring the patient into the high dose range and thereby cause a loss of effectiveness. MIF-I should be clinically studied in conjunction with narcotics to determine if it can be used to block the development of addiction and at the same time not interfere substantially with the analgesic effects of morphine. Such use of MIF-I might allow it to act as a methadone substitute in chronic narcotic addiction, as suggested by Walter *et al.* (1979).

The prognostic value of the TSH response to TRH in mental depression should be explored further. At the present time patients are continued for months and years on maintenance antidepressant therapy because there is no reliable prognostic indicator of continued remission or potential for relapse. In addition, the use of TRH as an antidote for both acute alcohol and barbiturate intoxication, as well as its use as a blocker of the development of alcohol tolerance and addiction, should be explored.

References

Barbeau, A. (1975). Potentiation of levodopa effect by intravenous 1-prolyl-1-leucyl-glycine amide in man. *Lancet*, **2**, 683

Bigelow, L. B., Gillen, J. C., Semal, S. and Wyatt, R. J. (1975). Thyrotropin-releasing hormone in chronic schizophrenia. *Lancet*, **2**, 869

Brambilla, F., Smeraldi, E., Sacchetti, E., Negri, F., Cocchi, D. and Müller, E. E. (1978). Deranged anterior pituitary responsiveness to hypothalamic hormones in depressed patients. *Arch. Gen. Psychiat.*, **35**, 1231

Breese, G. R., Cott, J. M., Cooper, B. R., Prange, A. J. and Lipton, M. A. (1974). Antagonism of ethanol narcosis by thyrotropin releasing hormone. *Life Sci.*, **14**, 1053

Caraceni, T., Parati, E. A., Girotti, F.. Celano, I., Frigerio, C., Cocchi, D. and Muller, E. E. (1979). Failure of MIF-I to affect behavioral responses in patients with Parkinson's disease under L-dopa therapy. *Psychopharmacology*, **63**, 217

Carroll, B. J. and Mendels, J. (1976). Neuroendocrine regulation in affective disorders. In E. J. Sachar (ed.), *Hormones, Behavior and Psychopathology*, pp. 193–224. (New York: Raven Press)

Chiu, S. and Mishra, R. K. (1979). Antagonism of morphine-induced catalepsy by L-prolyl-L-leucyl-glycinamide. *Eur. J. Pharmacol.*, **53**, 119

Coppen, A., Peet, M., Montgomery, S. and Baily, J. (1975). Thyrotropin-releasing hormone in the treatment of depression. *Lancet*, **2**, 433

Cox, B., Kastin, A. J. and Schneider, H. (1976). A comparison between a melanocyte-stimulating hormone inhibitory factor (MIF-I) and substances known to activate central dopamine receptors. *Eur. J. Pharmacol.*, **36**, 141

Crowley, T. J. and Hydinger, M. (1976). MIF, TRH and simian social and motor behavior. *Pharmacol. Biochem. Behav.*, suppl. 1, 79

Davis, K. L., Hollister, L. E. and Berger, P. A. (1975). Thyrotropin-releasing hormone in schizophrenia. *Am. J. Psychiat.*, **132**, 951

Davis, K. L., Kastin, A. J., Beilstein, B. A. and Vento, A. L. (1980). MSH and MIF in animal models of tardive dyskinesia. *Pharmacol. Biochem. Behav.*, **13**, 37

Ehrensing, R. H. and Kastin, A. J. (1978). Dose-related biphasic effect of prolyl-leucyl-glycinamide (MIF-I) in depression. *Am. J. Psychiat.*, **135**, 562

Ehrensing, R. H. and Kastin, A. J. (1977). TRH: clinical investigations for non-endocrine actions in man. In L. Martini and G. M. Besser (eds.), *Clinical Endocrinology*, pp. 133–142. (New York: Academic Press)

Ehrensing, R. H. and Kastin, A. J. (1974). Melanocyte-stimulating hormone release inhibiting hormone as an anti-depressant. A pilot study. *Arch. Gen. Psychiat.*, **30**, 63

Ehrensing, R. H., Kastin, A. J., Larson, P. F. and Bishop, G. (1977). Melanocyte-stimulating hormone release inhibiting factor-I and tardive dyskinesia. *Dis. Nerv. Syst.*, **38**, 303

Ehrensing, R. H., Kastin, A. J., Schalch, D. S., Friesen, H., Vargas, R. and Schally, A. V. (1974). Affective state and thyrotropin and prolactin responses after repeated injections of thyrotropin-releasing hormone in depressed patients. *Am. J. Psychiat.*, **161**, 714

Fischer, P. A., Schneider, E., Jacobi, P. and Maxion, H. (1974). Effect of melanocyte-stimulating hormone release inhibiting factor (MIF) in Parkinson's syndrome. *Eur. J. Neurol.*, **12**, 360

Friedman, E., Friedman, J. and Gershon, S. (1973). Dopamine synthesis: stimulation by a hypothalamic factor. *Science*, **182**, 831

Gerstenbrand, F., Poewe, W., Aichner, F. and Kozma, C. (1979). Clinical utilization of MIF-I. In Collu *et al.* (eds.), *Central Nervous System Effects of Hypothalamic Hormones and Other Peptides*, pp. 415–426. (New York: Raven Press)

Gold, P. W., Goodwin, F. K., Wehr, T. and Repar, R. (1977). Pituitary thyrotropin response to thyrotropin-releasing hormone in affective illness: relationship to spinal fluid amine metabolites. *Am. J. Psychiat.*, **134**, 1028

Hall, R., Besser, G. M., Schally, A. V., Coy, D. H., Evered, D., Goldie, D. J., Kastin, A. J., McNeilly, A. S., Mortimer, C. H., Rhenekos, D., Turnbridge, W. M. G. and Weightman, D. (1973). Action of growth-hormone-release inhibitory hormone in healthy men and in acromegaly. *Lancet*, **2**, 581

Inanga, K., Nakano, T., Nagata, T., Tanaka, M. and Ogawa, N. (1978). Behavioural effects of protirelin in schizophrenia. *Arch. Gen. Psychiat.*, **35**, 1011

Itil, T. M. (1976). Neurophysiological effects of hormones in humans: computer EEG profiles of sex and hypothalamic hormones. In E. J. Sachar (ed.), *Hormones, Behavior and Psychopathology*, pp. 31–40. (New York: Raven Press)

Kastin, A. J. (1967). Letter to the editor. *N. Engl. J. Med.*, **276**, 1041

Kastin, A. J. and Barbeau, A. (1972). Preliminary clinical studies with 1-prolyl-1-leucyl-glycine amide in Parkinson's disease. *Can. Med. Assoc. J.*, **107**, 1079

Kastin, A. J., Coy, D. H., Schally, A. V. and Meyers, C. A. (1978a). Activity of VIP, somatostatin and other peptides in the mouse vas deferens assay. *Pharmacol. Biochem. Behav.*, **9**, 673

Kastin, A. J., Ehrensing, R. H., Schalch, D. S. and Anderson, M. S. (1972). Improvement in mental depression with decreased thyrotropin response after administration of thyrotropin-releasing hormone. *Lancet*, **2**, 740

Kastin, A. J., Plotnikoff, N. P., Sandman, C. A., Spirtes, M. A., Kostrzewa, R. M., Paul, S. M., Stratton, L. O., Miller, L. H., Labrie, F., Schally, A. V. and Goldman, H. (1975). The effects of MSH and MIF on the brain. In W. E. Stumpf and L. D. Grant (eds.), *Anatomical Neuroendocrinology*, pp. 290–297. (Basel: Karger)

Kastin, A. J., Schally, A. V., Ehrensing, R. H. and Barbeau, A. (1974). Endocrine and extraendocrine studies of hypothalamic hormones in man. In K. Lederis and K. E. Cooper (eds.), *Recent Studies of Hypothalamic Function*, pp. 196–206. (Basel: Karger)

Kastin, A. J., Scollan, E. L., Ehrensing, R. H., Schally, A. V. and Coy, D. H. (1978b). Enkephalin and other peptides reduce passiveness. *Pharmacol. Biochem. Behav.*, **9**, 515

Kiely, W. F., Adrian, A. D., Lee, J. H. and Nicoloff, J. T. (1976). Therapeutic failure of oral thyrotropin-releasing hormone in depression. *Psychosom. Med.*, **38**, 233

Kirkegaard, C., Bjørum, N., Cohn, D. and Lauridsen, V. B. (1978). Thyrotropin-releasing hormone (TRH) stimulation test in manic-depressive illness. *Arch. Gen. Psychiat.*, **35**, 1017

Kirkegaard, C. and Smith, E. (1978). Continuation therapy in endogenous depression controlled by changes in the TRH stimulation test. *Psychol. Med.*, **8**, 501

Kostrzewa, R. M., Kastin, A. J. and Sobrian, S. K. (1978). Potentiation of apomorphine action in rats by L-prolyl-L-leucyl-glycine amide. *Pharmacol. Biochem. Behav.*, **9**, 375

Kostrzewa, R. M., Kastin, A. J. and Sprites, M. A. (1975). Alpha MSH and MIF-I effects on catecholamine levels and synthesis in various rat brain areas. *Pharmacol. Biochem. Behav.*, **3**, 1017

Loosen, P. T. and Prange, A. J. (1979). Behavioral changes in depression after TRH: antagonism by pre-treatment with thyroid hormones. Presented at the *10th International Congress of the Society for Psychoneuroendocrinology*, August 8–11, Park City, Utah

Loosen, P. T., Prange, A. J. and Wilson, I. C. (1979). TRH (protirelin) in depressed alcoholic men. *Arch. Gen. Psychiat.*, **36**, 540

Loosen, P. T., Prange, A. J. and Wilson, I. C. (1978). Influence of cortisol on TRH-induced TSH response in depression. *Am. J. Psychiat.*, **135**, 244

Maeda, K., Kato, Y., Ohio, S., Chihard, K., Yoshimoto, Y., Yamaguchi, N., Kuromaru, S. and Imura, H. (1978). Growth hormone and prolactin release after injections of thyrotropin-releasing hormone in patients with depression. *J. Clin. Endocrinol.*, **40**, 501

Plotnikoff, N. P. and Kastin, A. J. (1974). Pharmacological studies with the tripeptide prolyl-1-leucyl-glycinamide. *Arch. Int. Pharmacodyn.*, **211**, 211

Plotnikoff, N. P., Kastin, A. J., Anderson, M. S. and Schally, A. V. (1973). Deserpidine antagonism by a tripeptide, 1-prolyl-1-leucyl-glycinamide. *Neuroendocrinology*, **11**, 67

Plotnikoff, N. P., Kastin, A. J., Anderson, M. S. and Schally, A. V. (1972a). Oxotremorine antagonism by a hypothalamic hormone, melanocyte-stimulating hormone release-inhibiting factor, MIF. *Proc. Soc. Exp. Biol. Med.*, **140**, 811

Plotnikoff, N. P., Kastin, A. J., Anderson, M. S. and Schally, A. V. (1971). DOPA potentiation by MIF. *Life Sci.*, **10**, 1279

Plotnikoff, N. P., Minard, F. N. and Kastin, A. J. (1974). Dopa potentiation in ablated animals and brain levels of biogenic amines in intact animals after prolyl-leucyl-glycinamide. *Neuroendocrinology*, **14**, 271

Plotnikoff, N. P., Prange, A. J., Bresse, G. R., Anderson, M. S. and Wilson, I. C. (1972b). Thyrotropin releasing hormone: enhancement of DOPA activity by a hypothalamic hormone. *Science*, **178**, 417

Prange, A. J., Bresse, G. R., Cott, J. M., Martin, B. R., Cooper, B. R., Wilson, I. C. and Plotnikoff, N. P. (1974). Thyrotropin-releasing hormone: antagonism in pentobarbitol in rodents. *Life Sci.*, **14**, 447

Prange, A. J., Wilson, I. C., Lara, P. O., Alltop, L. B. and Breese, G. R. (1972). Effects of thyrotropin-releasing hormone in depression. *Lancet*, **2**, 999

van Ree, J. M. and de Wied, D. (1976). Prolyl-leucyl-glycinamide (PLG) facilitates morphine dependence. *Life Sci.*, **19**, 1331

van Ree, J. M., de Wied, D., Bradbury, A. F., Hulme, E. C., Smyth, D. G. and Snell, C. R. (1976). Induction of tolerance to the analgesic action of lipoprotein C-fragment. *Nature*, **264**, 792

Spitzer, R. L., Endicott, J. and Robbins, E. (1978). Research diagnostic criteria—rationale and reliability. *Arch. Gen. Psychiat.*, **35**, 773

Stratton, L. O., Gibson, C. A., Kolar, K. G. and Kastin, A. J. (1976). Neonatal treatment with TRH affects development, learning and emotionality in the rat. *Pharmacol. Biochem. Behav.*, **5** (suppl. 1), 65

Takahashi, S., Kondo, H., Yoshimura, M. and Ochi, Y. (1973). Thyrotropin response to TRH in depressive illness: relation of clinical subtypes and prolonged duration of depressive episode. *Folia Psychiat. Neurol. Jpn.*, **28**, 305

Walter, R., Ritzmann, R. F., Bhargava, H. N. and Flexner, L. B. (1979). Prolyl-leucyl-glycinamide cyclo (leucylglycine) and derivatives block development of physical dependence on morphine in mice. *Proc. Natl. Acad. Sci., USA*, **76**, 518

Wilson, I. C., Lara, P. P. and Prange, A. J. (1973). Thyrotropin-releasing hormone in schizophrenia. *Lancet*, **2**, 43

Voigt, K. H., Fehm, H. L., Lang, R. E., Beinert, K. E. and Pfeiffer, E. F. (1977). Suppression of ACTH secretion by synthetic MSH-release inhibiting factor PRO-LEU-GYL-NH$_2$ in Addison's disease. *Horm. Metab. Res.*, **9**, 150

Address for correspondence

Dr R. H. Ehrensing, Chairman, Department of Psychiatry, Ochsner Clinic, 1514 Jefferson Highway, New Orleans, LA 70121, USA

2.6
Neurohypophysial hormones and addiction

J. M. van REE

ABSTRACT

A common denominator for the occurrence of abuse with various psychoactive drugs is their reinforcing property. This can reliably be studied in experimental animals by using procedures for drug self-administration. Initiation, maintenance and cessation of self-administering behaviour is influenced by external and internal factors and by drug-induced alterations of homeostatic mechanisms in the organism. Among the internal factors which modulate the reinforcing efficacy of opiates are the neurohypophysial hormones and their fragments.

Animal experiments indicate that des-glycinamide[9], arginine[8], vasopressin (DGAVP) reduces acquisition of heroin self-administration, suggesting that this neuropeptide attenuates the reinforcing action of heroin. Treatment of heroin addicts with DGAVP facilitates their methadon detoxification. It is postulated that derangements in neurohypophysial hormone-containing systems may be critical factors in the development of drug-seeking behaviour. Analysis of the significance of various brain neuropeptide systems for experimental and human addictive behaviour may lead to a more goal-directed treatment of addiction in the future.

INTRODUCTION

A variety of naturally occurring substances has been used for many centuries to influence the brain function of healthy individuals. Some of them are (self-) administered to such an extent that a state of drug dependence is achieved, which is characterized by the drug user performing substantial amounts of behaviour leading specifically to further administration of the drug even when this requires the sacrifice of other behaviours (Kalant *et al.*, 1978). Severe degrees of dependence are commonly labelled as addiction, particularly in clinical practice.

The establishment of drug-seeking behaviour is controlled by variables determining the interaction between the drug, the organism and the environment. Although the external environmental factors markedly affect the initiation, maintenance and cessation of drug-seeking behaviour, the most important variable in drug dependence is the unique interaction between the drug and its substrate, which underlies the reinforcing capacity of the drug. A drug serves as a reinforcer when the occurrence of the behavioural pattern which is followed by drug administration increases or is maintained. Obviously, this reinforcing action is the common denominator for the occurrence of abuse with various drugs. It can be analysed reliably in self-administration experiments in animals as well as in humans. The self-administration techniques in animals have proved to be the most consistent predictor of human abuse potential. In fact, drugs with a high abuse potential are those which have properties leading to their self-administration under various conditions in experimental animals.

Using these models it has become increasingly clear that external environmental factors, e.g. the dose of the drug, the schedule of drug availability, stimulus control (conditioned stimuli, discriminative stimuli), social conditions and aversive conditions, specifically interact and even contribute to drug self-administration. The same holds for the drug-induced alteration of homeostatic mechanisms in the organism, including changes in mood (euphoria or dysphoria), in social, sexual and aggressive behaviour and in the development of tolerance and physical dependence. Predisposing variables ranging from genetic constitution to various historical variables, e.g. preexisting behaviour repertoire and the biochemical state, may be implicated in the mechanisms determining whether or not a drug-injection gains and maintains control over behaviour in a particular individual. However, only few data concerning the internal factors involved in drug self-administration are available. The endogenous C-fragment of β-lipotrophin (α-endorphin) has been shown to possess both positive reinforcing and discriminative stimulus properties similar to those of narcotic drugs (van Ree *et al.*, 1979b). These drugs may mimic certain of the actions of β-endorphin and thereby affect behaviour to the point that the integrity of the organism becomes conditional upon the narcotics, a phenomenon generally referred to as opiate abuse. This has led to the postulate that altered bio-availability of endorphins may be a critical factor in the development of narcotic abuse. Also, internal factors which modulate drug-induced reinforcing activity may be important for the initiation and cessation of self-administration. Among these factors are the neurohypophysial hormones and their fragments.

HEROIN SELF-ADMINISTRATION IN RATS

Neurohypophysial hormones (i.e. vasopressin and oxytocin) and their fragments modulate brain processes selectively to consolidate, retrieve and repress recently acquired information (van Ree et al., 1978a; de Wied, 1977). Since learning and memory processes play a critical role in the initial phase of a new behavioural pattern, it was postulated that these neuropeptides may modulate acquisition of self-administering behaviour. To test this hypothesis experiments were performed with intravenous heroin self-administration in rats. Heroin was selected for these studies because with this drug self-injecting behaviour develops relatively fast and is rather reproducible, at least under standard conditions (van Ree et al., 1978b). Daily subcutaneous treatment with des-glycinamide (van Beek-Verbeek et al., 1979), with arginine (Mello and Mendelson, 1979), and with vasopressin (DGAVP) appeared to reduce acquisition of heroin self-administration (van Ree and de Wied, 1977a). The effect of the peptide was clearly present in the second phase of testing. The influence of DGAVP in heroin self-administration is due to a central effect, is long-lasting, and is located in the ring-structure of vasopressin. Intracerebroventricularly applied specific vasopressin anti-serum markedly stimulated heroin self-administration (van Ree and de Wied 1977b), suggesting that vasopressin is physiologically involved in acquisition of heroin self-administration. Interestingly, the C-terminal tripeptide of oxytocin, prolyl-leucylglycinamide (PLG), affects heroin self-administration in a way opposite to that observed with DGAVP, i.e., this tripeptide facilitates acquisition of the behaviour. Since the amount of drug taken can serve as an index of the reinforcing efficacy of the reinforcer, i.e. drug injection (van Ree et al., 1978b), it was postulated that DGAVP attenuates and PLG enhances the reinforcing efficacy of heroin. This possibility is supported by data on intracranial self-stimulating behaviour. This behaviour is widely used to investigate the significance of certain brain structures with respect to reward (Wauquier and Ross, 1976). Administration of DGAVP attenuated and that of PLG enhanced self-stimulating behaviour elicited from electrodes implanted in the ventral tegmental–medial substantia nigra area, which contains the cell bodies of the mesolimbic and mesocortical dopaminergic pathways. Both peptides markedly modified the response rate of current intensities near the threshold for eliciting the behaviour, but no effect was noted at current intensities which evoked maximal response rates (Dorsa and van Ree, 1979).

The characteristics of the effectiveness of vasopressin in heroin self-administration are strikingly similar to those for enhancement of memory consolidation (van Ree et al., 1978a; de Wied, 1976). Assuming that DGAVP acts similarly in heroin self-administration and memory consolidation, it can be expected that the neuropeptide is only effective during the acquisition of the behaviour or when the behaviour is changed in response to variation in the reinforcement or environmental cues. Thus, the degree of reinforcement control over behaviour may be of importance with respect to the effectiveness of DGAVP. This is supported by the fact that DGAVP did not reduce morphine self-administration in well-trained monkeys, physically dependent on morphine and with a long history of self-administration (Mello and Mendelson, 1979). The drug-seeking behaviour of these monkeys may be fixed, in that all environmental and internal cues present in or induced by the test situation had received a certain and stable value. Moreover, the ability of DGAVP to interact with electrical self-stimulation at low and not at high current intensities is further evidence for the postulate that the effect of DGAVP on reward mechanisms depends on the degree of reinforcement control over behaviour. This fits well with the assumption that neuropeptides may exert their effects on behavioural adaptation by modulation of ongoing activity in the brain and thus function as neuromodulators (Barchas *et al.*, 1978).

HEROIN ADDICTS

The outcome of the experimental drug self-administration suggests the relevance of animal models for human addiction. Apart from the prediction of abuse liability, qualitatively as well as quantitatively, other commonalities in human and in infra-human drug self-administration have been described. Particularly similar effects were obtained when various external environmental factors were varied (Griffiths and Bigelow, 1978). The same may hold for the drug-induced changes in the organism and for predisposing variables, although data on these factors are scarce, especially in human addiction.

Since the most important factor in drug abuse is the reinforcing activity of the drug, it seems worthwhile for treatment of addicts to eliminate or to decrease this activity. The practice of giving the narcotic antagonist naloxone to narcotic addicts is an example of blocking the reinforcing effects of narcotics. Although this principle of treatment is valid, the actual outcome to date has not been impressive. There are three possible reasons for this: (a) the opiate abstinence syndrome can be severe, (b) the action of the drug is too short-lived, (c) the drug may be insufficiently potent. Somewhat more successful, though still in only a limited number of patients, is treatment with methadone, as used in methadone detoxification programmes and methadone maintenance schedules. Methadone seems to possess a lower reinforcing efficacy than heroin and by replacing heroin with methadone, and as a consequence changing the drug-seeking behaviour, the reinforcing control over behaviour seems to be decreased. The partial success of the methadone detoxification programme for patients with a moderate degree of heroin addiction, which comprises gradually decreasing the daily methadone dose, may be at least partly due to weakening the reinforcing control over behaviour, since a lower drug dose is less reinforcing than a higher dose (van Ree *et al.*, 1978b).

Since the animal data suggest that DGAVP decreases the reinforcing action of heroin, it was deemed of interest to investigate whether DGAVP might exert a similar action in human addicts. As the effectiveness of DGAVP may be most pronounced in situations in which the behaviour is changed in response to alterations in the reinforcement, the influence of DGAVP on drug intake was studied in human addicts during the initial phase of the methadone detoxification therapy. The standard methadone detoxification programme comprises daily oral treatment with methadone followed, after two to three weeks, by a gradual decreasing of the daily methadone dose in an out-patient clinic. Patients who were considered for this programme had a moderate heroin addiction, according to current criteria, and wanted to drop the addiction habit. Beneficial effects of the methadone treatment are best judged from the time course of attendance at the clinic and from the number of morphine (a metabolite of heroin) free urine samples. Twelve patients starting with the detoxification programme in the Jellinek Center in Amsterdam received, for five days, a sublingual tablet containing DGAVP or placebo simultaneously with the methadone administration following a double-blind design (van Beek-Verbeek *et al.*, 1979). It appeared that DGAVP treatment facilitated the methadone detoxification of heroin addicts as could be judged from the longer time course of attending the clinic and from the lower percentage of urine samples with detectable morphine in patients treated with DGAVP compared to those receiving placebo. Moreover, the medical attendant judged the methadone detoxification of the DGAVP treated patients to have been more successful than that of the patients on placebo. The beneficial effect of DGAVP was present not only during treatment with this neuropeptide, but also in the period following cessation of DGAVP administration. These preliminary findings indicate once more the predictive value of experimental drug self-administration for human addiction. The decrease of heroin intake in patients treated with DGAVP supports the hypothesis that this neuropeptide attenuates the reinforcing efficacy of heroin. However, it remains to be seen whether DGAVP also has a beneficial effect in heroin addicts when given at times other than during the initial phase of the methadone detoxification programme.

CONCLUSIONS

Drug self-administration is a very complex behavioural pattern which is influenced by many external and internal variables and is attended by alterations in peripheral and brain homeostatic mechanisms. Once established, this behavioural pattern is powerfully controlled by the reinforcing action of the drug injection. It is accompanied by social and psychic dysfunctioning of the drug user and is only slightly responsive to treatment. The main problem of treatment is the persisting craving for the effects of the drug even after successful detoxification. It is associated with a high probability of relapse, particularly induced by intero- and exteroceptive stimuli. Moreover, treatment is generally symptomatic, since our knowledge about the underlying mechanism of drug addiction is limited. In particular little, if anything, is known about disturbances in the brain which may be important for the process by which drug injections gain control over behaviour in a particular individual.

The data reviewed here may suggest that neuropeptide systems are implicated in drug addiction, e.g. the altered bio-availability of endorphins may contribute to the development of narcotic abuse. Moreover, reward mechanisms triggered by heroin and involved in the acquisition and maintenance of drug-seeking behaviour may be modulated by neurohypophysial hormones and their fragments. Thus, disturbances in brain and/or pituitary neurohypophysial hormone-containing systems or in the generation of neuropeptides from these hormones may lead to a state in which drug-seeking behaviour may be elicited. Treatment of these disturbances either by replacing a deficient entity or by the attentuation of the effect of a relative or absolute excess of another entity may decrease the probability that addictive behaviour will develop. Unfortunately. treatment generally starts when drug-seeking behaviour has already existed for a long period of time. During this period the incentive for repeated administration of drugs may have changed, since many factors, including drug-induced alterations of homeostatic mechanisms in the organism, may alter the reinforcing properties of self-administered drugs. The subjective and objective effects induced by the drug may even themselves reinforce drug-seeking behaviour. Thus, treatment of persisting drug-seeking behaviour may be quite different from that when the behaviour is of recent origin. Since there are various pituitary–brain neuropeptide systems which more or less contribute to the adaptation of the individual to the environment, these systems may be differentially concerned in the subsequent stages of addictive behaviour. Even the functioning of a particular neuropeptide may change from one stage to another. That neuropeptides other than those related to neurohypophysial hormones may influence drug-seeking behaviour can be inferred from findings in rats showing that $ACTH_{4-10}$ interferes selectively with the discriminative internal stimuli elicited by narcotic injections (Colpaert et al., 1978) and that the neuroleptic-like peptide des-tyrosine-γ-endorphin attenuates the acquisition of heroin self-administration (van Ree et al., 1979a).

The beneficial effect of DGAVP on the methadone detoxification of heroin addicts justifies detailed analysis of the significance of the activity of various neuropeptide systems during acquisition, maintenance and extinction of experimental drug-seeking behaviour and, if possible, of human addiction. The demonstration of disturbances in neuropeptide systems contributing to the development and maintenance of addictive behaviour, and the subsequent identification and correction of these disturbances in the human addict, may lead to a more goal-directed treatment of addiction in the future.

References

Barchas. J. D.. Akil. H.. Elliott. G. R.. Holman. R. B. and Watson. S. J. (1978). Behavioural neurochemistry: neuroregulators and behavioural states. *Science.* **200**. 964

van Beek-Verbeek. G., Fraenkel. M.. Geerlings. P. J.. van Ree. J. M. and de Wied. D. (1979). Desglycinamide-arginine-vasopressin in methadon detoxification of heroin addicts. *Lancet* (In press)

Colpaert, F. C.. Niemegeers, C. J. E.. Janssen. P. A. J.. van Ree. J. M. and de Wied. D. (1978). Selective interference of ACTH$_{4\ 10}$ with discriminative responding based on the narcotic cue. *Psychoneuroendocrinology*. **3**. 203

Dorsa. D. M. and van Ree. J. M. (1979). Modulation of substantia nigra self-stimulation by neuropeptides related to neurohypophyseal hormones. *Brain Res..* **172**. 367

Griffiths, R. R. and Bigelow. G. E. (1978). Commonalities in human and infrahuman drug self-administration. In J. Fishman (ed.). *The Bases of Addiction,* p. 157. (Berlin: Dahlem Konferenzen)

Kalant, H., Engel, J. A., Goldberg. L.. Griffiths. R. R.. Jaffe, J. H.. Krasnegor, N. A., Mello. N. K., Mendelsohn, J. H.. Thompson. T. and van Ree. J. M. (1978). Behavioral aspects of addiction—Group Report. In J. Fishman (ed.). *The Bases of Addiction,* p. 463. (Berlin: Dahlem Konferenzen)

Mello, N. K. and Mendelson, J. H. (1979). Effects of the neuropeptide DGAVP on morphine and food self-administration by dependent rhesus monkey. *Pharm. Biochem. Behav..* **10**, 415

van Ree, J. M., Bohus. B.. Versteeg. D. H. G. and de Wied. D. (1978a). Neurohypophyseal principles and memory processes. *Biochem. Pharmacol..* **27**. 1793

van Ree. J. M.. Bohus, B. and de Wied. D. (1979a). Similarity between behavioral effects of des-tyrosine-γ-endorphin and haloperidol and of α-endorphin and amphetamine. *Proceedings International Narcotics Research Conference 1979.* (In press)

van Ree, J. M., Slangen, J. L. and de Wied. D. (1978b). Intravenous self-administration of drugs in rats. *J. Pharmacol. Exp. Ther.,* **204**, 547

van Ree, J. M., Smyth, D. G. and Colpaert, F. (1979b). Dependence creating properties of lipotropin C-fragment (β-endorphin): evidence for its internal control of behaviour. *Life Sci.,* **24**, 495.

van Ree, J. M. and de Wied, D. (1977a). Modulation of heroin self-administration by neurohypophyseal principles. *Eur. J. Pharmacol.,* **43**, 199

van Ree, J. M. and de Wied, D. (1977b). Heroin self-administration is under control of vasopressin. *Life Sci.,* **21**, 315

de Wied, D. (1977). Peptides and behaviour. *Life Sci.,* **20**, 195

de Wied, D. (1976). Behavioural effects of intraventricularly administered vasopressin and vasopressin fragments. *Life Sci..* **19**. 685

Wauquier, A. and Ross, E. T. (1976) (eds.). *Brain Stimulation Reward.* (New York: American Elsevier/North-Holland)

Address for correspondence

Dr J. M. van Ree, Rudolf Magnus Instituut voor Farmacologie, Medische Faculteit, Rijksuniversiteit Utrecht, Vondellaan 6, 3521 GD Utrecht, The Netherlands

2.7
Androgens and behaviour

R. M. ROSE

ABSTRACT

This paper reviews findings from a number of studies designed to assess the joint contribution of hormonal and social factors to sexual and aggressive behaviours. Studies with male rhesus monkeys have shown that exposure to receptive females results in increased plasma testosterone and copulatory behaviour, while defeat experiences with or without wounding result in decreased testosterone and a decrease in all forms of social behaviour. Studies of human males under conditions of combat threat or arduous training show parallel androgen suppression and a decrease in covert use of sexual imagery. However, the data are generally strongest in studies involving environmental manipulation with nonhuman primates and highlight considerable individual dissociation between androgen levels and sexual or aggressive behaviours. This lack of concurrence for individual animals can be understood in terms of differences in social factors such as status within the group and the seasonal nature of social relationships. Male rhesus monkeys show a significant increase in testosterone during the breeding season, but the frequency of their sexual behaviour appears largely determined by dominance rank in the group. Similarly, males show testosterone increases when introduced to a group of females, but frequency of sexual behaviours depends largely upon the females' acceptance of the males as a more dominant member of the group. Little behavioural change after HCG induced testosterone increase in males with a constant social structure lends further credence to the importance of social factors in determining sexual and aggressive behaviours. Studies with rhesus male adolescents suggest that sexual and aggressive behaviours increasing during the third and fourth years may not parallel the increase in testosterone. although these behaviours appear to be influenced by changing androgen secretion. In humans, however. data relating androgens with sexuality and aggression are largely inconclusive. Thus while androgens may permit the expression of sexual or aggressive behaviours. the actual occurrence of such behaviours seems to depend on other factors. particularly on the relationship of an individual animal with other members of the group. A focus of interest on such psychosocial variables in addition to biological parameters is suggested for future research.

INTRODUCTION

There are problems in communication between behavioural scientists and endocrinologists working in psychoendocrinology, parallel to those observed in other fields of psychobiology. Many behavioural scientists de-emphasize or minimize the role of biological factors, such as androgens, in influencing behaviour. At the same time, many workers in endocrinology are overly reductionistic and over-emphasize the role of hormones in determining behaviour, such that the presence of androgens is the only major variable determining the expression of aggression or sexual behaviour.

This paper will focus primarily on studies done with male rhesus monkeys in collaboration with Irwin Bernstein and Tom Gordon at the Yerkes Field Station in Georgia, in which various environmental manipulations were performed and changes observed in both testosterone and behaviour. Our goal was to study psychosocial influences on androgen secretion as well as what effect changes in testosterone had on subsequent behaviour, i.e. both sides of the behavioural–endocrine relationship. A few comments on some work with humans will follow, albeit brief because of the scarcity of comparable psychoendocrine data in man.

The review will emphasize major dissociations between levels or changes in levels of androgens, primarily testosterone, and sexual or aggressive behaviour. This is not to minimize the influence of testosterone, but to clarify how other factors such as status in a group of social relationships influence the appearance of both sexual and aggressive behaviour.

The goal of this review is to dissuade the reader of the view that if you raise testosterone or compare those with higher endogenous levels of testosterone, you will induce or observe more frequent sexual or aggressive behaviour and if you lower testosterone or study those with lower levels, there is usually less sexual or aggressive behaviour. There are so many exceptions to this conclusion that such a review is warranted to re-emphasize how important psychosocial factors are in modifying any influence of androgens on sexual or aggressive behaviour.

In our early work we were initially impressed with how changes in behaviour paralleled changes in testosterone. In later studies we came to appreciate the importance of social rank and past history in modifying testosterone's influence on sexual or aggressive behaviour.

FEMALE INFLUENCES ON TESTOSTERONE

In 1972 we observed that females act as a very powerful stimulus to male rhesus monkeys to increase testosterone and to increase the frequency of sexual behaviour (Rose *et al..* 1972). Male rhesus who were released from individual cages and placed with receptive females showed a very brisk and substantial rise in testosterone in a very short period of time, less than 24 hours, and maintained this elevation for several days. Males were observed to copulate very frequently with the females during this same period of time.

We also observed that. parallel to some preliminary observations in man,

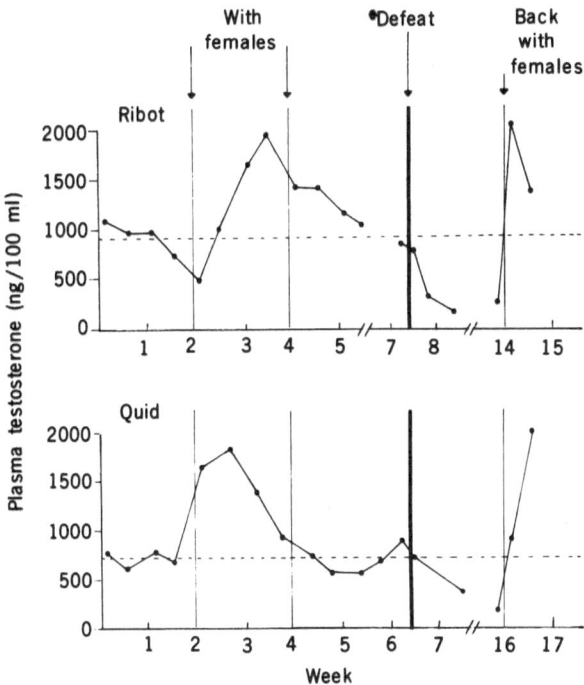

Figure 1 Plot of the plasma testosterone responses for two males for approximately 4 months. Values on discontinuous weeks are not connected. After defeat. both males showed a drop below baseline levels, depicted as horizontal broken lines, which were determined from weeks 1 and 2 prior to access to the females. Within 2 to 4 days after reintroduction to the females both animals showed a rise in plasma testosterone equivalent to what they had initially experienced

various stresses such as defeat functioned as a very powerful stimulus to inhibit testosterone. We were also surprised to observe that defeat, complicated by wounding, led to prolonged suppression of testosterone, as long as animals were kept socially isolated following the experience. Testosterone levels in several animals were observed to be low for several months following defeat. We found that this inhibition was not physiologically based, i.e. the inability of the pituitary or testis to respond to appropriate trophic stimuli, in that these same males showed a rapid rise in testosterone upon re-exposure to receptive females. We concluded that the low testosterone was primarily a consequence of central inhibition following the stress of defeat. These findings are summarized in Figure 1.

EFFECTS OF DEFEAT

In a later study published in 1975 we were able to replicate the effects of defeat on testosterone without the added complication of wounding in the defeated animal (Rose *et al.*, 1975). We also observed that after testosterone fell in the four defeated animals there was a decline in social interactions between these males and the rest of the social group. The defeated males assumed a very peripheral status in the social group, interacting little with other animals and engaging in very infrequent sexual behaviour, as well as showing very infrequent agonistic behaviour during the period of lower testosterone.

These studies with rhesus males reinforced our impressions derived from studies with human subjects, i.e. that psychological stress tended to inhibit testosterone secretion and one consequence of diminished testosterone in both species was a fall in sexual behaviour or libido.

In studying men under the threat of attack in Viet Nam, or engaged in basic combat training in the army, we found that androgen metabolites including testosterone glucuronide, androsterone and etiocholanolone were significantly diminished during these experiences (Rose *et al.*, 1969). Anecdotal observations of these men indicated the absence of sexual thoughts or imagery along with a general fall in sexual libido during these periods of time.

Later work (Kreuz *et al.*, 1972) involving men studied during officer candidate training confirmed these observations using plasma levels of testosterone rather than urinary metabolites as the index of gonadal activity. These men were observed to have significantly depressed levels of testosterone early in training which returned to normal levels in the weeks prior to graduation and at the conclusion of the training period. It was also observed that there was a significant diminution of sexual interests and libido in these young men during the training period when testosterone was significantly depressed.

The work reviewed so far supports the conclusion that a suppression of testosterone is a major factor leading to diminished sexual activity in rhesus monkeys and diminished sexual libido in human males. Further work, however, indicated that the relationship was not so clear cut and other variables could override the influence of testosterone on sexual behaviour.

SEASONAL INFLUENCES

In 1976 we reported a seasonal rhythm in plasma testosterone levels in male rhesus monkeys living in a social group, observed over a three-year period of time (Gordon *et al.*, 1976). The seasonal variation of plasma testosterone showed a significant increase in testosterone to levels of approximately 1000–1200 ng/dl, which occurred in the early to late fall, i.e. September, October and November. Levels fell following this to reach a low during the birth season, i.e. April, May, June and July. The increase in testosterone was coincident with the breeding season when animals engaged in frequent consort behaviour and copulation. *For the group* there was a close relationship

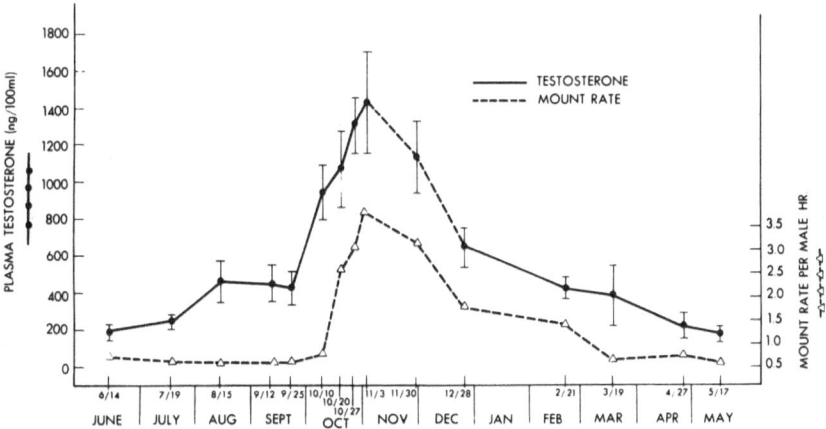

Figure 2   Mean plasma testosterone value ± the SE and mean mount rate per hour for seven sexually mature male members of a rhesus monkey breeding colony at each of 15 sample points in a 12-month span

observed between the mount rate and plasma testosterone levels, as shown in Figure 2. To this point we might conclude, as in previous studies, that there was a very close and tight relationship between testosterone and sexual behaviour. However, when the relationship between testosterone levels and the mount rate was observed for *individual* animals, a great deal of dissociation occurred. It was found, as indicated in Table 1, that all the males had elevated levels of testosterone during the three days they were studied in October and November as compared to their own levels during the summer months. However, there was no correlation between each animal's testosterone and the frequency of mounting, although all the males experience a

Table 1   Total mounts and ejaculations displayed by each subject during three 12-hour observation sessions, and the corresponding testosterone concentration (ng/100 ml) as assayed from a sample obtained the following morning

Subject	October 19: October 20	October 26: October 27	November 2: November 3
RGd	17(3):1135	80(5): 803	4(0): 740
RRe	1(0):1577	258(2):1790	32(1): 705
RPe	2(0): 482	86(5):1062	13(2):2274
RSe	7(1):1470	75(4): 808	169(0):2290
ROb	1(0): 473	0(0):1592	0(0): 669
RKd	1(0):1795	1(0):1605	1(0):1795
RQe	0(0): 668	3(2):1529	8(4):1567

significant rise in testosterone at this time. What appeared to be the major factor in determining the frequency of mounts and ejaculations was not the absolute level or even relative increase of testosterone, but rather the rank of the animal in the group. The males are listed in rank order and it can be seen that the three lowest ranking subjects (ROb, RKd, RQe) had the lowest mount rates while the higher ranking, more dominant animals showed more frequent mounting although not necessarily higher testosterone levels. One can conclude from these data that the breeding season serves as a stimulus to increase testosterone but the frequency of sexual behaviour for any given male was actually determined by other factors. Testosterone, it might be concluded, served to increase the set or propensity for increased mounting and copulation but did not actually determine the frequency of such behaviour.

It has been known for some time that the dominance rank of monkeys is greatly influenced by the relationship of that animal to other males and females living in the group (Bernstein et al., 1974). Females have been observed to support males in establishing their dominance rank and to support them during subsequent agonistic encounters to maintain their rank. The role of females in influencing rank may in part parallel their ability to serve as a stimulus to increase testosterone. We observed that for the males who were defeated in the formation of a new social group (Rose et al., 1975) their integration into the group in subsequent breeding seasons was facilitated by the development of consort behaviour with various females and it was only during these latter breeding seasons that these males began to engage in more frequent copulations, showed increased agonistic behaviour, rose in dominance rank while experiencing the appropriate seasonal increase in testosterone; all in the context of the developing social relationship with adult females resident in the group.

NATURE OF FEMALES AS STIMULI

More experimental evidence of the influence of social relationships on both testosterone and sexual behaviour was obtained in a study published in 1977

(Bernstein *et al.*, 1977). We observed previously that males did not engage in very frequent copulations except during the breeding season, when the females were receptive. We also had observed that when the females were receptive, i.e. in behavioural oestrus, not only was there a significant increase in copulation, but the females accepted the males as the more dominant member of the social group. In this study we introduced six males, one at a time, to a group of eight females during late October in the middle of the breeding season and again in June at the end of the birth season. Significant differences were observed. In June the males were not accepted as a member of the social group, let alone the dominant member, were frequently threatened by the females, and showed a high frequency of submissive responses. No copulations were observed and there was a very low frequency of mounts by the males during this non-breeding season.

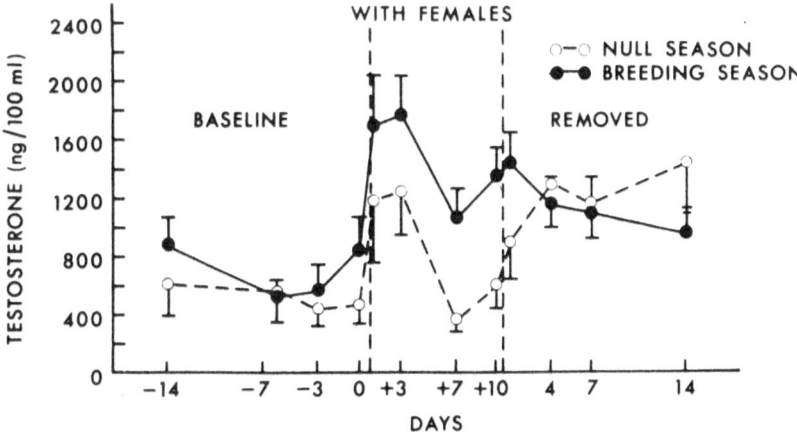

Figure 3   Mean testosterone levels of the males before. during and after introductions to females

When these same males were introduced during the breeding season they were threatened only for a very short time by the females, showed much fewer submissive responses and quickly were accepted as the dominant animal. After the first hour following introduction there was a significant number of mounts and copulations. The plasma testosterone levels in these males increased on both occasions although the increase during the non-breeding season was significantly less than that observed during the breeding season when the animals actually engaged in copulations with the females. These results are shown in Figure 3.

These findings may be interpreted to show that the presence of females serves as a stimulus to increase testosterone regardless of the subsequent consequences, i.e. whether or not the males engage in copulations, but social variables such as acceptance by the females determine whether sexual behaviour actually occurs. This would be consistent with the observation that females serve as a major stimulus to increase testosterone in all males in the social group during the breeding season. The theory that females act as a general stimulus to increase testosterone regardless of whether or not copulation occurs, was further tested in a study reported in 1979 (Gordon et al., 1979). In this study we permitted seven adult male rhesus living by themselves in an all-male group, to observe all social interactions, including copulation between males and females living in an adjacent, well-established breeding group. These males were housed in a compound approximately 6–7 metres away from the breeding group, which provided visual, auditory and possibly olfactory but no physical contact, i.e., through a chain-link fence. The animals in the all-male group showed just as great a rise in testosterone as the males in the breeding group who were engaging in frequent copulatory behaviour during the months of the breeding season. This demonstrated that females themselves, without contact, served as powerful stimuli to increase testosterone in adult males. These males who were so stimulated also showed a large increase in male to male mounting during this period of time when they observed the other males mount the females and themselves were experiencing a large increase in testosterone. There was also a significant dissociation between testosterone levels and the frequency of mounting behaviour among these seven males, parallel with that we described earlier in male mounting of females during the breeding season (Gordon et al., 1976).

MALE TO MALE SEXUAL BEHAVIOUR

It is of interest that these sexually aroused male rhesus monkeys, in the absence of female partners, engaged in male to male sexual behaviour which mimicked typical heterosexual behaviour. The males during this period of visual stimulation engaged in sexual behaviour characterized by a series of mounts by one male to a second male, which culminated in ejaculation by the male during the mounting period. Not all the animals exhibited this behaviour and those that did seemed to form stable pairs. However, we have not observed male to male sexual behaviour terminating with ejaculation in heterosexual groups, even when some hormonally aroused males do not have frequent access to female sexual partners.

The all-male group was then removed to an isolated compound where they had no visual or auditory access to any females of the genus Macaca. During the second breeding season these isolated males showed an increase in testosterone to approximately 600 ng/dl, or one-half of what was observed during the previous breeding season. We concluded that the season itself had some stimulating effect which is intensified by the presence of females, even without sexual contact with females. These findings are shown in Figure 4.

The relationship between changes in testosterone and the changes in aggressive behaviour is less clear. Although we reported earlier that milder forms of aggressive behaviour, in the form of non-contact aggression such as threat or chase behaviour, vary seasonally, this finding was not replicated in the study just reviewed. Again, the differences may be accounted for by the fact that in smaller social groups, and in groups where females are absent or immature males are absent, the number of potential social partners is mini-

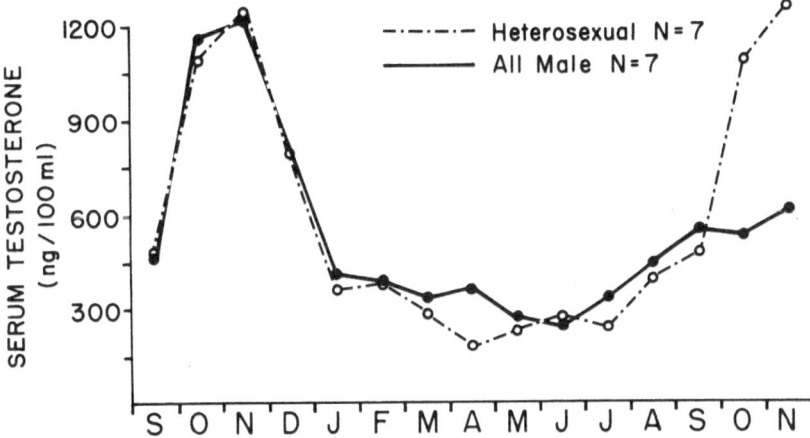

Figure 4 Mean monthly testosterone concentrations for seven male rhesus monkeys maintained in an all-male social group (All Male) during a 15-month span compared with testosterone values obtained from seven male rhesus maintained in a breeding group (Heterosexual) and studied concomitantly. The all-male group was housed in proximity to the breeding group during the first three months, and isolated from all contact with female rhesus thereafter

mized. Although we did observe some increase in aggressive behaviour during various scoring sessions, it was apparent from wounding data which occurs only sporadically even during the breeding season, that serious fighting did increase in November, albeit very sporadically, when the males were stimulated while observing other males and females.

HCG STIMULATION OF TESTOSTERONE

In a recent study we increased testosterone levels in four of seven adult males living in the same social group to see if we would find significant changes in behaviour secondary to alterations in androgen level (Gordon et al., 1979). We did not manipulate any social variables, such as introducing new females or males, but rather kept the social environment constant.

Four out of the seven males, the two highest and two lowest in the dominance hierarchy, received 1000 units of HCG intramuscularly twice weekly for four weeks. Testosterone levels increased approximately ten-fold to a peak of about 10 000 ng/dl. There was no change in the dominance hierarchy and no change in the direction of agonistic and submissive behaviour during the period of increased testosterone levels. The two most dominant animals received increase in aggression from the other males during the period of stimulated testosterone levels. In general, behavioural changes accompanying the rise in testosterone were not predictable, but appeared consistent with the behaviour of the animals prior to treatment, i.e. an intensification of existing behavioural patterns. The elevated testosterone led to an increase in aggressive behaviour in only one animal, the number two ranking male who displayed the most frequent aggressive behaviour before hormonal stimulation. The aggressive behaviour was directed toward subordinate animals, as it had been previously, so there was no change in direction of aggression. The male lowest in the dominance hierarchy, the omega male, showed no changes in either sexual or aggressive behaviour during the period of time when his testosterone was elevated. The stability of the dominance hierarchy and social relationships within the group despite dramatic changes in the hormonal state of four monkeys are indications of the persistent influence of the social structure on individual behaviour.

ADOLESCENCE

Further evidence of the potential dissociation between testosterone and behaviour or, stated differently, the influence of other variables, was obtained in a study of juvenile male rhesus during adolescence. We found that in juvenile males there is a rise in testosterone occurring during the third year, coincident with the breeding season, which increases to adult levels during the breeding season of the fourth year (Rose et al., 1978). When one compares the second year with the third year, there is a fall in play behaviour during the third year with an increase in sexual behaviour as shown in Figure 5. However, such a change in behaviour is not necessarily mediated by testosterone, despite the fact that testosterone shows significant increases in year three. We had several juvenile monkeys in various groups who were observed to 'miss' the rise in testosterone in their third year, but showed an increase parallel to age mates by their fourth year. In one juvenile male this was associated with him breaking his leg prior to the onset of the breeding season in his third year, while another animal was blinded in one eye during the same period of time. However, for both these juveniles, we observed the age specific change in behaviour, i.e. fall in play and increase in sexual behaviour, predominantly mounting of sub-adult females, despite the fact that they failed to show any rise in testosterone.

We have also found that the onset of adolescence, both with respect to the rise in testosterone and changes in behaviour, can be significantly influenced by other social factors. In the previous study just referred to (Rose et al., 1978) we observed significant differences in the rise in testosterone in males living in different social groups. In the groups with few adult males there was a large increase in testosterone compared to an absence of any rise in juvenile males living with large numbers of adult males and females. In a subsequent study, not yet published, we found that the crucial variable in determining whether or not three-year-old juvenile males showed a rise in testosterone with the associated fall in play and increase in sexual behaviour, was the rank of the adolescent male. For two different groups of juveniles the three-year-old

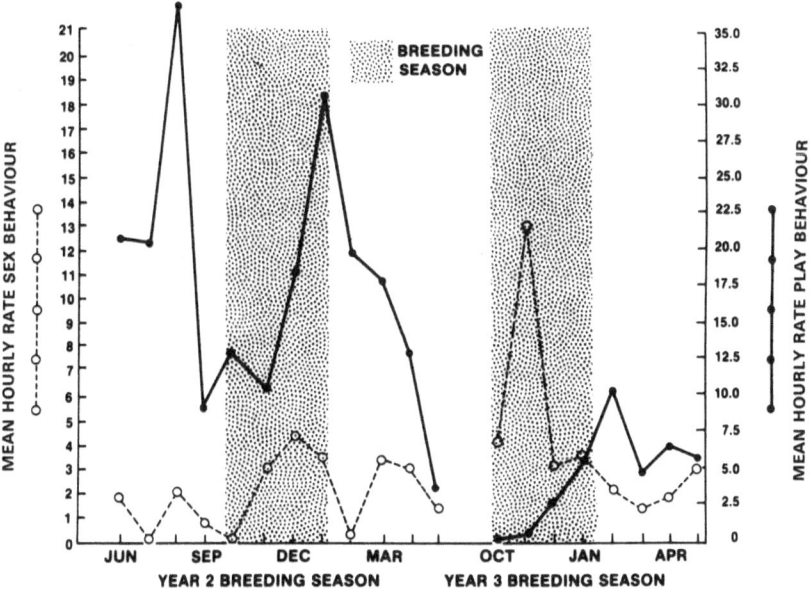

Figure 5   Mean hourly rate of sex and play behaviour for four males throughout their second and third years of development. The breeding seasons are shown as a hatched area

males who were high in dominance in the group showed a large increase in testosterone during the breeding season of their third year, while their lower ranking age mates failed to show such an increase. It has been observed from other studies that the position in the dominance hierarchy of the juvenile male is in large part a reflection of his mother's dominance status and thus one might conclude that the timing of adolescence is greatly influenced by social relationships, especially those associated with the matrilineal line.

HUMAN STUDIES

Our understanding of the influence of androgens on sexual and aggressive behaviour in humans has been hampered by many factors. Until recently, sexual behaviour has been reported more anecdotally than scientifically.

Aggressive behaviour is difficult to define and measure, and is usually under-reported in non-criminal populations. Thus, only recently have we become aware of the true prevalence of interpersonal violence. Furthermore, most work in humans has focused either on behaviour or endocrine variables separately, and rarely have both been reported in the same population. Even when behavioural and endocrine data are available, these studies have usually been done among institutionalized, criminal populations.

As other reviews in this volume focus on the relationship between the androgens and sexual behaviour, this review will be limited to those few studies which report both measures of androgens and assessment of aggressive behaviour in human males.

In general, there is consensus that castration in man does not lead to a fall in *aggressive* behaviour, despite the reduction observed in sexual libido or sexual activity (Rose, 1977).

Among institutionalized males, there are conflicting reports as to the relationship of testosterone and aggressive behaviour. One study reported that aggressive and socially dominant males had higher levels of testosterone compared to other prisoners (Ehrenkranz *et al.*, 1974), while another study failed to find a correlation between aggressive behaviour in prison and plasma testosterone levels (Kreuz and Rose, 1972). In a similar vein, studies of aggressive behaviour in normal males usually measured by self-report and not observed behaviour, have yielded inconsistent findings. However, a recent study on college hockey players did report a significant correlation between serum levels of testosterone and the coach's rating of one of six items designed to measure aggressive behaviour (response to threat) (Scaramella and Brown, 1978). Thus, data are still too sparse to comment definitely, or to estimate the magnitude of influence of androgens on aggressive behaviour in humans.

CONCLUSIONS

From this information it is clear that testosterone does influence sexual and aggressive behaviour, although the data are much stronger for non-human primates than man. However, the relationship is far from unitary. It does appear that stimuli that stimulate sexual behaviour also increase testosterone. However, there is no close relationship for an individual between the level of testosterone and subsequent sexual or aggressive behaviour. Thus, testosterone might be viewed as having a permissive influence in which it increases the propensity to behave sexually or aggressively, but other factors, especially the relationship to other members in the social group, seem to determine the final expression of any sexual or aggressive behaviour. Future research will necessitate not only measurements of testosterone but a careful examination of other psychosocial variables before we can clarify the relationship between the androgens, sexuality and aggression.

References

Bernstein. I. S.. Gordon. T. P. and Rose. R. M. (1974). Aggression and social controls in rhesus monkey (Macaca mulatta) groups revealed in group formation studies. *Folia Primatol.*. **21.** 81

Bernstein, I. S., Rose, R. M. and Gordon. T. P. (1977). Behavioural and hormonal responses of male rhesus monkeys introduced to females in the breeding and non-breeding seasons. *Anim. Behav.*, **25**, 609

Ehrenkranz, J.. Bliss, E. and Sheard, M. (1974). Plasma testosterone: correlation with aggressive behaviour and social dominance in man. *Psychosom. Med..* **36.** 469

Gordon, T. P., Bernstein, I. S. and Rose. R. M. (1978). Social and seasonal influences on testosterone secretion in the male rhesus monkey. *Physiol. Behav..* **21.** 623

Gordon, T. P., Rose, R. M. and Bernstein, I. S. (1979). Effects of increased testosterone secretion on the behaviour of adult male rhesus living in a social group. *Folia Primatol.* (In press)

Gordon, T. P., Rose, R. M. and Bernstein, I. S. (1976). Seasonal rhythm in plasma testosterone levels in the rhesus monkey (Macaca mulatta): a three-year study. *Horm. Behav..* **7.** 229

Kreuz, L. E. and Rose, R. M. (1972). Assessment of aggressive behaviour and plasma testosterone in a young criminal population. *Psychosom. Med..* **34.** 321

Kreuz, L. E., Rose, R. M. and Jennings, J. R. (1972). Suppression of plasma testosterone levels and psychological stress: longitudinal study of young men in officer candidate school. *Arch. Gen. Psychiat.*, **26**, 479

Rose. R. M. (1977). Neuroendocrine correlates of sexual and aggressive behaviour in humans. In M. A. Lipton, A. DiMascio and K. F. Killam (eds.). *Psychopharmacology: a Generation of Progress.* (New York: Raven Press)

Rose, R. M., Bernstein, I. S. and Gordon. T. P. (1975). Consequences of social conflict on plasma testosterone levels in rhesus monkeys. *Psychosom. Med..* **37.** 50

Rose, R. M., Bernstein, I. S., Gordon. T. P. and Lindsley. J. G. (1978). Changes in testosterone and behaviour during adolescence in the male rhesus monkey. *Psychosom. Med.*, **40**, 60

Rose, R. M., Bourne. P. G., Poe. R. O.. Mougey. E. H.. Collins. D. R. and Mason, J. W. (1969). Androgen responses to stress: II. Excretion of testosterone. epitestosterone. androsterone and etiocholanolone during basic combat training and under threat of attack. *Psychosom. Med.*, **31.** 418

Rose, R. M., Gordon, T. P. and Bernstein. I. S. (1972). Plasma testosterone levels in the male rhesus: influences of sexual and social stimuli. *Science.* **178.** 643

Scaramella, T. J. and Brown, W. A. (1978). Serum testosterone and aggressiveness in hockey players. *Psychosom. Med..* **40.** 262

Address for correspondence

Professor R. M. Rose, Department of Psychiatry and Behavioral Sciences. University of Texas Medical Branch, Galveston, TX 77550, USA

2.8
Female hormones and brain function

H. KOPERA

ABSTRACT

Animal studies and the limited available experiences in the human have shown that female sex hormones and similarly-acting substances exert profound influences on the brain. This paper reviews the data published to date and some of the assumptions made concerning the physiological and pharmacological significance of these substances. After discussion of uptake, distribution and binding in the central nervous system, the effects of oestrogenic and of progestational compounds on brain mechanisms such as respiration, water, electrolyte and protein metabolism, and enzyme activities, and on neurotransmitters are summarized. An account is then given of the effects of these substances on brain functions, including their effects on ovulation, posture, locomotion, body temperature and respiration, as well as on brain excitability, electrical activity and sleep. Finally, consideration is given to the influences of female sex hormones and of their pharmacological equivalents on sexual and non-sexual behaviour in animals and in man, and on psychic functions in the human. It is concluded that very little of the highly interesting findings is, as yet, applicable for therapeutic medicine, the use of these substances for substitution purposes in cases of deficiency being the only exception.

INTRODUCTION

This paper—necessarily an incomplete, subjective selection of facts and assumptions from the literature—deals not only with the female sex hormones, i.e. oestrogens and progesterone, but also with all substances employed in respective studies having pronounced oestrogenic or progestational effects. Hence, results with natural parent oestrogens and catechol oestrogens, with (half)synthetic steroidal and non-steroidal oestrogens and with natural gestagens as well as with progestagens (oestranes and pregnanes) will be considered, in most instances without explicit differentiation. The effects of oestrogens combined with progestins will not be discussed in detail. However, very frequently there is such an inextricable interaction between oestrogens and progestins and also with other hormones (e.g. androgens and peptide hormones) that the effects of any single hormone are usually not distinguishable. The great majority of data comes from animal experiments, mainly with rats, less frequently with monkeys, and the question of their importance for all species and the human in particular has to remain unanswered for the time being in most instances. Finally, it should be remembered that the interrelationship between the nervous and endocrine systems is so very complex that a brief review cannot but touch on just a few of the processes involved.

The literature cited is mainly restricted to a few books and reviews. These, particularly those marked with an asterisk, contain most of the relevant references for further reading.

Before discussing the effects of oestrogens and progestins on brain function, a short summary of a few relevant details on hormone uptake and distribution, the mechanisms of action and the influences upon brain development seems appropriate.

HORMONE UPTAKE, DISTRIBUTION AND BINDING

Most information has been obtained using measurements of labelled hormones. After the injection of oestradiol, radio-activity in all brain regions exceeds blood levels by a factor of 3 or more, but oestrogens are taken up and distributed differentially in various areas of the CNS (Eisenfeld, 1972). The specific accumulation of eostrogens is greatest in the anterior pituitary, in the hypothalamus and in the limbic system. In rats one hour after intravenous administration the concentration of oestrogens in the anterior pituitary is about 100 times greater than in plasma. The hormone is taken up to a greater extent by the neurons. Oestrogens attach to protein containing macromolecules, and specific nuclear and cytosol receptors have been identified in various areas of the brain including the hypothalamus, the anterior pituitary and the pre-optic area. The anterior pituitary has a 60-fold, and the hypothalamus at least a 10-fold, higher concentration of specific binding macro molecules than, for example, the cerebrum or cerebellum. A potent competition by catechol oestrogens for oestrogen receptors of the pituitary and hypothalamus has been reported, which can possibly be of physiological significance. The concentration of catechol oestrogens in hypothalamus and pituitary has been found to be at least 10 times higher than for the parent oestrogens (Paul and Axelrod, 1977).

There is a clear relation between the plasma hormone levels and the levels in the cerebrospinal fluid (CSF). It has been reported that the levels in the CSF are in agreement with the calculated unbound, i.e. the physiologically active, oestrogen plasma fraction.

Progesterone also seems to be taken up into the brain rather rapidly. Apparently it accumulates in the midbrain rather than in the hypothalamus, cerebral cortex and hippocampus. The rat brain contains one progestin receptor system in the hypothalamus and pre-optic area which is oestrogen regulated, and another in the midbrain and cerebral cortex which is insensitive to elevated plasma oestrogen (MacLusky and McEwen, 1978). Progesterone has no effect on the hypothalamic oestradiol binding capacity. In contrast to other target organs, uptake of female sex hormones in neural tissues is not influenced by the age of the animal nor by the adrenals. However, hormone-priming can enhance hormone retention in some brain areas. It is assumed that, in the rat, the effects of progesterone in regulating the timing of ovulation and sexual behaviour are related to the effect on oestradiol retention in the CNS (Lisk and Reuter, 1977).

EFFECTS ON BRAIN MECHANISMS

The mechanism of action of sex steroids in the brain at the molecular level is unknown.

Respiration and metabolism of brain tissue

Effects of sex hormones on the metabolism of the CNS have not been extensively studied in man. Data obtained in animal experiments indicate, with a few exceptions, very little effect at least in the mature individual.

Large doses of progestins have a powerful anaesthetizing action and some progestational compounds produce in man a profound reduction in cerebral blood flow, oxygen and glucose consumption comparable to that of barbiturate anaesthesia. Parallels between the anaesthetic action of steroids and their ability to inhibit glucose oxidation of rat brain homogenates have been found for progesterone and α-oestradiol. but not for stilboestrol. This non-steroidal oestrogen is less anaesthetic but it is the most potent brain respiration inhibitor; it may exert its effect by competing with cytochrome C as a hydrogen acceptor for lactic dehydrogenase. The elevated cerebral oxygen consumption found in castrated pre-pubertal rats is restored to normal *in vivo* by the administration of progesterone, but not by 17β-oestradiol. The steep fall in cerebral metabolic rate at puberty is possibly the result of the increased production of steroid hormones such as androgens and corticosteroids.

Water and electrolytes

Perhaps one of the primary important effects of sex hormones is the one directly concerned with the regulation of water and electrolyte metabolism. Most hormones affect calcium metabolism directly or indirectly, and in this way are thought to exert important effects on brain maturation, excitability and behaviour. Effects on calcium metabolism have been demonstrated for oestrogens in a variety of species. However, brain excitability is thought to be influenced by oestrogens not only via electrolyte changes but also through other mechanisms.

Protein metabolism

Hormones can influence protein metabolism of nervous tissues via enzymes directly involved in protein synthesis or via indirect effects on RNA metabolism. They increase RNA synthesis or synthesis of selective RNAs at least in peripheral organs concerned with reproduction. Hormones may also affect the transport or metabolism of amino acids or influence the energy metabolism of the cell. Little is known in this respect of the effects of female hormones. Oestrogens have been found to increase protein synthesis in the cerebral cortex of oophorectomized guinea-pigs.

Effects on brain enzyme activities and neurotransmitters

Oestrogens counteract the increase of monoamine oxidase (MAO) in oophorectomized rats and decrease MAO activity in various brain regions in a dose-dependent manner. Plasma and platelet MAO activities in humans have been shown to vary during the menstrual cycle and can be reduced by oestrogens. Choline acetylase is influenced by oestrogens in an opposite manner. Various other enzymes, such as catechol-O-methyltransferase (COMT), glucose-6-phosphate dehydrogenase, isocitrate dehydrogenase, and malate dehydrogenase, as well as neurotransmitters, such as noradrenaline, serotonin (5-HT), and dopamine, are also influenced by oestrogens. The levels of these substances vary during the cycle, in pregnancy, after gonadectomy and perhaps also after hypophysectomy. These effects, particularly on brain amines, may be mediated by gonadotrophins, but direct effects on turnover, increased amine synthesis and decreased uptake of noradrenaline and 5-HT, have also been reported for oestrogens and for the aromatizable testosterone. Since female hormones affect amine metabolism and behaviour, these two may be linked. In male and female mammals the depression of 5-HT activity in the CNS induces sexual behaviour. The elevation of dopamine levels in males and their depression in females has a similar effect. Changes of adrenaline or noradrenaline have little effect on behaviour. However, the question as to whether or not there is indeed a causal relationship between these alterations in brain amines and sexual behaviour remains to be answered. A possible beneficial effect of oestrogens on drug-induced dyskinesia is thought to be related to their assumed antidopaminergic activity. Hormone dependent changes have also been observed in tryptophan and γ-aminobutyric acid (GABA) metabolism.

Progesterone is reported to influence serotonin; it reduces 5-HT uptake, increases 5-HT turnover, lowers the brain GABA content, and counteracts the increase of GABA after oophorectomy. It has also been suggested that progesterone activates a noradrenergic system in the hypothalamus by causing a release of noradrenaline or by sensitizing noradrenaline receptors in postsynaptic membranes. Some data indicate that progesterone may activate dopaminergic systems; thus, inhibition of lordosis could be due to a dopamine-induced increase in locomotor activity (Feder and Marrone, 1977).

EFFECTS ON BRAIN DEVELOPMENT, MORPHOLOGY AND DIFFERENTIATION

Sex hormones exert regulatory influences on the CNS particularly during 'critical' periods in the rapidly developing embryonic, fetal and postnatal brain. They result in sexual differentiation and profound modification of both sexual and non-sexual behaviour and of endocrine function in the adult animal. Female and male brains differ with respect to gonadotrophin regulation and behaviour. Males secrete FSH and LH constantly, females have a cyclic discharge. Aromatizable androgens are converted during infancy into oestrogens by central neuroendocrine tissues in localized areas related to reproductive function (Naftolin et al., 1975). Many recently-published data support the concept that in the period of hypothalamic differentiation oestrogens are essential for sexual differentiation, i.e. for the suppression of the female patterns of gonadotrophin secretion and sexual behaviour, and for the central organization of normal patterns of male sexual behaviour (Booth, 1978). In mammals a lack of oestrogens results in a cyclic schedule of gonadotrophin secretion and in female sexual behaviour because the basic pattern of differentiation in the absence of fetal gonads is female (it is masculine in birds). Administration of androgens to females during the first few days after birth prevents ovulation at maturity. Neonatally androgen-treated females appear not to respond to oestrogens as well as normal females; they show less frequently the behaviour pattern characteristic for oestrogens — assuming a lordotic position when mounted by a male. Possibly the reduced responsiveness is due to a defective oestrogen-binding. In some species, centres sensitive to the action of sex hormones and responsible for the control over sexual behaviour have been located. Presumably these have to be primed prenatally to enable steroids to act on them in the adult animal. The differentiation of such centres seems to depend on the concentrations of the oestrogens rather than on the type of the hormone. Pre- and neonatally oestrogens cause a pronounced proliferation of these hormone sensitive centres, increasing the number of neurons and dendritic synapses. Sex hormones continue to modify the structure of the hypothalamus until puberty and in appropriate amounts may even affect the structures in adult life; in the rat persistent oestrus and polycystic ovaries are associated with an oestrogen-induced disconnection of the circuit responsible for cyclic drive of gonadotrophin secretion.

Little research has been done concerning the interactions of progesterone with the brain. The results reported do not indicate a specific progesterone interaction in the rat.

Knowledge of the effects of prenatal and early postnatal hormone exposure in the human is restricted to observations in subjects exposed to abnormally high or low levels of sex hormones because of endocrine abnormalities of the fetus, hormone-producing tumours in the mother, or hormone treatment during pregnancy (Ehrhardt, 1978; Meyer Bahlburg, 1978). Some such experiences have been used for claims that exposure to natural hormones or synthetic equivalents in the first trimester of pregnancy can have long-term effects on IQ (very much disputed), on educational attainments (Dalton, 1976), and on personality and/or temperament (Reinisch and Karow, 1977). Others, taking heed of evidence from animal experiments, have emphasized the possible dangers of hormone treatment in pregnancy because, administered during critical stages of development, sex hormones can play a major role in determining the rate of maturation and differentiation of the CNS.

EFFECTS ON BRAIN FUNCTIONS

Regulation of ovulation

A high sensitivity to the negative feed-back actions of sex steroids probably controls prepubertal gonadotrophin secretion. In the rat a sudden change in the hypothalamic threshold to the gonadotrophin-inhibiting effect of oestrogens over a narrow range of time near the onset of puberty has been observed. This decline in sensitivity is the principal factor initiating puberty.

Sex hormones modulate hypothalamic releasing factors and pituitary gonadotrophins by direct action on the pituitary (oestrogens) and by feedback mechanisms (oestrogens and gestagens). The elevated mid-cycle plasma oestrogen level provokes, presumably via a discharge of LHRF synchronized with an increased pituitary sensitivity to LHRF, the pre-ovulatory surge of LH and FSH secretion which is most probably responsible for ovulation.

Posture and locomotion

In castrated adult female rats oestrogens promote a typical receptive behaviour pattern: when mounted by a male they assume a lordotic position. This effect on sexual receptivity can also be produced in castrated males, be it only with much higher doses. Areas in the anterior hypothalamus and the preoptic region are thought predominantly responsible for this oestrogen-induced lordosis, and involvement of changes of MAO activity might be of relevance. Progesterone can either facilitate or reduce this oestrogen effect depending on the sequence of administration of the hormones.

Oestrogens may activate both excitatory and inhibitory neural substrates for locomotion. There seems to be a fundamental relationship between lordosis and locomotion and between these two phenomena and the limbic–hypothalamic system.

The decreased tonus and electromyographic activity of abdominal muscles during pregnancy or following treatment with progestins might be caused by a central action of these steroids. This action is thought to favour development of compensatory lordosis in pregnancy.

Taste, smell, hearing and food intake

Clinical observations indicate effects of changes in gonadal and adrenal function on thresholds for taste, smell and hearing. Detailed respective investigations performed with adrenocortical steroids show that the thresholds for taste, smell and hearing are significantly decreased in adrenocortical insufficiency. This can be restored to normal by glucocorticoid administration, but not, however, by gonadal steroids. Food intake shows cyclic variations and oestrogens have been found to reduce food intake.

Body temperature regulation

Data suggest a close relationship between the temperature regulating mechanisms and the endocrine system. There is a rise in body temperature in women at the time of ovulation persisting until menstruation, and in pregnancy the body temperature remains elevated during the first half of gestation. This thermogenetic action is also seen after the administration of progestins to non-ovulating women and to men. It is most likely caused by a direct or indirect effect on a thermogenetic centre in the hypothalamus. The 5β-OH steroid hormone metabolites. etiocholanolone. pregnenolone and 11-keto-pregnanolone. also cause a rise in body temperature in humans, though the fever-producing action of these steroid metabolites seems to be highly species-specific.

Respiration

The CO_2 sensitivity of the respiratory centre increases in the normal cycle after ovulation and in the second half of pregnancy. Respiratory stimulation can likewise be produced by the administration of progesterone or progestagens both in women and in men. Similar effects have also been observed with oestrogens.

The biological clock

Various recurring rhythmic biological and behavioural events such as ovulation and the menstrual cycle are regulated by mechanisms more primitive than homeostasis. These suggested 'biological clock mechanisms' are hardly affected by internal and external influences with the exception of light. Endocrinological changes, such as gonadectomy, mating, pregnancy, lactation or hypophysectomy, have been reported to be without effect on the 'biological clock'.

ELECTROPHYSIOLOGICAL EFFECTS

Brain excitability

Brain excitability is markedly and differentially influenced by sex hormones. Oestrogens have an excitatory effect. The electroshock threshold (EST) is lower in female rats than in males and it fluctuates with the phases of the menstrual cycle, reaching the lowest level at ovulation. A decrease in EST can be produced in a dose-dependent fashion by oestrogen administration. This effect is assumed to be mediated by mechanisms other than electrolyte changes since EST has been found to be lowered by oestrogen in spite of elevated plasma sodium concentrations and increased extracellular/intracellular sodium ratio in the cerebral cortex. The micro electroshock seizure threshold in different parts of the brain reacts differently to oestrogens, increasing in some parts, decreasing in others.

Various steroid hormones including progesterone (Selye, 1941) have an anaesthetic effect in a number of animals. Large doses produce deep anaesthesia. In man, progesterone has a soporific effect. It has been shown that the CNS depressant effect of progesterone surpasses that of short-acting barbiturates, and that the related 5β-pregnane derivatives are even more potent than hydroxydione and pentobarbital in depressing arousal from reticular formation stimulation. The anaesthetic activity of these steroids can be dissociated from the hormonal activity by structural modification of the molecule.

An increased epileptogenic activity has been observed after injection and after cortical application of oestrogen. Progesterone raises the EST. The threshold of cortical EEG arousal on direct stimulation of the hypothalamus is much increased by progesterone, while the elevation of the threshold on stimulation of the reticular formation is not as large. In patients with partial epilepsy, a very low number of generalized seizures has been found when progesterone levels are high, whereas many seizures occur during the follicular phase and after a rapid decrease of the progesterone level following menstruation. This is in accordance with the repeatedly supposed beneficial effect of progesterone on seizures and the claimed epileptogenic effect of oestrogens in epileptics. Progesterone seems to be an anticonvulsive agent.

Electrical activity and sleep

A number of pre- and post-ovulatory differences in the EEG observed in animals and in man may be linked with effects of sex hormones. The reported observations, however, are far from uniform. Under oestrogen treatment driving response rates to photic stimulation have been found to be inhibited in amenorrhoeic and in depressed women, a reaction similar to the one observed after treatment with adrenergic substances. A possible relationship with suppression of increased MAO activity has been suggested.

Power spectral analysis of the EEG shows that the α-rhythm is slightly but significantly accelerated in the luteal phase with a maximum shortly before menstruation (Itil et al., 1976). Some investigators have observed changes in the ratio between theta waves and total activity of the frontal lobes during the menstrual cycle with the lowest ratio during the luteal phase. It has also been reported that sufficient slowing of the EEG occurs in association with menstruation to convert a normal EEG to an abnormal one. In the final weeks of pregnancy when progesterone levels are high, the EEG is low compared to post-partum tracings. However, the post-menopausal EEG is not significantly altered by progestins or stilboestrol.

Oestrogen effects in the quantitative pharmaco-electroencephalogram (CEEG) are similar to those of tricyclic antidepressants, whereas progestagens caused changes of the CEEG profile resembling those of minor tranquillizers (Herrmann and Beach, 1978a and 1978b).

In guinea-pigs hormone-induced oestrus has been seen to be accompanied by a decrease in the amounts of both paradoxical (REM) and slow wave sleep; in rabbits oestrogens increased total sleeping time and REM sleep, while in the intact cat large doses of oestrogens produced no significant changes in cortical electrical activity. Peri-menopausal women treated with oestrogens show more REM sleep, significantly reduced intervening wakefulness and frequency of wakenings.

Electrical activity—single neurons

In the lateral anterior hypothalamic areas oestrogens enhance the inhibitory responsiveness to pain, cold and cervical stimuli, whereas in the septum the number of inhibitory responses is decreased. Exogenous or endogenous progesterone selectively depresses the excitation of hypothalamic neurons by stimuli from the genital tract, an effect which may be related to that of progesterone on 5-HT metabolism (Ladisich, 1977).

EFFECTS ON BEHAVIOUR

Human behaviour results from the interaction of physiological, psychological and social factors. The part played by female sex hormones in the direct control of overt human behaviour is—compared with that found in lower mammals—slight and less easy to define. These hormones, though necessary for the maintenance of libido and sexual behaviour, seem to control the intensity of such behaviour rather than the direction. Their most pronounced influences on behaviour are perhaps on psychological (emotional rather than intellectual) and sociological aspects (Eayrs and Glass, 1962). In fetal or neonatal life sex hormones organize the sexually undifferentiated brain with regard to neuroendocrine function and patterns not only of sexual but also of non-sexual behaviour.

In castrated male rats oestrogens inhibit the production of sexual excitement by androgens. In sufficiently high doses oestradiol activates the complete male copulatory pattern including ejaculation; it also makes castrated male rats exhibit female sexual behaviour (lordosis). Oestrogens—like aromatizable androgens—augment mating behaviour in oophorectomized rhesus monkeys by increasing proceptivity (female's willingness to initiate copulation), but are without effect on receptivity (active co-operation with the male's initiation of copulation). They stimulate aggressiveness, not only in relation to mating behaviour but also towards a third individual and inanimate objects. Additional progesterone decreases aggressiveness in relation to mating behaviour, and in particular the aggressiveness towards a third individual. Oestrogens decrease fearfulness, influence conditioned taste aversion, delay extinction and counteract some behavioural effects of d-amphetamine in rodents.

Insufficient research has been undertaken into the effects of physiological concentrations of female sex hormones on psychic function in man. Certainly there are significant fluctuations in mood, mental content, and outlook during the menstrual cycle. These are thought to be related to concomitant hormonal changes. It is assumed that oestrogens account, at least in part, for the increased well-being, alertness and vigour found in the first half of the menstrual cycle, at which time an active extrovert heterosexual drive with an ovulatory peak in sexual attractiveness and both female initiated autosexual and heterosexual activity has also been demonstrated (Adams *et al.*, 1978). However, there is no convincing evidence that the administration of oestrogens would appreciably increase sexual drive in the normal woman. This is consistent with the observation that neither physiological ovarian failure at menopause nor ovariectomy alters sexual behaviour dramatically; this is only the case when all sources of endogenous androgens and oestrogens are removed by additional adrenalectomy.

Recent studies indicate that children prenatally exposed to more oestrogens than progestins show effects on the personality in that they are more group-oriented and group-dependent, less individualistic and less self-sufficient than other children; they are more 'outer' or 'other' directed (Reinisch and Karow, 1977).

There seems to be a physiological predisposition towards hyperoestrogen-ism in puberty, and in some individuals prolonged mental stress can produce this condition. In such subjects deterioration in school achievement, social hyperactivity, hypochondria, inhibited aggression, sexual problems, increased sensitivity and, after prolonged intrapsychic conflict, psychic exhaustion have been reported. In men treated with high doses of oestrogens for diseases such as prostatic carcinoma, a loss of sexual desire and potency, a longing for asexual tenderness, mood changes towards depression, reduced drive and inactivity are observed; hyperactivity and euphoria to explosiveness are less often recorded. In trials to improve mental functioning in conditions such as cerebral thrombosis or atherosclerosis high doses of oestrogens have not led to pronounced beneficial effects. Recently high doses of oestrogens have been claimed to exert an antidepressant effect comparable to that of tricyclic antidepressants (Herrmann and Beach, 1978a). Whether or not they are indeed therapeutically useful in relieving chronic severe intransigent states of depression by influences upon central adrenergic functioning has still to be confirmed.

Oestrogen deficiency, as found in women with inadequately developed sexual organs such as Turner's syndrome, causes psychosexual infantility. The psychological features of these patients are described as warm and friendly, they are naive, lack aggression and obtain little satisfaction from sexual activity. These symptoms respond to oestrogen administration. In castrated women the psychological changes caused by the oestrogen deficiency are usually more regular but of shorter duration and less severe than those in the climacteric woman in whom oestrogen production gradually diminishes. In neither instance is a sudden reduction in active sexual behaviour observable, though a variety of psychic disturbances accompany the post-menopausal years. Obviously, many of these disturbances are not connected with the progressive oestrogen deficiency. However, in some the hormonal imbalance seems to be of importance. This can be deduced from a number of recent investigations in which reproducible psychometric methods have been employed. The observations clearly indicate a beneficial prophylactic and therapeutic effect of oestrogens on some psychic functions. Improvements have been set in psychomotor co-ordination, concentration, attention, information processing capacity, irritability, anxiety, and in some parameters of alertness. A few reports suggest that oestrogens improve social behaviour and prevent expected deterioration of mental performance, such as some perceptual, attentional and memory processes, but others dispute such effects. Some investigations suggest that oestrogens display effects usually associated with psychostimulants (Herrmann and Beach, 1978a). However, the most beneficial and frequently observed therapeutic action of oestrogens is a mood-elevating psychotonic effect which often causes a sense of extreme well-being and vigour, most probably due to the restorement of somatic efficiency and psychic equilibrium.

In a wide variety of non-primates oestrogens activate female behaviour. A similar effect of progesterone varies markedly among species, can be absent altogether and in some non-primates progesterone actually suppresses female sexual behaviour. Thus animal experiments indicate that progesterone can have either facilitory or inhibitory influences on female sexual behaviour (Feder and Marrone, 1977). It may interact with oestrogens in facilitating sexual responses in different temporal sequences in different species, but can also cause inhibition of sexual behaviour depending on whether the oestrogen conditioning is complete and accompanied by a low level of progesterone (sequential) or incomplete and accompanied by a high level of progesterone (concurrent). Oestrogens promote the female's sexual attractiveness; progesterone makes the females sexually less attractive. Progestins can delay extinction of conditioned avoidance in the rat. Cats under long-term administration of a progestagen are more docile and easier to trap.

There is some indication that noradrenergic mechanisms are involved in the facilitation of sexual behaviour by progesterone, but other neurotransmitters are also likely to be of importance. The inhibitory effects of progestins on oestrogen-dependent processes are thought to be indirect. They appear to depend more on transference of information from progesterone-responsive cells to oestrogen-responsive cells than on direct impedance of intranuclear programming processes in oestrogen-sensitive cells (Feder and Marrone, 1977).

The available evidence concerning the psychological changes thought to be associated with progestins in man is very incomplete and conflicting. Based on observations during the menstrual cycle, in pregnancy, and on administration of progestational substances, one could conclude that these compounds decrease libido and activity, induce tiredness, a lowering of the incidence of emotional instability, impulsiveness and irritability, that they might be involved in pre-menstrual tension, and that they provoke tension, anxiety, depression and occasionally even psychotic episodes. These common beliefs have, however, been questioned by opposite findings. Some psychopharmacological studies in the luteal phase or with progestins have indicated an increase in reaction time, performance speed and quality, an anti-anxiety effect and a favourable influence on instinctive maternal tendencies, as expressed in dreams. Progestagens used as anti-androgens in the treatment of sex offenders have a mood-stabilizing, mildly sedative effect. Progestagens block the impairment of performance caused by LSD via a mechanism which is not yet clear. Studies with the CEEG suggest that some progestins have a profile similar to that of a minor tranquillizer. This is consistent with the observation that progestins have sedative–tranquillizing properties and in high intravenous doses an anaesthesia-like effect. It is also in agreement with the assumption that progesterone has a protective effect against stress reactions (Ladisich, 1977), and is compatible with the repeated observation that progestagens can diminish aggressive behaviour and can have a mood equilibrating effect. The claim that prenatal administration of progesterone enhances intelligence and improves educational attainments (Dalton, 1976) meets much criticism and is still a matter of debate (Sachar, 1976). It seems, however, that prenatal exposure to mainly progestagens affects personality; children of mothers given progestagens for the maintenance of at-risk pregnancies have been found to be significantly more independent, sensitive, individualistic, self-assured and self-sufficient than other children; they are more 'inner' or 'self' directed (Reinisch and Karow, 1977), and show less athletic skills.

The evidence reported so far of psychic effects of female sex hormones is certainly insufficient to permit final conclusions to be drawn. This also holds true for the numerous and conflicting respective observations in women using contraceptive preparations which contain a progestin or a combination of an oestrogen with a progestagen as the active compounds. In this field the methodological difficulties are formidable, hence a large amount of literature with contradictory viewpoints exists on the subject. Nevertheless, the majority of data supports the conventional idea that oestrogens are rather stimulating, activity inducing, cause irritability and worsen pre-menstrual tension, while progestins seem to cause passivity, mood changes towards depression and to relieve pre-menstrual irritability. However, the great diversity of partly unidentifiable factors contributing to the net result of psychic influences of female sex hormones prevents the isolation of the effect of any single hormonal substance.

CONCLUDING REMARKS

Studies with animals, but also experiences in man, indicate that the brain is certainly one of the target organs of female sex hormones. Hormone uptake, distribution and binding are differential in various areas of the CNS. Specific receptors for oestrogens and progestins have been identified in the brain. The mechanism of action at the molecular level is still obscure, however, some data are available on the effects on respiration and metabolism of brain tissue, on water and electrolyte balance, protein metabolism, enzyme activities and on neurotransmitters. The influence of female gonadal hormones on the brain in pre- and perinatal periods is responsible for sexual differentiation and endocrine functions of the CNS. In postnatal life sex steroids regulate ovulation, affect posture, locomotion, temperature regulation and respiration. Sex hormones interfere with the excitability and electrical activity of the brain and with sleep. Undoubtedly, female gonadal hormones and their pharmacological equivalents exert profound influences on brain functions. With our present knowledge it seems rather hazardous, however, to predict a therapeutic applicability of these effects for pathological conditions with the exception of their use to supplement deficiencies. This is equally valid for the proposal to use female hormones in psychiatry, as well as for the speculation that the availability of catechol oestrogens, which have virtually no uterotropic activity but could have an important role in neuroendocrine regulation (Fishman, 1977) would open new therapeutic possibilities.

References

* The books and reviews marked with an asterisk contain most of the relevant references for further reading on this subject.

Adams, D. B., Gold, A. R. and Burt, A. D. (1978). Rise in female-initiated sexual activity at ovulation and its suppression by oral contraceptives. *N. Engl. J. Med.*, **299**, 1145

*Bäckström, T. (1977). Oestrogen and progesterone in relation to different activities in the central nervous system. *Acta Obstet. Gynecol. Scand.*, 66 (Suppl.), 1

Booth, J. E. (1978). Effects of the aromatization inhibitor androst-4-ene-3,6,17-trione on sexual differentiation induced by testosterone in the neonatally castrated rat. *J. Endocrinol.*, **79**, 69

Dalton, K. (1976). Prenatal progesterone and educational attainments. *Br. J. Psychiat.*, **129**, 438

Eayrs, J. T. and Glass, A. (1962). The ovary and behaviour. In S. Zuckerman, A. M. Mandl and P. Eckstein (eds.), *The Ovary*. (New York: Academic Press)

*Editorial (1979). Sexual behaviour and the sex hormones. *Lancet*, **2**, 17

Ehrhardt, A. A. (1978). Behavioural effects of oestrogen in the human female. *Pediatrics*, **62**, 1166

Eisenfeld, A. J. (1972). Interaction of oestrogens, progestational agents, and androgens with brain and pituitary and their role in the control of ovulation. In S. H. Snyder (ed.), *Perspectives in Neuropharmacology*. (New York: Oxford University Press)

Feder, H. H. and Marrone, B. L. (1977). Progesterone: its role in the central nervous system as a facilitator and inhibitor of sexual behaviour and gonadotropin release. *Ann. N.Y. Acad. Sci.*, **206**, 331

Fishman, J. (1977). The catechol oestrogens. *Neuroendocrinology*, **22**, 363

*Herbert, J. (1977). Hormones and sexual behaviour in adulthood. In J. Money and H. Musaph (eds.). *Handbook of Sexology*, pp. 375–492 (Amsterdam: Excerpta Medica)

Herrmann, W. M. and Beach, R. C. (1978a). The psychotropic properties of oestrogens. *Pharmakopsychiat.*, **11**, 164

Herrmann, W. M. and Beach, R. C. (1978b). Experimental and clinical data indicating the psychotropic properties of progestogens. *Postgrad. Med. J.*, **54**, 2 (Suppl.), 82

*Itil, T. M., Laudahn, G. and Herrmann, W. M. (1976) (eds.). *Psychotropic Action of Hormones*. (New York: Spectrum)

*Junkmann, K. (1968) (ed.). *Handbuch der Experimentellen Pharmakologie. Die Gestagene.* Vol. XII/1. (Berlin: Springer)

*Junkmann, K. (1969) (ed.). *Handbuch der Experimentellen Pharmakologie. Die Gestagene.* Vol. XII/2. (Berlin: Springer)

*Kopera, H. (1973). Oestrogens and psychic function. In P. A. van Keep and C. Lauritzen (eds.). *Ageing and Oestrogens.* Front. Hormone Res.. vol. 2. pp. 118–133. (Basel: Karger)

Ladisich, W. (1977). Influence of progesterone on serotonin metabolism: a possible causal factor for mood changes. *Psychoneuroendocrinology*, **2**, 257

Lisk, R. D. and Reuter, L. A. (1977). *In vivo* progesterone treatment enhances (^{3}H) estradiol retention by neural tissue of the female rat. *Endocrinology.* **100**. 1652

MacLusky, N. J. and McEwen. B. S. (1978). Oestrogen modulates progestin receptor concentrations in some rat brain regions but not in others. *Nature.* **274**. 276

Meyer Bahlburg, H. F. L. (1978). Behavioural effects of oestrogen treatment in human males. *Pediatrics*, **62**. 1171

Naftolin, F., Ryan, K. J., Davies. I. J.. Reddy. V. V.. Flores. F.. Petro, Z. and Kuhn, M. (1975). The formation of oestrogens by central neuroendocrine tissues. In R. O. Greep (ed.). *Recent Progress in Hormone Research.* Vol. 31. (New York: Academic Press)

Paul, S. M. and Axelrod, J. (1977). Catechol oestrogens: Presence in brain and endocrine tissues. *Science*, **197**, 657

*Porter, R. and Whelan, J. (1979) (eds.). *Sex. Hormones and Behaviour.* Ciba Foundation Symposium 62 (new series). (Amsterdam: Excerpta Medica)

Reinisch, J. M. and Karow, W. G. (1977). Prenatal exposure to synthetic progestins and oestrogens: effects on human development. *Arch. Sex. Behav.*, **6**, 257

*Sachar, E. J. (1976) (ed.). *Hormones, Behaviour and Psychopathology.* (New York: Raven Press)

*Sawyer, C. H. and Gorski, R. A. (1971) (eds.). *Steroid Hormones and Brain Function.* (Berkeley: University of California Press)

Selye, H. (1941). Anaesthetic effect of steroid hormones. *Proc. Soc. Exp. Biol. Med..* **46**. 116

*Tausk, M. and de Visser, J. (1971). Various other effects of progesterone. In M. Tausk (ed.). *Int. Encyclopaed. Pharmacol.*, **48**, pp. 375–387 (Oxford: Pergamon Press)

*Vernikos-Danellis. J. (1972). Effects of hormones on the central nervous system. In S. Levine (ed.). *Hormones and Behaviour.* (New York: Academic Press)

Address for correspondence

Dr H. Kopera, Clinical Pharmacology Unit, Department of Experimental and Clinical Pharmacology, Universität Graz, Universitätsplatz 4, A-8010 Graz, Austria

2.9
Hormones and sexual impotence

J. J. LEGROS, P. CHIODERA, C. MORMONT,
J. SERVAIS and P. FRANCHIMONT

ABSTRACT

A review of recent studies on the roles of testosterone and prolactin, the two hormones most specifically involved in human male sexuality, reveals that much research work remains to be done in this field. Whilst it is clear, for instance, that androgens variously affect the human male in all life phases, their effects are not completely understood particularly where sexual problems are concerned. In the adult it is now clear that androgen plasma levels are not a reliable guide to sexual orientation. A complicating factor appears to be a disturbed gluco-lipidic function, even one not implying severe diabetes; it now seems likely that impotence in such cases stems not from a lack of androgens but rather from a peripheral arteriolar or neurological problem. The effect of prolactin on the brain and its action via 5α-reductase and/or through an influence on the dopamine hypothalamic turnover needs to be further investigated. It is hypothesized that a confirmation of an action of prolactin on androgen metabolism in the brain would suggest that some psychosexual disturbances may be caused by an excess of cerebral oestrogens; this, in turn, leads to the speculation that treatment with an oestrogen antagonist could be of therapeutic value. Much research is needed, however, before this stage is reached.

INTRODUCTION

In this paper we shall consider the effects of the two hormones which seem to be specifically involved in male sexuality in mammals, i.e. testosterone and prolactin. We shall not deal here with impotence occurring in conjunction with general endocrine diseases such as hypothyroidism and diabetes, as in these cases the impotence is part of the effect of the disease on the organism as a whole. Furthermore, as our group is mainly involved in clinical research, we shall confine our consideration to the effects of these two hormones in the human species.

TESTOSTERONE AND ITS METABOLITES

In man, testosterone is often associated entirely and only with sexually oriented behaviour. It seemed to us only partially correct that it should be, and we therefore decided to systematically analyse the influence of this steroid on human psychosocial and sexual behaviour. Numerous studies have been undertaken in this connection in animals, but extrapolation from these to man is difficult (a) because of species differences, (b) because of the fact that the doses used in the animal studies lead to hormone blood levels vastly different from normal physiological conditions, and (c) because of the fact that in man social factors predominate over biological ones.

Androgen action on the central nervous system

Testosterone, a 17β-hydroxysteroid, is the principal androgen secreted by the testicular Leydig cells. Its secretion, which is dependent on the hypophysial luteinizing hormone (LH), has minor circadian variations, minimal values being found at the end of the day (de Lacerda et al., 1973). Testosterone circulates in the blood, bound for the most part (95–99%) to a plasma globulin (testosterone binding globulin). Only the free form is metabolically active. When its target organs, in particular the brain, are reached, the testosterone is transformed under the influence of the enzyme 5α-reductase into dihydro-testosterone (DHT), or aromatized into oestrogens (Martini, 1978).

Testosterone and DHT are fixed to a specific cellular receptor which eventually brings about variations in cellular DNA synthesis. As androgens, these substances have numerous metabolic actions influencing, among others, the muscular osseous, pilary and gluco-lipidic systems. Of more interest in the present instance is the fact that the central nervous system is also a target organ for androgens, the presence at this level of specific cellular steroid receptors and of 5α-reductase being indirect proof of this fact. The influence of endogenous and of exogenous testosterone on the hypothalamic modulation of LH synthesis and/or liberation is a direct neuroendocrinological proof of this action. In the fetus, and possibly also in the adult, testosterone is responsible for an increase in the process of neuronal myelinization, which may partially explain its action at the level of the embryonic hypothalamus.

Androgens and sexual behaviour

Androgen action on the genital system

Androgens influence the external genital system from the fetus to senility. However, different actions occur in different life phases. During the pre-natal period, testicular androgens have a morphogenic action; they induce the formation of a masculine external genital system through an action on the genital tubercle and folds of the fetus. In the absence of androgens a female-type genital system will develop. During the pre-pubescent period the androgens, which are secreted in increased quantity compared to the infantile period, induce a hypertrophy of the genital system and the appearance of secondary sexual characteristics (morphotype, pilosity, voice, etc.). In adult life the androgens' role at the level of the genital system is purely trophic. An insufficiency, seen for example in certain patients presenting with a destructive hypophysial tumour, results only in a moderate genital hypotrophy.

Androgen effect on sexual behaviour

The effect of androgens on human sexual behaviour is a matter of controversy. Again it seems that the hormonal effects are different at different times of life. During the peri-natal period, the weeks preceding and following birth, androgens have a clear effect on the hypothalamus. They 'masculinize' it, so that at puberty a masculine type of hypothalamic endocrine sexual regulation develops (tonic regulation of gonadotrophin secretion, as opposed to the cyclical type observed in the female). It is, in effect, at this time that the infant's later sexual conduct is imprinted. Preliminary studies show that direct or indirect ingestion (through the mother's milk) of a substance competing for cerebral androgen receptors can induce a defect in masculinization in the newborn male. It has been hypothesized that this could be the basis of certain sexual difficulties, such as homosexuality (Ziviani, 1972). During puberty the androgens reveal the sexual behaviour imprinted in infancy. Certain authors have compared this action to the process of photographic impression and development (Signoret, 1971). In adulthood androgens appear to play only an accessory role. Castration of an adult animal or man does not always lead to an absence of sexual behaviour. When such a problem does exist, it is thought to be more a function of the psychological impact of castration than the result of an hormonal deficit. However, the deficit of genital trophism, which can by itself induce mechanical difficulties, must not be under-estimated. Finally, it has been demonstrated that in senility there is a variable diminution of androgenic impregnation (Vermeulen *et al.*, 1972). Free testosterone diminishes in a more constant fashion than total plasma testosterone. This deficit can lead to trophic modifications.

Androgens and male sterility

In the bull a liberation of LH leading to an elevation of plasma testosterone levels occurs after copulation (Katongole *et al.*, 1971). No such phenomenon occurs in man, as has been shown by a study in which LH and plasma testosterone levels were carefully measured, beginning within minutes of sexual intercourse (Stearns *et al.*, 1973). A previous paper giving results obtained by less precise methods, such as observations on the rate of beard growth and the measurement of urinary testosterone excretion, had already given rise to suspicions about the existence of such a phenomenon (Ismael *et al.*, 1970).

Mean plasma testosterone levels have been found to be abnormally low in patients suffering from psychogenic impotence (Servais *et al.*, 1976; Legros *et al.*, 1973a) whilst other hormonal parameters, such as urinary 17-keto-steroid excretion, are normal (Legros *et al.*, 1973b). This fact has been confirmed by some authors (Ismael and Harkness, 1967), but not by others (Benkert, 1975; Racey *et al.*, 1973).

In a recent study we found hyperinsulinic glucose intolerance in 30% of patients presenting with erective impotence (patients suffering from severe diabetes were excluded from this calculation) (Legros *et al.*, 1978). In this study the mean plasma testosterone level of these patients (470 ± 23 ng per 100 ml) was significantly lower than in the impotent patients with a normal gluco-lipidic function (575 ± 77 ng per 100 ml, $p < 0.05$), and circulating LH levels were higher (5.5 ± 5 mIU/ml, compared to $3.5 + 0.3$ mIU/ml, $p < 0.001$). These data suggest a testicular insufficiency in the patients suffering from gluco-lipidic dysfunction; this likelihood is reinforced by the fact that the FSH levels were higher in these patients than in the impotent group with normal gluco-lipidic function (7.5 ± 0.9 mIU/ml compared to 5.1 ± 0.6 mIU/ml).

We believe that in these patients suffering from gluco-lipidic dysfunction, the impotence stems not from a lack of androgens but rather from some peripheral arteriolar or neurological problem. Tests have revealed a paradoxical situation in such patients in that the higher their androgen levels the greater their tendency, when assessed by means of the Minnesota Multiphasic Personality Inventory, towards a 'feminine-type' orientation (Figure 1). This is not so with impotent patients with normal gluco-lipidic function (Figure 1). It is clear from this that certain patients suffering from impotence, totally or partially secondary to a neurological or vascular affliction, have sexual orientations contrary to what one would expect from their androgen plasma levels.

In this connection it is interesting to recall the work of Keith *et al.* (1974),

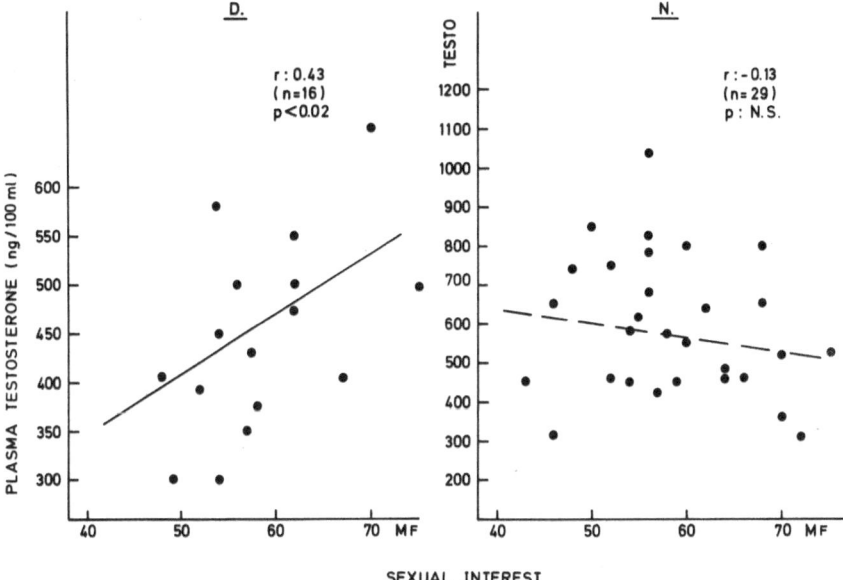

Figure 1 Relationship between plasma testosterone and sexual interest (MF. MMPI score) in two groups of impotent males. D = intolerance to glucose. N = no intolerance to glucose (Legros *et al..* 1978)

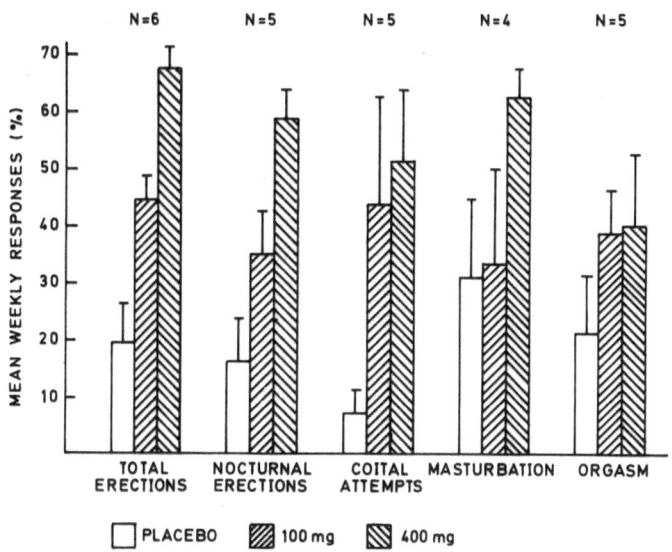

Figure 2 Sexual activity reported by 6 patients suffering from organic androgen deficiency but receiving i.m. injections of testosterone enanthate (100 mg and 400 mg) and placebo in a blind study (Davidson *et al.*, 1979)

who found higher plasma testosterone levels in homosexuals than in hetero-sexuals. Sachar *et al.* (1973), however, found no important relationship between androgen levels and the depressive phenomena for which 15 male patients were hospitalized. Such a relationship was very evident, however, in a recent blind study of Davidson *et al.* (1979) in which a group of six patients suffering from a primary androgen deficiency received intramuscular injections of placebo and of testosterone enanthate (100 mg and 400 mg). The results of this study, the patients' self reports of masturbation, nocturnal erections, and coital attempts, showed a clear dose-related increase of sexual activity following androgen replacement therapy (Figure 2).

At the present time, therefore, the findings of various studies being conflicting, the relationship between androgen levels and male sexuality remains unclear.

Androgens and psychosexual behaviour

Although sexual conduct may be minimally influenced by androgens in adult life, it seems that this is not the case for a series of vaguely defined characteristics which are generally attributed to the masculine gender. Money (1966) has proposed that these, grouped together, could form an entity of tertiary sexual characteristics. Among these, aggressiveness has been studied the most frequently.

In the normal individual there exists a relationship between the importance of aggressive behavioural components, as evaluated by various psychologic tests, and androgen secretion (Ehrenkranz *et al.*, 1974; Persky *et al.*, 1971). This has been indirectly confirmed by Kreuz and Rose (1972), who found that in a population of prisoners incarcerated for various reasons, plasma testosterone levels were significantly higher in those imprisoned for violent crimes such as homicide and armed assault, than in those imprisoned for non-violent crimes such as theft.

Lederer (1974) has shown that anti-androgen treatment (cyproterone acetate) in cases of sexual perversion can result not only in a sedation of the sexual perversion but also in a clear character modification, oriented, according to the author, towards its 'softening'. In our opinion it is probable that the influence of this drug is the result of its action on a component of aggressiveness rather than on true sexual behaviour. Further studies are needed in this domain.

It should be noted, however, that not all authors agree about the existence of a relationship between androgenic function and aggressiveness. The study of Meyer-Bahlburg *et al.* (1974). for instance. did not confirm Persky's results (1971) in an analogous normal population, though it must be said that a slightly modified protocol was used. Similarly, Eaton and Resko (1974) found no correlation between testosterone secretion and aggressiveness or social dominance in a group of Japanese macaque monkeys.

PROLACTIN

Since the advent of the specific RIA for prolactin in the human, the role of this hormone in the reproductive cycle and in behaviour has appeared more and more important.

(We shall not discuss here the role of prolactin in the female, in whom its excess is said to be accompanied by, or perhaps the cause of, a variety of difficulties, among them frigidity, menstrual disturbances, galactorrhoea and mental problems.)

Interest of prolactin study in men

The study of prolactin secretion in sexual disturbances in men is interesting for two main reasons. Firstly, prolactin secretion is controlled by a double neurotransmitter mechanism (serotoninergic stimulatory and dopaminergic inhibitory) which is opposite to the one controlling sexual behaviour, mainly erection (serotoninergic inhibitory and dopaminergic stimulatory). Hence it would seem that a study of the prolactin secretion in clinical practice could give a good index of hypothalamic (or brain?) neuromediator balance in sexual disorders. Secondly, prolactin itself affects brain metabolism either by its action on 5α-reductase or by increasing dopamine hypothalamic turnover.

Prolactin secretion in sexual impotence

Prolactin adenoma

Sexual impotence can be the *only* symptom of pituitary prolactin microadenoma. This has been clearly described by Besser's group (Besser and Thorner, 1975). In our multi-disciplinary group, such an adenoma has been found in 1 to 2% of patients whose only complaints were a loss of erectile capacity and a loss of sexual drive (Legros *et al.*, 1978). Other groups have reported a similar incidence (Buvat *et al.*, 1978). On the other hand, in a group of 29 patients with raised prolactin levels secondary to pituitary tumours, Franks and his co-workers found only six patients without any impairment of sexual function (Franks *et al.*, 1978). Functional hyperprolactinaemia, secondary to major neuroleptic therapy, appears sometimes to result in sexual problems. In clearly hyperprolactinaemic patients neurosurgical treatment and/or bromocriptine (dopamine agonist) or serotonine antagonist therapy appears to induce an increase in sexual behaviour.

Prolactin secretion in so-called 'psychogenic' sexual impotence

Since hyperprolactinaemia is so clearly related to impotence in man, it was of interest to us to test prolactinic function and antiprolactinic treatment in patients suffering from 'psychogenic' impotence.

We have previously described our study in a group of patients with low testosterone and low LH blood levels, the combination of which is likely to foster 'hypothalamic disturbances' leading to an alteration of the classic gonadal hypothalamic feed-back (Legros et al., 1978). In these patients there was an inverse relationship between basal plasma testosterone and TRH-induced prolactin release, although both were within the normal range. This led us to hypothesize that endogenous prolactin may play a role in such disturbances. We therefore began a double-blind study with bromocriptine. Unfortunately the preliminary results neither confirmed nor refuted our hypothesis. However, detailed endocrine evaluations of the patients in this study revealed a tendency towards higher adrenal androgen excretion (DHEA. etiocholanolone, androsterone) indicating that the disturbances found in this group may be primarily caused by adrenal gland overproduction with a consequent inhibition of the hypothalamo-gonadal axis. This second hypothesis awaits investigation.

In a recent study Buvat et al. (1978) compared basal and TRH-stimulated prolactin release in 11 normal men, 19 patients with idiopathic impotency, 10 suffering from anejaculation, and 12 with premature ejaculation. The responses were normal in the impotent patients and in those with premature ejaculation, whereas in patients suffering from anejaculation the response was significantly decreased (although still within the normal range). An emotional increase of α-adrenergic stimulation (which also inhibits prolactin release) could presumably explain these results.

The lack of a significant increase in prolactin secretion in the impotent male in this study is in accordance with the poor clinical results obtained with dopamine agonist therapy (bromocriptine). Buvat et al. (1978) and Ambrosi et al. (1977) reported no significant improvements with this therapy, the latter group finding, in 47 patients, 44% good results with placebo and 52% with bromocriptine. This proportion is very similar to the one observed in a double-blind study of our own group in males suffering from sexual impotence and an intolerance to glucose, in which 6/14 patients responded to placebo. and 9/16 responded to bromocriptine (Legros et al.. 1980).

INTERRELATIONSHIP BETWEEN PROLACTIN SECRETION AND ANDROGEN METABOLISM

It is clear that there is an interrelationship between prolactin action and androgen metabolism, though the matter of the precise site (or sites) of action is still controversial.

Most patients suffering from chronic hyperprolactinaemia (pituitary adenoma, functional origin) have low testosterone blood levels. The lowering of the prolactin levels by transphenoidal neurosurgery or by bromocriptine therapy induces a normalization of testosterone levels in about one-third of such cases. In contrast to chronic hyperprolactinaemia, *acute* hormonal hypersecretion, obtained either by sulpiride injection or by TRH infusion, increases the functional endocrine capacity of the ovaries or testes. It appears therefore that the *duration* of hyperprolactinaemia is of fundamental import-ance for its action on steroid and androgen synthesis. Such a difference would best be explained by an action of prolactin either on LH receptors or on central dopamine metabolism.

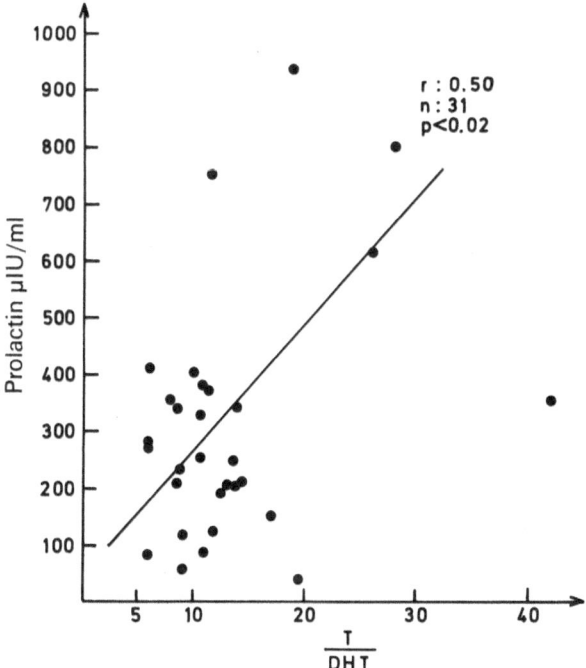

Figure 3 Correlation between basal prolactin serum levels and the ratio of plasma testosterone to DHT in 31 impotent patients suffering from glucose intolerance (Chiodera and Legros. 1980)

It is also thought that prolactin may act at the 5α-reductase level, by decreasing its capacity to transform testosterone to its active form, DHT. We have recently obtained clinical results which appear to support this hypothesis (Legros *et al.*, 1980). In a group of 31 impotent patients with glucose intolerance, we found a significant relationship between prolactin and the testosterone/DHT ratio: the higher the prolactin the higher the ratio (Figure 3). There was no correlation, however, between prolactin and testosterone or DHT individually, or between prolactin and 17β-oestradiol. Although the prolactin was within the normal range, it was slightly higher in these patients than in a group of controls with no sexual problems. Circulating DHT, however, was lower and 17β-oestradiol higher in the impotent glucose-intolerant patients than in the controls (Figure 4). This indicates a decrease of testosterone transformation to DHT and an increase in its aromatization into oestrogens.

It is also noteworthy that the patients who responded clinically either to

Table 1   Comparison of testosterone, DHT, 17μ-oestradiol and prolactin blood levels before and after one month of treatment with placebo or bromocriptine in 29 patients suffering from psychogenic impotence and glucose-intolerance. Patients are divided according to their clinical responses into 'responders' (n = 15) and 'non-responders' (n = 14). The figures for placebo and bromocriptine treatment are pooled in both groups. Statistical analyses were made using paired *t* test, M ± SD (Legros *et al.*, 1980)

	Responders (n = 15)			Non-responders (n = 14)		
	Before	p	After	Before	p	After
Testosterone ng per 100 ml	497 ± 196	N.S.	543 ± 149	502 ± 187	N.S.	485 ± 138
DHT ng per 100 ml	38 ± 12	< 0.05˙	47 ± 20	43 ± 24	N.S.	51 ± 22
17β-oestradiol µg per 100 ml	6.8 ± 2.3	N.S.	8.2 ± 3.2	6.7 ± 2.7	N.S.	7.3 ± 3.1
Prolactin µIU/ml	372 ± 250	< 0.005	178 ± 150	333 ± 118	N.S.	257 ± 157

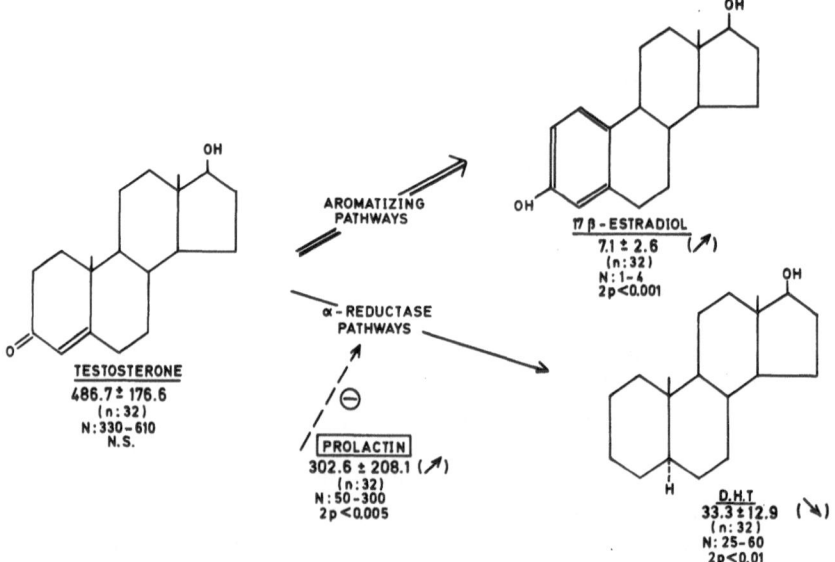

Figure 4   Scheme of the two pathways of metabolization of testosterone in the brain (Martini, 1978). Blood levels observed in a group of 32 impotent patients suffering from glucose intolerance are given; values found in a group of 11 normal males (N) are shown for comparison. Units: testosterone, ng per 100 ml; DHT, ng per 100 ml; 17β-oestradiol, µg per 100 ml; prolactin µIU/ml (Chiodera and Legros, 1980)

bromocriptine or to placebo showed a decrease of basal prolactin concentrations, whereas those who responded to neither showed no such decrease (Table 1). This raises the interesting possibility of the 'effect' of placebo being elicited through the central dopaminergic pathway (Legros *et al.*. 1980). In the responder group the decrease of prolactin was concomitant with an increase in DHT, a change which was not seen in the non-responder group. No change in circulating 17β-oestradiol was seen in either group.

A confirmation of the action of prolactin on androgen metabolism in the brain would mean that some psychosexual disturbances may be caused by an excess of cerebral oestrogens. In the group of impotent glucose-tolerant patients referred to above, the levels of 17β-oestradiol were higher in the patients suffering from a decrease in 'sexual drive' than in those without this complaint. If the hypothesis of an action of prolactin on androgen metabolism was proved, one could speculate than an oestrogen antagonist, such as clomiphene, would be capable of restoring a normal libido and hypothalamic feed-back.

CONCLUSIONS

Androgens play a major role in initiating and maintaining sexual function in man. A deficit of androgens induces a decrease of sexual potency, but this is reversible by replacement therapy. Prolactin also plays a role in this respect: a small concentration facilitating steroid biosynthesis, a high concentration for a long period of time seeming to antagonize the androgen biosynthesis through either a peripheral or a central mechanism.

In contrast to patients suffering from endocrine diseases, patients suffering from 'psychogenic impotence' show subtle hormonal changes which could be either the peripheral reflection of modifications in hormonal metabolism in the brain or the neuroendocrine expression of some neuromediator modifications related to psychological troubles.

Acknowledgement

The authors wish to thank Mrs F. Louis, Neuroendocrinology Section, Institute of Medicine, University of Liège, for her helpful technical assistance in connection with the work described in this paper.

References

Ambrosi. B., Bara. R., Travaglini, P., Weber, G., Beck Peccoz, P., Rondena, M., Elli, R. and Faglia, G. (1977). Study of the effects of bromocriptine on sexual impotence. *Clin. Endocrinol.*, 7, 417

Benkert, R. (1975). Studies on pituitary hormones and releasing hormones in depression and sexual impotence. In W. H. Gispen, T. B. van Wimersma Greidanus, B. Bohus and D. de Wied (eds.). *Hormones, Homeostasis and the Brain*, pp. 25–36. (Amsterdam: Elsevier)

Besser, G. M. and Thorner, M. O. (1975). Prolactin and gonadal function. *Pathol. Biol.*, **23**, 779

Buvat, J., Asfour, M., Buvat-Herbaut, M. and Fossati, P. (1978). Prolactin and human sexual behaviour. In C. Robyn and M. Harter (eds.). *Progress in Prolactin Physiology and Pathology*. (Amsterdam: Elsevier/North-Holland Biomedical Press)

Chiodera, P. and Legros, J. J. (1980). La fonction androgénique chez les patientes soufraut d'impuissance sexuelle et d'intolérance en glucose: absence de corrélations avec la libération d'insuline loin de l'HGPO. *Acta Psychiatr. Belg.* (In press)

Davidson, J. M., Camargo, C. A. and Smith, E. R. (1979). Effects of androgen on sexual behaviour in hypogonadal men. *J. Clin. Endocrinol.*, **48**, 955

Eaton, G. G. and Resko, J. A. (1974). Plasma testosterone and male dominance in a Japanese macaque (malaca fuscata) troop compared with repeated measures of testosterone in laboratory males. *Horm. Behav.*, **4**, 251

Erhenkranz, J., Bliss, E. and Sheard, M. H. (1974). Plasma testosterone: correlation with aggressive behaviour and social dominance in man. *Psychosom. Med.*, **36**, 469

Franks, S., Jacobs, H. S., Martin, N. and Nabarro, J. D. N. (1978). Hyperprolactinemia and impotence. *Clin. Endocrinol.*, **8**, 277

Ismael, A. A. A., Devidson, D. W., Lorraine, J. A., Cullen, D. R., Irvine, W. J., Cooper, A. J., and Smith, C. G. (1970). Assessment of gonadal function in impotent men. In J. Irvine (ed.). *Reproduction Endocrinology*, pp. 138–147. (Edinburgh: Livingstone)

Ismael, A. A. A., and Harkness, R. A. (1967). Urinary testosterone excretion in man in normal and pathological conditions. *Acta Endocrinol. (Kbh)*, **56**, 469

Katongole, C. B., Naftolin, F. and Short, R. V. (1971). Relationship between blood levels of luteinizing hormone and testosterone in bulls, and the effects of sexual stimulation. *J. Endocrinol.*, **50**, 457

Keith, H., Brodie, H., Gartrell, N., Doering, G. and Rhue, T. (1974). Plasma testosterone in heterosexual and homosexual man. *Am. J. Psychiat.*, **131**, 82

Kreuz, L. E. and Rose, R. M. (1972). Assessment of aggressive behaviour and plasma testosterone in a young criminal population. *Psychosom. Med.*, **34**, 321

de Lacerda, L., Kowardski, A., Johanson, A. J., Athanasiou, R. and Migeon, C. J. (1973). Integrated concentration and circadian variation of plasma testosterone in normal men. *J. Clin. Endocrinol.*, **36**, 366

Lederer, J. (1974). Le traitement des déviations sexuelles par l'acétate de cyprotérone. In *Le Cerveau et les Hormones*, pp. 249–260. (Paris: Expansion Editeur)

Legros, J. J., Chiodera, P., Mormont, C. and Servais, J. (1980). A psychoneuroendocrinological study of sexual impotence in patients with abnormal reaction to glucose tolerance test: influence of bromocriptine therapy. In J. Mendlewicz and H. M. van Praag (eds.). *Psychoneuroendocrinology and Abnormal Behaviour. Advances in Biological Psychiatry*, vol. 5, pp. 117–124. (Basel: Karger)

Legros, J. J., Franchimont, P., Palem-Vliers, M. and Servais, J. (1973a). FSH–LH and testosterone blood level in patients with psychogenic impotence. *Endocrinol. Exp.*, **7**, 59

Legros, J. J., Mormont, C. and Servais, J. (1978). A psychoendocrine study of erectile 'psychogenic impotence'. A comparison between normal patients and patients with abnormal glucose tolerance tests. In L. Carenza, P. Pancheri and L. Zichella (eds.). *Clinical Psychoneuroendocrinology in Reproduction*, pp. 301–319. (New York: Academic Press)

Legros, J. J., Palem-Vliers, M., Servais, J., Margoulies, M. and Franchimont, P. (1973b). Basal pituitary gonadal function in impotency evaluated by blood testosterone and LH essays. In K. Lissak (ed.). *Hormones and Brain Function*, pp. 527–529. (New York: Plenum Press)

Legros, J. J., Servais, J. and Mormont, C. (1975). A preliminary psychoendocrine study in patients suffering from psychogenic impotence. *Psychoneuroendocrinology*, **1**, 203

Martini, L. (1978). Testosterone metabolism in the brain and the control of sexual behavior. In L. Carenza, P. Pancheri and L. Zichella (eds.). *Clinical Psychoneuroendocrinology in Reproduction*, pp. 271–279. (New York: Academic Press)

Meyer-Bahlburg, H. F. L., Boon, D. A. and Sharma, M. (1974). Aggressiveness and testosterone measures in man. *Psychosom. Med.*, **36**, 269

Money, J. (1966). *Sex Research, New Developments.* (New York: Holt, Rinehart and Winston)

Persky, H., Smith, K. D. and Basu, G. K. (1971). Relation of psychogenic measures of aggression and hostility to testosterone production in man. *Psychosom. Med.*, **33**, 265

Racey, P. A., Ansari, M. A., Rowe, P. H. and Glover, T. D. (1973). Testosterone in impotent men. *J. Endocrinol.*, **59**, 23

Sachar, E. J., Halpern, F., Rosenfeld, R. S., Gallagher, R. F. and Hellman, L. (1973). Plasma and urinary testosterone levels in depressed man. *Arch. Gen. Psychiat.*, **28**, 15

Servais, J., Mormont, C. and Legros, J. J. (1976). L'impuissance: aspects diagnostiques et thérapeutiques. *Rev. Med. Psychosom. Psycho. Med.*, **3**, 263

Signoret, J. P. (1971). Le comportement sexuel des mammifères. *La Recherche*, **2**, 845

Stearns, E. L., Winter, J. S. and Fairman, C. (1973). Effect of coitus on gonadotropin prolactin and sex steroid levels in man. *J. Clin. Endocrinol.*, **37**, 687

Sy Lim, V. and Fang, V. S. (1976). Restoration of plasma testosterone levels in uremic men with clomiphens citrate. *J. Clin. Endocrinol.*, **43**, 1370

Vermeulen, A., Rubens, R. and Verdonck, L. (1972). Testosterone secretion and metabolism in male senescence. *J. Clin. Endocrinol.*, **34**, 730

Ziviani, N. (1972). Endocrinological aspects of homosexualism. Potential risk of homosexualism in sons of pregnant women taking barbiturates and antibiotics. *Hormones*, **3**, 56

Address for correspondence

Dr J. J. Legros, Université de Liège, Département de Clinique et de Pathologie Médicales, C.H.U., local 4/12, Sart Tilman, 4000 Liège, Belgium

Section 3
Psychopathology
as a Consequence of
Hormone Dysfunction

3.1
Amphetamines and psychosis

I. MUNKVAD, A. RANDRUP and R. FOG

ABSTRACT

At the present stage of knowledge it seems reasonable to assume that every normal thought process or normal behaviour has one neurobiological correlate, and that every abnormal form of function—even if induced by the environment—has another. The neurobiological correlate of schizophrenia has been the object of much speculation and research, and during the last fifteen years interesting information, summarized in the dopamine hypothesis, has emerged, mainly from studies with amphetamines and neuroleptic drugs. These drugs have, respectively, a psychotogenic and an anti-psychotic effect, both of which appear to be mediated mainly via actions on brain dopamine. Many new details about brain dopamine have been discovered recently, including information about the dopamine receptors and about the interactions of dopamine with other substances in the brain, i.e. with γ-aminobutyric acid (GABA) and with endorphins. These findings raise hopes that new anti-psychotic drugs can be created, including the ideal anti-schizophrenic drug, one which would not only antagonize psychotic behaviour but also bring about its replacement by normal behaviour.

INTRODUCTION

Recent research makes it obvious that both genetic and environmental variables operate in the transmission of schizophrenia. Modern molecular biology shows that a genetic disturbance will be reflected in a biochemical abnormality. It is realistic, therefore, to assume that one form or another of biochemical abnormality exists in the schizophrenic patient, probably in his brain. Modern molecular biology operates with physical and chemical processes and generally refutes the existence of a soul as an independent agent. According to this, it could be stated that every normal thought process or normal behavioural function must have one form of neurobiological correlate, and that every abnormal form of function, even if it is induced by the environment, must have another. Nevertheless, the so-called 'brain–mind' problem still exists and is open for discussion in psychiatry.

It is, however, very difficult to describe mental processes and behaviour, normal as well as abnormal, in neurobiological and/or neurobiochemical terms.

Concerning the schizophrenic process, many investigators have tried to localize a (hypothetical) abnormal process in the brain of the schizophrenic patient hoping that this would be reflected in some form of abnormality in, perhaps, blood, urine or spinal fluid. An 'inborn error' in the form of an enzymatic deficiency has also been postulated in relation to many enzymatic systems, but nothing has been established with any degree of certainty.

To continue in so-called biological terms, there is also the possibility that a hypothetical abnormal activity in the schizophrenic brain does *not* demonstrate itself in blood, urine or spinal fluid, but that it runs on a microneurobiological level inside certain brain areas—on a, so to say, molecular level.

In 1962 our laboratory, taking account of these considerations, and inspired also by numerous reports of schizophrenia-like psychoses in relation to abuse of amphetamines, attempted to establish an animal model of schizophrenia.

There is much evidence in the literature that non-psychotic persons develop a temporary psychosis after taking large doses of amphetamines (*d*-amphetamine, methamphetamine, phenmetrazine) (Randrup *et al.*, 1980; Segal and Janowsky, 1978; Randrup and Munkvad, 1974 and 1967a). Most authors have observed these psychotic symptoms in addicts, but cases of psychosis resulting from a single dose or from a few doses taken within less than 24 hours have also been reported (Segal and Janowsky, 1978; Randrup and Munkvad, 1974 and 1967a). The symptoms of the amphetamine psychosis differ among individuals but in many cases they are very similar to those seen in certain forms of schizophrenia, particularly the paranoid form. The similarity can be so pronounced that misdiagnoses are made. Sometimes these schizophrenia-like psychoses are of long duration—up to several months—even when the intake of amphetamine is stopped upon admission to hospital. Some cases of amphetamine psychoses have been reported to be reminiscent of manic-depressive psychosis, hypomania or agitated depression, or to have mixed manic-depressive and schizophrenic symptomatology. In the beginning this was regarded as an unexplained complication, detracting from the value of the

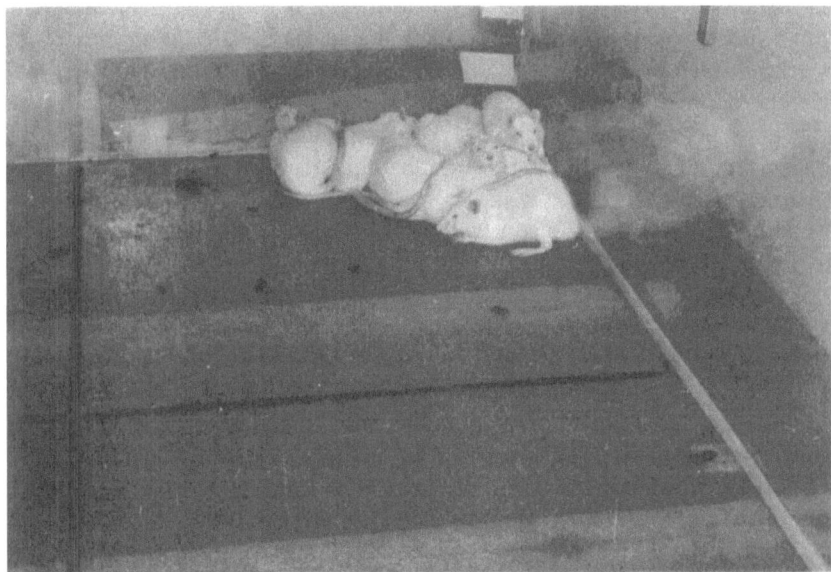

(A)

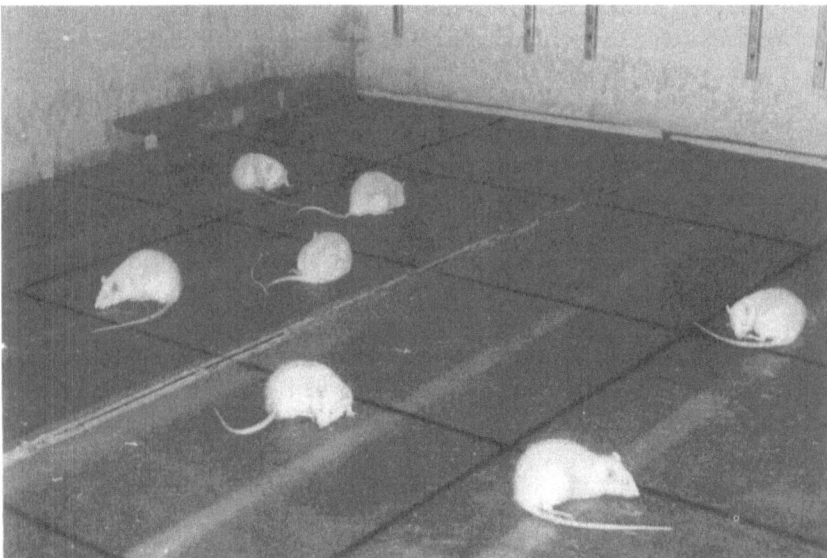

(B)

Figure 1 Rats injected with (A) placebo and (B) 5 mg/kg *d*-amphetamine sulphate s.c. The amphetamine rats are constantly sniffing, licking or biting at the floor, and all normal activities, such as social grouping, are completely absent. (From Schiørring and Randrup, 1971)

amphetamine model, but more recent evidence indicates that the amphetamine model is valid both for schizophrenia and for affective psychoses, brain dopamine being the common link. This newer development has been discussed in detail in recent reviews (Randrup et al., 1980, 1979 and 1975b; Segal and Janowsky, 1978; Murphy, 1977). For the sake of brevity we shall here concentrate on the value of the amphetamine model in connection with schizophrenia.

From the above-mentioned it will be clear that the amphetamine-induced toxic psychosis is, in our opinion, the best model of schizophrenia in man. In 1962 we began injecting animals with amphetamine and related compounds in milligram per kilogram doses which were comparable with the intake of abusers. In all mammals tested (rats, mice, guinea-pigs, rabbits, pigs, cows, horses, sheep, cats, dogs, squirrel monkeys, vervet monkeys, chimpanzees and humans) amphetamine-like compounds caused the development of stereotypies, continuous repetitive movements without any aim accompanied by abolition of normal behaviour and movements (Sharman, 1978; Lewander, 1977; Andersen et al., 1975; Randrup et al., 1975a; Randrup and Munkvad, 1968 and 1967a). An experiment with rats is illustrated in Figure 1.

We looked for an anatomical as well as a biochemical background for the stereotypy phenomenon, and, in short, there is strong evidence that stereotypy is produced by an effect of amphetamines on the transmitter dopamine or dopamine receptors in the nigrostriatal system in the brain. The evidence is of biochemical nature, via an analysis of dopamine and its metabolites and of other amines in the brain, and of an anatomical nature, the result of the study of microinjections and lesions in the nigrostriatal system (Lewander, 1977). Bilateral lesions of corpus striatum in rats are, for example, able to inhibit or modify amphetamine-stereotypy and from a biochemical point of view stereotypy can be prevented by pre-treatment with α-methyl-tyrosine and other inhibitors of the synthesis of dopa, the precursor of the brain dopamine. Many investigations in our laboratory confirm these findings (Randrup and Mogilnicka, 1976; Andersen et al., 1975; Randrup et al., 1975a; Randrup and Munkvad, 1968).

The phenomenon of stereotypy per se is interesting, but isolated it has not so much to do with schizophrenia. It was only when it was demonstrated that neuroleptics antagonize stereotypy behaviour induced by amphetamine that its potential relevance became apparent. In the clinic neuroleptics have a proven anti-schizophrenic effect (and also an anti-manic one). All known neuroleptics also have an anti-dopaminergic effect (Christensen, 1979; Hyttel, 1979; Kebabian and Calne, 1979; Randrup et al., 1980 and 1975b; Matthysse, 1977; Randrup and Mogilnicka, 1976).

The dopamine hypothesis concerning schizophrenia is well established. It is, in brief, that schizophrenia is partly linked to some form of hyperactivity of the dopaminergic system in the brain—in the corpus striatum, cortex and/or the meso-limbic system (Randrup et al., 1979; Randrup and Munkvad, 1974,

1968 and 1967a; Fog et al., 1967). It is a very complex matter. A delicate balance between the adrenergic and cholinergic mechanisms appears to play an important role, but exactly what and how is not yet clear. The postulated hyperactivity of the dopaminergic system in schizophrenic patients has not so far been proved biochemically or neurophysiologically, nor have the different clinical effects of individual neuroleptics yet been fully explained.

The antagonism between the action of neuroleptics and stereotypies in animals is clear. It should be mentioned, however, that although neuroleptic drugs can cause the disappearance of stereotypies, we have not yet found one which is then able to normalize, more than partially, the social behaviour of amphetamine-dosed animals. Figures relating to experiments with verbet monkeys are given in Table 1.

Table 1   Suppression of social interaction in pairs of vervet monkeys ($\male$ and $\female$) by amphetamine, and its partial prevention by neuroleptics.

Neuroleptic	Doses (mg/kg) s.c.	Monkey pairs	Average number of social interactions			Number of experiments		
			Placebo (P)	Amphetamine 0.37 mg/kg s.c. (A)	Neuroleptic + amphetamine (N+A)	P	A	N+A
Haloperidol	0.015 to 0.04	Jo + Ju	32.5	0.3	6.4	13	4	9
		G + V	42.6	1.0	3.8	9	3	6
		A + B	32.4	13.0	3.0	5	2	3
		An + Ana	38.7	0	5.7	7	4	3
Chlorpromazine	0.2 to 0.6	O + So	48.2	16.8	36.4	12	4	8
		A + B	41.0	0	0.7	8	2	6
		G + V	73.0	0	9.4	9	2	7
Pimozide	0.03 to 0.06	O + So	28.3	12.0	12.0	9	3	6

Each experiment comprised three or four (always the same number within one horizontal line) 30-minute observation periods distributed between ¼ and 3½ hours after the injection of amphetamine. Haloperidol and chlorpromazine were injected ½ hour and pimozide 3 hours before the amphetamine. A placebo experiment was performed the day before each drug experiment. The social acts studied were: grooming of the other monkey, stretching to be groomed, touching the other monkey with the hand,   presenting rear to $\male$, mounting, fighting and biting. The number of times these social acts were performed in each observation period were totalled and the averages are shown in the table. The time spent on these activities was also recorded and shows the same trend as the figures in the table. The data are from experiments performed by Kjellberg and Randrup (Randrup et al., 1980 and 1976).

It is also notable that in normal animals (those not given amphetamines) neuroleptics may disrupt social interaction (Hecht, 1979; Randrup et al., 1980). These observations can be of relevance in the clinic. In the schizophrenic patient neuroleptics work best on productive symptoms (hallucinations, paranoid ideas, restlessness and so on), but sometimes then leave the patient with deep autism. In popular terms: the patient's internal television has been switched off and he is left in social isolation. This result of neuroleptic treatment is sometimes forgotten in the after-care of schizophrenic patients.

It has also been demonstrated in animal experiments in our laboratory that chronic administration of neuroleptics decreases the ability of the animal to perform previously learned behaviour (Nielsen, 1977; Seiden and Dykstra, 1977). If parallels can be drawn in the clinic, this clearly means a drawback for non-psychopharmacological therapies—forms of behavioural treatment, for instance—when these are used in combination with neuroleptic therapy.

As a (so to say) derivative of the dopamine hypothesis in relation to psychoses, is the idea that the anti-psychotic action of most neuroleptics given for a long period of time may depend on a form of hypersensitivity in the dopamine receptors in the brain. The background for this postulate is a special animal model—gnawing behaviour induced by central stimulant agents—and the study of neuroleptics on this gnawing behaviour (Christensen, 1979; Hyttel, 1979). It is not yet known, however, if the clinical effect of neuroleptics is related to this hypersensitivity, to an inhibition of the nigrostriatal or of other dopaminergic systems in the brain, or to a combination of both effects.

In recent years it has been shown that there are at least two, but perhaps more, types of dopamine receptors in the brain (Kebabian and Calne, 1979; Randrup and Mogilnicka, 1976). Some investigators believe there to be what they call a 'multidopaminergic receptor system'. This indicates that the whole problem of brain function in relation to dopamine is more complicated than was earlier imagined, and opens up many problems of discussion. In this connection it should be remembered that the so-called receptor (which is in reality a complex molecular and not a diagram model) is a dynamic structure and not a static-mechanistic one. One might also ask whether special dopamine receptors are not related to certain psychotic states.

Dopamine receptors in the brain—in corpus striatum, mesolimbic system and cortex—have connections with many other transmitter systems; in some respects the brain must be regarded as a unit in the structuralistic sense, where interference with known and with unknown transmitter systems can take place.

Recently our laboratory in connection with others has become interested in the GABA-system in relation to schizophrenia (Krogsgaard-Larsen et al., 1979). GABA, γ-aminobutyric acid, is now widely accepted as a central nervous system transmitter and is generally considered to be the principal inhibitory brain transmitter. Its present status and role in normal brain function and in various pathological brain diseases are still far from being completely understood. It is realized, however, that GABA participates in human motor co-ordination, endocrine and higher integrative cortical functions. There is thus a malfunction of GABA in Huntington's chorea and Parkinsonism. The hypothesis that GABA system dysfunction occurs in schizophrenic illness earlier gained some support from studies of central nervous system tissues obtained at autopsy, which indicated an increased dopamine level and reduced glutamic acid decarboxylase (GAD) activity in nucleus accumbens and other brain regions in schizophrenic patients. More recently, however, serious doubt has been cast on the validity of these earlier findings (Krogsgaard-Larsen *et al.*, 1979).

In our laboratory we have become interested in the interactions among the various central dopamine/GABA systems as a topic relevant not only for Huntington's chorea and Parkinsonism but also for schizophrenia. From a recently developed animal model the results indicate that the connection between the GABA and dopamine systems is more complex than was previously thought. Our data show that certain dopaminergic effects are increased by GABA (stereotyped gnawing activity) whereas others are decreased (locomotion activity) (Krogsgaard-Larsen *et al.*, 1979; Scheel-Krüger and Christensen, 1979; Scheel-Krüger *et al.*, 1978). In human studies, muscimol, the only GABA agonist tested clinically to date, has not been found to improve psychotic symptoms in patients with chronic schizophrenia (Tamminga *et al.*, 1978), and, although it appears that the GABA system may be involved in cognitive processes (Krosgaard-Larsen *et al.*, 1979), any direct link with the pathogenesis of schizophrenia now seems relatively unlikely.

In the hypothalamus there is a system of short dopamine neurons, and the secretion of prolactin from the pituitary gland is influenced by dopamine (Kebabian and Calne, 1979). Anti-psychotic drugs elevate prolactin concentration in blood, but there does not appear to be a clear relationship between this concentration and the clinical effect of neuroleptics.

The role of endorphins in cases of schizophrenia is currently a theme of great interest (Jørgensen *et al.*, 1979; Lehmann *et al.*, 1979; de Wied, 1979). Few data are available on the interaction between endorphins and catecholaminergic transmission in the brain; it seems though that α-endorphin affects dopamine turnover in some brain areas, including the caudate nucleus and globus pallidus. It also seems that des-tyrosine-γ-endorphin may interfere with neurotransmission in the nigrostriatal system. These preliminary findings relate the hypothesis based on an inborn error in the generation of des-tyrosine-γ-endorphin, and perhaps other endorphins, to the dopamine hypothesis of schizophrenia (Meites *et al.*, 1979; de Wied, 1979).

Other recent results in our laboratory indicate that an increased release of dopamine in striatum is able to reduce the level of dopamine receptors (Nielsen *et al.*, 1979); as mentioned above, amphetamine releases dopamine from dopamine nerve terminals in corpus striatum, and in schizophrenia some form of hyperactivity of the dopaminergic system appears to exist. Receptor studies in the brain could be of great value in this connection, and in relation to the dopamine hypothesis of schizophrenia. Such studies in the human brain are, however, very difficult to perform, not only because of the changes which quickly occur upon death, but primarily because at the time of death most schizophrenic patients are being treated with neuroleptics.

CONCLUSIONS

In this short paper we have been able to do little more than sketch an outline of the dopamine hypothesis in relation to schizophrenia. We feel that if there is a key to the mystery of schizophrenia, it is likely that this will be found in pharmacological agents which have structures and properties rather different from those known at present. It is likely that useful knowledge will be gained by analysing the pharmacological actions of such drugs in relation to the amphetamine model and comparing the results with the clinical effects. Experience has shown that the ideal anti-schizophrenic drug would be one which would not only antagonize psychotic behaviour, but which would also, either alone or in conjunction with other therapies, bring about its replacement by normal behaviour.

References

Andersen. H.. Braestrup. C. and Randrup, A. (1975). Apomorphine-induced stereotyped biting in the tortoise in relation to dopaminergic mechanisms. *Brain, Behav. Evol.*. **11**, 365

Christensen. A. V. (1979). Adaptation i dopamin neuroner efter enkel og gentagen dosering med neuroleptika. Thesis. The Royal Danish School of Pharmacy, Copenhagen

Fog, R., Randrup, A. and Munkvad, I. (1967). Dependence of the amphetamine excitatory response upon amines in the corpus striatum. IVth World Congress of Psychiatry, Madrid. *Excerpta Medica International Congress Series*, no. 117

Hecht, A. (1979). Behavioural effects produced by long-term administration of a neuroleptic drug (flupenthixol) upon social interaction in a group of eight rats. *Psychopharmacology*. **62**, 301

Hyttel, J. (1979). Neurochemical effects of neuroleptic drugs. Thesis. University of Copenhagen

Jørgensen, A., Fog, R. and Veilis, B. (1979). Synthetic enkephalin analogue in treatment of schizophrenia. *Lancet*, **1**, 935

Kebabian, J. W. and Calne, D. B. (1979). Multiple receptors for dopamine. *Nature*. **277**, 93

Krogsgaard-Larsen, P., Scheel-Krüger, J. and Kofod, H. (eds.)(1979). *GABA-Neurotransmitters*. (Copenhagen: Munksgaard; New York: Academic Press)

Lehmann, H., Nair, N. P. V. and Kline. N. V. (1979). β-endorphin and naxolone in psychiatric patients: clinical and biological effects. *Am. J. Psychiatry*. **136**, 762

Lewander, T. (1977). Effects of amphetamine in animals. In R. Martin (ed.). *Drug Addiction*. vol. 2, pp. 33–46. (Berlin: Springer)

Matthysse, S. W. (1977). The role of dopamine in schizophrenia. In E. Usdin, D. A. Hamberg and J. D. Barchas (eds.). *Neuroregulators and Psychiatric Disorders*. pp. 3–13. (New York: Oxford University Press)

Meites, J., Bruni, J. F., van Vugt, D. A. and Smith. A. F. (1979). Relation of endogenous opioid peptides and morphine to neuroendocrine functions. *Life Sci.*, **24**, 1325

Murphy, D. L. (1977). Animal models for mania. In I. Hanin and E. Usdin (eds.). *Animal Models in Psychiatry and Neurology*, pp. 211–223. (Oxford: Pergamon Press)

Nielsen. E. B. (1977). Long-term behavioural and biochemical effects following prolonged treatment with a neuroleptic drug (flupenthixol) in rats. *Psychopharmacology*. **54**, 203

Nielsen, M., Nielsen. E. B.. Ellison. G. and Braestrup, C. (1979). Modification of dopamine receptors in brain by continuous amphetamine administration to rats. In C. Ballus (ed.). *Proceedings of 2nd World Congress of Biol. Psychiat.*. Barcelona 1978

Randrup, A. and Mogilnicka. E. (1976). Spectrum of pharmacological actions on brain dopamine. Indications for development of new psychoactive drugs. *Pol. J. Pharmacol. Pharm.*. **28**, 551

Randrup. A.. Kjellberg, B.. Schiørring. E.. Scheel-Krüger. J.. Fog. R. and Munkvad. I. (1980).

Stereotypies and their relevance for testing neuroleptics. In F. Hoffmeister and G. Stille (eds.). *Antipsychotics and Antidepressants.* (Heidelberg: Springer). (In press)

Randrup, A. and Munkvad, I. (1974). Evidence indicating an association between schizophrenia and dopaminergic hyperactivity in the brain. In R. Cancro (ed.). *Annual Review of the Schizophrenic Syndrome*, vol. 3, pp. 130–136. (New York: Brunner/Mazel)

Randrup, A. and Munkvad, I. (1968). Behavioural stereotypies induced by pharmacological agents. *Pharmakopsychiatrie Neuro-Psychopharmakologie*, **1**, 18

Randrup, A. and Munkvad, I. (1967a). Stereotyped activities produced by amphetamine in several animal species and man. *Psychopharmacologia (Berl.).* **11**, 300

Randrup, A. and Munkvad, I. (1967b). Stereotype behaviour produced by amphetamine and other substances. Investigations on the mechanism of action. In Proceedings of the Vth International Congress of the Collegium Internationale Neuropsychopharmacologicum. *Excerpta Medica International Congress Series*. no. 129

Randrup, A., Munkvad, I., Fog, R. and Ayhan, I. H. (1975a). Catecholamines in activation. stereotypy, and level of mood. In A. J. Friedhoff (ed.). *Catecholamines and Behaviour*, vol. 1. pp. 89–107. (New York: Plenum Press)

Randrup, A., Munkvad, I., Fog, R., Braestrup, C. and Molander, L. (1979). The case for involvement of dopamine in depression and mania. Presented at the *11th C.I.N.P. Congress*. July 9–14, Vienna. (Oxford: Pergamon Press)

Randrup, A., Munkvad, I., Fog, R., Gerlach, J., Molander, L., Kjellberg, B. and Scheel-Krüger. J. (1975b). In W. B. Essman and L. Valzelli (eds.). *Current Developments in Psychopharmacology*, vol. 2, pp. 205–248. (New York: Spectrum)

Randrup, A., Munkvad, I., Fog, V., Kjellberg, B., Lyon, M., Nielsen, E., Svennild, I. and Schiørring, E. (1976). Behavioural correlates to antipsychotic efficacy of neuroleptic drugs. In G. Sedvall, B. Uvnäs and Y. Zotterman (eds). International symposium on *Antipsychotic Drugs, Pharmacodynamics and Pharmacokinetics*, Stockholm, pp. 33–41. (Oxford: Pergamon Press)

Scheel-Krüger, J. and Christensen, A. V. (1979). The role of GABA in acute and chronic neuroleptic action. Presented at the international symposium on *Advances in Psychopharmacology*, Monte Carlo. (New York: Raven Press). (In press)

Scheel-Krüger, J., Christensen, A. V. and Arnt, J. (1978). Muscimol differentially facilitates stereotypy but antagonizes motility induced by dopaminergic drugs: a complex GABA-dopamine interaction. *Life Sci.*, **22**, 75

Schiørring, E. and Randrup, A. (1971). Social isolation and changes in the formation of groups induced by amphetamine in an open-field test with rats. *Pharmakopsychiatrie Neuro-Psychopharmakologie*, **4**, 2

Segal. D. S. and Janowsky. D. S. (1978). Psychostimulant-induced behavioural effects: possible models of schizophrenia. In M. A. Lipton, A. DiMascio and K. F. Killan (eds.). *Psychopharmacology: a Generation of Progress*, pp. 1113–1123. (New York: Raven Press)

Seiden, L. S. and Dykstra, L. A. (1977). *Psychopharmacology. A Biochemical and Behavioural Approach.* (New York: Van Nostrand Reinhold)

Sharman, D. F. (1978). Brain dopamine metabolism and behavioural problems of farm animals. In P. J. Roberts. G. N. Woodruff and L. L. Iversen (eds.). *Advances in Biochemical Psychopharmacology*, vol. 19, pp. 249–254. (New York: Raven Press)

Tamminga, C. A., Crayton, J. W. and Chase. T. N. (1978). Muscimol: GABA agonist therapy in schizophrenia. *Am. J. Psychiat.*, **135**. 6

de Wied, D. (1979). Schizophrenia as an inborn error in the degradation of bêta-endorphine: an hypothesis. *Trends Neurosci..* **2**. 79

Address for correspondence

Dr I. Munkvad. Sct. Hans Hospital. Dept. E. DK-4000 Roskilde. Denmark

3.2
Endorphins and pain

L. TERENIUS

ABSTRACT

Pain is the behavioural response to external or internal noxious stimuli. Clinical pain is very different from experimental pain and it is proposed that pain forms a hierarchy starting with activation of sensory fibres or internal clues and terminating with processing in the CNS at various levels. It is the affective component of pain which is influenced by morphine, and not the sensory thresholds. Endorphins should be expected to have an action similar to morphine, and experimental evidence is in keeping with this contention.

Three different areas relating to endorphins and pain are reviewed. Firstly, evidence is given that endorphins may be responsible for adaptation to pain, either congenital or acquired, as well as to diurnal changes in pain sensitivity. It is possible, in fact, that endorphins have a more general role in sensory adaptation. Secondly, some evidence suggests that endorphins are released in acute trauma and may play a protective role, for instance in parturition. Finally, endorphins seem to be involved in chronic pain. Patients with chronic neurogenic pain frequently show low levels of endorphins in their cerebrospinal fluid. These low levels may be raised by acupuncture with pain relief as a result. The relief of pain is reversed by the narcotic antagonist naloxone. These observations converge on one point, that endorphins play an important modulatory role and inadequate endorphin activity leads to pathologic changes.

INTRODUCTION

The phenomenology of pain is not simple. Phasic pain may be considered as one of the senses, like touch and vision, and is a signal for the rapid withdrawal from the source of injury. It is of short duration and serves an important role as a defence mechanism. More protracted pain is a sign of discomfort, not so very different from thirst and hunger. It may turn to a condition, which causes the individual to react by disposing behaviour in an attempt to return to a non-painful situation. At this stage symptomatic therapeutic remedies are given. The emotional component of acute and particularly chronic pain is always considerable. It should also be emphasized that pain is a rather specific sensation. For instance, severe injury may occur without concomitant pain, indicating a high degree of specialization of those receptors involved in pain sensation (Wall, 1979). On the other hand, pain of sufficient strength will affect the central nervous system in a very general way. For instance, studies of humans in severe pain, have revealed marked increases in the blood flow in almost all brain regions (Lassen *et al.*. 1978).

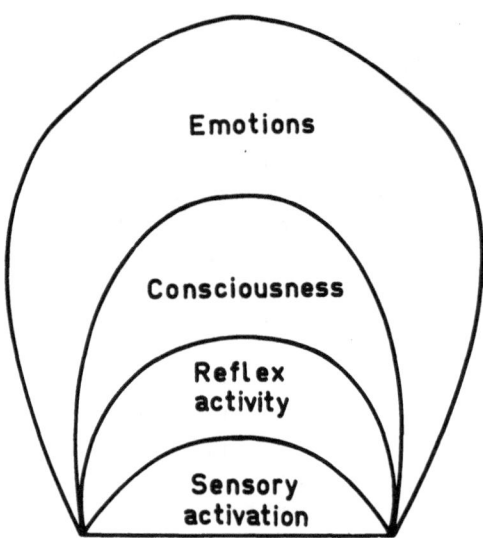

Figure 1   Schematic representation of the different levels in the pain hierarchy

One may classify pain and the reaction to pain in terms of its integration within the central nervous system. The diagram in Figure 1 includes the whole sequence of events from the simple activation of the primary sensory afferents to the higher mental events relating to suffering and mental distress. Viewed in this way, it is clear that pain is not a single phenomenon and that some mental and behavioural consequences of pain may have much in common with mental distress in general. This aspect will be considered later.

The functional advantage of pain is obvious. In fact, the absence of pain feeling, congenital analgesia, is a serious disorder (Thrush, 1973). Recent studies have shown that there is also a physiological system modulating pain and acting on receptors previously only known to be affected by morphine and allied substances. The endogenous substances have been named endorphins and their role in pain modulation is gradually being clarified (Terenius, 1978). In addition, there may be other pain modulating systems (Liebeskind and Paul, 1977). The present paper will deal only with endorphins and pain and some possible consequences of endorphinergic pain modulation.

It is now customary to name opiates and endorphins with a collective term, opioid. An opioid acts on opioid receptors. Those receptors which are of interest in relation to pain modulation seem to be naloxone sensitive. At least operationally, opioid receptors will here be defined as receptors which are antagonized by naloxone. Such receptors have been studied extensively with biochemical techniques and their distribution in the CNS has been mapped by autoradiography (Snyder and Simantov, 1977). The distribution of these receptors is quite widespread, including all levels of the spinal cord, the brain stem, and the midbrain, as well as higher brain centres. Opioid receptors are also present in all parts of the CNS which have been considered to be involved in pain transmission and processing. The endorphins are also ubiquitous. The pentapeptides, called enkephalins, show the widest distribution including all levels where opioid receptors have been identified (Hökfelt et al., 1977). The distribution of the long-chain β-endorphin peptide is different, involving a bundle of fibres which originates in the hypothalamus and projects rather diffusely via septal areas against the third ventricle (Watson and Akil, 1980; Bloom et al., 1978). Anatomically, it is therefore possible to identify en-kephalin fibres at all levels where pain signals may be modulated, such as in the substantia gelatinosa, the raphe nuclei and in the periaqueductal grey matter. β-endorphin terminals are present in the vicinity of the periaqueductal grey matter. It is also known that microinjection of morphine into the peri-aqueductal grey matter (Tsou and Jang, 1964) or into the raphe nuclei (Hertz et al., 1970) will produce strong analgesia, as will intrathecal administration (Yaksh and Rudy, 1976). Thus, we have the anatomic basis for the presence of endorphin neurons and receptors in areas of interest in pain modulation and we also know that morphine will show strong pharmacological effects in the same areas.

Most of the work mentioned in the preceding paragraph refers to animal work. Morphine is, of course, the favoured drug to combat severe pain in humans. However, it should be noticed that clinically used doses in the human are comparatively low (typically 10–15 mg i.v., while a pharmacological dose for analgesia in rats is 5–15 mg/kg). Morphine is used clinically to treat pains with strong emotional overtones of anxiety and suffering. In such conditions it is highly effective. However, if morphine is given in therapeutic doses to a healthy individual, there is practically no effect on experimental pain thresholds (Jaffe, 1975). Under such model conditions the 'pain' sensation hardly reaches emotional dimensions at all. We may in an analogous fashion expect that endorphins play no or little role in phasic pain while there may be release of endorphins in stressful pain and in pain with strong emotional components. In a more general way, we may also expect endorphins to be involved in similar mental events as those occurring in severe pain. In the following sections of this paper three possible aspects of the importance of endorphins will be considered: pain adaptation, acute pain, and chronic pain.

ENDORPHINS AND PAIN ADAPTATION

Sensitivity to pain is a highly individual phenomenon. Differences in pain sensitivity have been observed in relation to ethnic origin, sex and birth order (Melzack, 1973). It seems likely that these differences are acquired during early life. There may even be genetic components. Such questions are hard to study in humans. Unfortunately, animal studies are practically non-existent. One preliminary study indicates that exposure of a pregnant rat to naloxone during days 17–21 of pregnancy and for a further 3 days during lactation, renders the offspring supersensitive to morphine when studied 40 days later (Hetta and Terenius, 1979). Endorphins during early and later life may

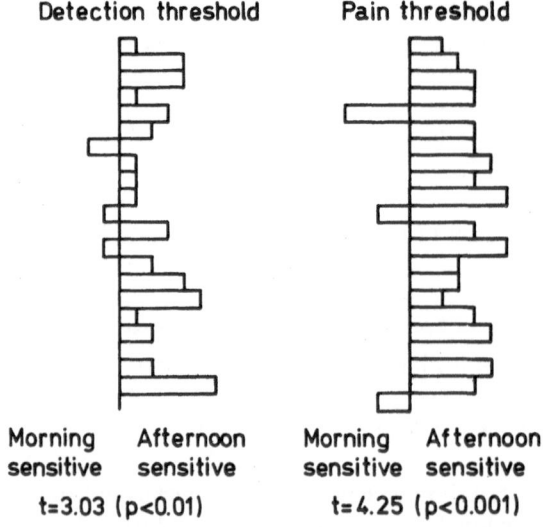

Figure 2   Diurnal variation in pain sensitivity. Twenty-two healthy volunteers were tested on six separate days with respect to detection thresholds and pain thresholds. Each horizontal bar represents one individual classified as morning or afternoon sensitive on each test day. The length of the bar is proportional to the number of times the criterion was reached. (Rogers and Vilkin, 1978. Reproduced with permission.)

therefore form a constitutional. characteristic pain adaptability and a certain preparedness to tolerate pain.

Another aspect of pain adaptation relates to the diurnal variation in pain sensitivity. This is a common clinical observation, in that patients with chronic pain are usually worse at the end of the day (Glynn et al., 1976). In healthy volunteers there is also a diurnal pattern in the sensitivity to experimental pain (Figure 2) (Rogers and Vilkin. 1978). Most individuals are afternoon-sensitive. To what extent are these diurnal differences endorphin-mediated? A recent study by Buchsbaum and co-workers (Davis et al., 1978) suggests that endorphins are responsible for the phenomenon. Naloxone given in the morning was found to increase pain sensitivity in the individuals and to increase the evoked responses to painful stimuli. However, in the afternoon. there was no significant effect of naloxone on either criterion. The conclusion would therefore be that early in the active period there is significant endorphin activity. while by the afternoon the activity is largely absent. Animal studies are confirmatory. endorphin activity being highest in the early part of the active period in mice (Frederickson et al., 1977).

ACUTE PAIN

It is definitely not easy to evaluate the role of endorphins in acute pain. Pain suffering is very difficult to quantify and self-judgement scales can only give the characteristic of the individual which may not be translatable to another individual. It has also been held that pain memory does not exist or at least is very vague. making it difficult for an individual to judge a change in suffering and its direction. Probably the only way to objectively evaluate pain suffering in a paradigm which allows interindividual comparison, is to use self-titration with narcotics. In this set-up, narcotics may be taken at will (with restrictions to protect from overdosage) to an extent which keeps the patient comfortable. If corrected for pharmacokinetic differences, this method would allow a titration end-point for the active concentration at the receptor level. This set-up has been developed to assist patients in post-operative pain. Certainly, the free access to an active pain remedy relieves some of the anxiety of the post-operative phase. Still there are considerable differences in the administration rate which can hardly be explained by the differences in trauma. Whether or not the endorphin systems can contribute to the observed inter-individual differences is at present being studied. Only a few studies in the literature address the problem of endorphin activation in acute pain. Levine et al. (1978b) used naloxone in a double-blind cross-over design during the post-operative phase in patients undergoing molar extraction. and found that naloxone caused a significantly steeper increase in reported pain than placebo. The same group has also studied whether placebo treatment, which in itself may have considerable clinical value, acts through endorphin activation. The results are seemingly positive, in that naloxone significantly reduces placebo-induced pain relief (Levine *et al.*, 1978a). However, the interpretation of these experiments is not easy. Certain individuals tend to be placebo-reactors, others not. It is often difficult to predict who is going to react. Recently it was shown that the apparent severity of pain may be one factor, those suffering most severely showing the best placebo response (Levine *et al.*, 1979). Tentatively, we may therefore assume that placebo reactivity is a function of the pain status, but it may also be a characteristic of the individual.

Although the evidence so far is rather incomplete, it still seems likely that endorphins are released in severe pain and stress. This could certainly be of a considerable survival value. In mammals, parturition is both a stressful and a painful act. Our studies indicate that naloxone administered to rats during the parturition period will decrease the survival rate of the offspring (Hetta and Terenius. 1979). It should also be remembered that the copulation act in several animal species (e.g. dog, cat) is painful. Again, endorphin release may play a protective role. Finally, a number of induced changes in attention or altered consciousness are known to attenuate the sensation of pain. In a very strong concentration. such as in trance or in certain sporting activities, an almost analgesic state can be induced. To date it has not been investigated to what extent this phenomenon relates to endorphin activation.

CHRONIC PAIN

Chronic pain syndromes have a great personal, social and economic impact. It has been estimated that in the United States the annual expenditure on chronic pain is in the order of 60 billion U.S. dollars (Bonica, 1979). Despite the considerable clinical problem of chronic pain, there has been comparatively little interest in the study of basic mechanisms. One contributing factor is the difficulty of establishing laboratory models. Experimental trauma in higher species is hardly ethically permissible, while work in lower species raises questions as to its relevance to the clinical situation. One model which has recently been established holds some promise. It uses rats which are subjected to extensive rhizotomy (Lombard *et al.*, 1979). The animals react by strong discomfort, dysesthesia, which may have parallels in chronic pain. So far, no functional or pharmacological studies have been done. It may also be questioned whether an animal model could give the information wanted. Perhaps the human being is a unique species in having an insight of suffering and its consequences and in demanding treatment. There is no evidence that an animal has an insight into problems of chronicity in a disease situation, or for that matter, in death. Thus, the reactive component, which is always present in a clinical, chronic pain syndrome, may be absent in animals. From what has been inferred earlier, it is probably this component which endorphins affect in humans. It may also be that the human being is particularly susceptible to chronic pain syndromes, which frequently may relate to difficulties in a personal or social context, rather than to the constant presence of painful stimuli. Although this aspect has not been studied extensively, the clinical impression that acute traumatic pain is more severe than chronic pain is probably correct. This ought to be analysed in terms of, for instance, effects on the hypothalamic–pituitary–adrenal axis or in sympathetic activity.

Some years ago, at a time when the chemical structure of endorphins was still not known, I decided that a study of endorphin levels in patients with chronic pain might give some insight into this syndrome. A method was developed which allowed the measurement of endorphin-like material in the cerebrospinal fluid (CSF) of patients. The method was based on affinity measurements for opioid receptors. Our results indicated that patients with severe trigeminal neuralgia had lower endorphin levels than other patients (Terenius and Wahlström, 1975). The study has now been extended and amplified. Essentially two basic questions have been asked: (1) is there some characteristic abnormality in the endorphin system of these patients? and (2) are these abnormalities corrected or affected by treatment?

Table 1   Distribution of endorphin Fraction 1 levels in patients with chronic pain as compared with healthy volunteers

Patient category	Fraction 1 (pmol/ml) *	
	⩽0.6	>0.6
Chronic pain, positive neurology	12	2
Chronic pain, negative neurology	2	21
Healthy volunteers	3	16

*Calculated as if due to methionine-enkephalin

An extensive study was designed to evaluate the first of these problems. The subjects were a series of chronic pain patients attending the Neurologic Clinic at the University of Umea. No selection of patients was done, except for the exclusion of those where old age, brain damage, or drug-use might have confused the picture. Routine diagnostic examination and X-ray, EMG and biopsy verifications of the diagnosis were carried out. The patients were then classified as having mainly neurogenic or non-neurogenic pain. Every patient was also seen by a psychiatrist and scored for selected items on the CPRS scale. Experimental pain thresholds and pain tolerance limits as well as evoked potentials to visual stimuli (V.EP) were also recorded. Most of the patients were also evaluated in personality inventories (the Eysenk personality scale and the Zuckerman sensation seeking scale). Finally a sample of lumbar CSF was obtained and analysed for endorphin content and for the content of monoamine metabolites. The results of endorphin measurements in relation to diagnosis are summarized in Table 1. Apparently patients with neurogenic pain tend to have very low endorphin levels in comparison with healthy volunteers, whilst patients with non-neurogenic pain have levels within the normal range. A number of variables seem to correlate with the endorphin levels (Table 2). It may not be unexpected that there is a correlation with pain measures and with sensory evoked potentials. The correlation with ratings in the CPRS system and with personality inventories is intriguing and supports the hypothesis that endorphins have a much more general role than solely as modulators of sensory input, notably pain.

Table 2   Relation between endorphin Fraction 1 levels and various clinical and laboratory variables in chronic pain patients ($n = 44$)

Positive correlation with:	pain threshold and pain tolerance (von Knorring et al., 1978), depression scores (Almay et al., 1978), monoamine (5HIAA) CSF levels (Almay et al., 1979)
Negative correlation with:	duration of pain (neurogenic group) (Almay et al., 1978)
Correlation with:	EEG responses to visual stimuli (V.EP) (von Knorring et al., 1979), personality variables (Johansson et al., 1979)
No correlation with:	sex, age, self-rated severity of pain (Almay et al., 1978)

The subnormal levels in patients with neurogenic pain indicate that these patients may be endorphin deficient. These are the patients who are particularly assisted by transcutaneous nerve stimulation (TNS), a method which is rapidly gaining clinical reputation. It is of considerable interest that the pain relief induced by these procedures seems to depend on endorphin activation. Pain returns on the administration of naloxone (Sjölund and Eriksson, 1979) and the pain relief is accompanied by increasing CSF endorphin levels (Sjölund et al., 1977). Thus, the endorphin systems are intrinsically powerful and can inhibit severe clinical pain.

CONCLUSION

Full understanding of these observations requires further work. For the moment many questions remain to be answered. For instance, are low levels of endorphins a consequence of a pain syndrome or do they characterize the 'pain prone' patient? Certainly, chronic pain should be regarded as a disease state which deeply influences the behaviour and personality of the patient. If, however, low endorphin levels are secondary to a long period of pain suffering, we should expect them in every patient with chronic pain, independent of aetiology. Since this is not the case, it could be that low endorphin levels are of fact primary in chronic neurogenic pain and therefore directly involved in the disease process. It then remains to be explained why patients with non-neurogenic pain have normal or even supernormal endorphin levels. There are several possibilities. There may be lesions in central endorphinergic mechanisms which are too small to be observed through analysis of lumbar CSF. It is also possible that these pain syndromes have an aetiology not directly involving the endorphin system.

Acknowledgement

This work is supported by the Swedish Medical Research Council.

References

Almay, B. G. L., Johansson, F., von Knorring, L., Sedvall, G. and Terenius, L. (1980). Relationships between CSF levels of endorphins and monoamine metabolites in chronic pain patients. *Psychopharmacology*, **67**, 139

Almay, B. G. L., Johansson, F., von Knorring, L., Terenius, L. and Wahlström, A. (1978). Endorphins in chronic pain. I. Differences in CSF endorphin levels between organic and psychogenic pain syndromes. *Pain*. **5**. 153

Bloom, F., Battenberg, E., Rossier, J., Ling, N. and Guillemin, R. (1978). Neurons containing β-endorphin in rat brain exist separately from those containing enkephalin: Immunocytochemical studies. *Proc. Natl. Acad. Sci. (Wash.)*. **75**. 1591

Bonica, J. J. (1979). Paper presented at the *International Symposium on Pain*. June 11–15. Sorrento

Davis, G. C., Buchsbaum, M. S. and Bunney. W. E., Jr. (1978). Naloxone decreases diurnal variation in pain sensitivity and somatosensory evoked potentials. *Life Sci.*. **23**. 1449

Frederickson, R. C. A., Burgis, V. and Edwards, J. D. (1977). Hyperalgesia induced by naloxone follows diurnal rhythm in responsivity to painful stimuli. *Science*. **198**. 756

Glynn, C. J., Lloyd, J. W. and Folkard, S. (1976). The diurnal variation in perception of pain. *Proc. R. Soc. Med.*, **69**, 369

Hertz, A., Albus, L., Metys, J., Schubert, P. and Teschemacher. H. (1970). On the central sites for the antinociceptive action of morphine and fentanyl. *Neuropharmacology*. **9**. 539

Hetta, J. and Terenius, L. (1980). Prenatal naloxone affects survival and morphine sensitivity of rat offspring. *Neurosci. Lett.*, **16**, 323

Hökfelt, T., Ljungdahl. Å., Terenius, L. Elde. R. and Nilsson. G. (1977). Immunohistochemical analysis of peptide pathways possibly related to pain and analgesia: Enkephalin and substance P. *Proc. Natl. Acad. Sci. (Wash.)*, **74**, 3081

Jaffé, J. H. (1975). Drug addiction and drug abuse. In L. S. Goodman and A. Gilman (eds). *The Pharmacological Basis of Therapeutics*. pp. 284–324. (London: Macmillan)

Johansson, F., Almay, B. G. L., von Knorring, L., Terenius, L. and Åström, M. (1979). Personality traits in chronic pain patients related to endorphin levels of CSF. *Psychiatr. Res.*, **1**, 231

von Knorring, L., Almay, B. G. L., Johansson, F. and Terenius, L. (1979). Endorphins in CSF of chronic pain patients in relation to augmenting-reducing response in visual averaged evoked response. *Neuropsychobiology*, **5**, 322

von Knorring, L., Almay. B. G. L., Johansson. F. and Terenius. L. (1978). Pain perception and endorphin levels in cerebrospinal fluid. *Pain*. **5**. 359

Lassen, N. A., Ingvar. D. H. and Skinhøj. E. (1978). Brain function and blood flow. *Sci. Am.*, **239**. 50

Levine, J. D., Gordon, N. C., Bornstein, J. E. and Fields, H. L. (1979). The role of pain in placebo analgesia. *Proc. Natl. Acad. Sci. (Wash.)*, **76**, 3528

Levine, J. D., Gordon, N. C. and Fields, H. L. (1978a). The mechanism of placebo analgesia. *Lancet*, **2**, 654

Levine, J. D., Gordon, N. C., Jones. R. T. and Fields. H. L. (1978b). The narcotic antagonist naloxone enhances clinical pain. *Nature*. **272**, 826

Liebeskind, J. C. and Paul, L. A. (1977). Psychological and physiological mechanisms of pain. *Ann. Rev. Psychol.*, **28**, 41

Lombard, M. C., Nashold, B. S. and Albe-Fessard. D. (1979). Deafferentation hypersensitivity in the rat after dorsal rhizotomy: A possible animal model of chronic pain. *Pain*. **6**, 163

Melzack, R. (1973). *The Puzzle of Pain*. (New York: Basic Books)

Rogers, E. J. and Vilkin, B. (1978). Diurnal variation in sensory and pain thresholds correlated with mood states. *J. Clin. Psychiatry*, **39**, 431

Sjölund, B. H. and Eriksson, M. B. E. (1979). The influence of naloxone on analgesia produced by peripheral conditioning stimulation. *Brain Res.*, **173**, 295

Sjölund, B., Terenius, L. and Eriksson, M. (1977). Increased cerebrospinal fluid levels of endorphins after electro-acupuncture. *Acta Physiol. Scand.*. **100**, 382

Snyder, S. H. and Simantov, R. (1977). The opiate receptor and opioid peptides. *J. Neurochem.*, **28**, 13

Terenius, L. (1978). Endogenous peptides and analgesia. *Ann. Rev. Pharmacol. Toxicol.*. **18**. 189

Terenius, L. and Wahlström, A. (1975). Morphine-like ligand for opiate receptors in human CSF. *Life Sci.*, **16**, 1759

Thrush, D. C. (1973). Autonomic dysfunction in four patients with congenital insensitivity to pain. *Brain*, **96**, 591

Tsou, K. and Jang, C. S. (1964). Studies on the site of analgesic action of morphine by intracerebral microinjection. *Sci. Sinica*. **8**, 1099

Wall, P. D. (1979). On the relation of injury to pain. *Pain*. **6**. 253

Watson, S. J. and Akil, H. (1980). On the multiplicity of active substances in single neurons: β-endorphin and α-melanocyte stimulating hormone as a model system. In D. de Wied and P. A. van Keep (eds.). *Hormones and the Brain*. (Lancaster: MTP Press)

Yaksh, T. L. and Rudy, T. A. (1976). Analgesia mediated by a direct spinal action of narcotics. *Science*, **192**, 1357

Address for correspondence

Professor L. Terenius, Institutionen för Farmakologi, Uppsala Universitets, Biomedicinska Centrum, Box 573, S-751 23 Uppsala, Sweden

3.3
Central vasopressin function in affective illness

P. W. GOLD, F. K. GOODWIN, J. C. BALLENGER,
H. WEINGARTNER, G. L. ROBERTSON and R. M. POST

ABSTRACT

This paper reports preliminary findings which show that in drug-free manic-depressive patients, both the cerebrospinal fluid levels of arginine vasopressin (AVP) and the plasma AVP response to hypertonic saline are reduced in depression compared with mania. When depressed patients were given sustained administration of 1-deamino-D-arginine vasopressin (DDAVP), a synthetic analogue of AVP, some showed enhancements of cognitive function and amelioration of depressive symptomatology. These findings are compatible with an hypothesis of relatively diminished AVP function in depression compared with mania.

INTRODUCTION

It is well established that integrative communication within the central nervous system proceeds not only by classical chemical neurotransmission, but also by interactions between brain and hormonal factors originating in the hypothalamic–pituitary axis. Many of these hormones appear to be extensively distributed in brain either by the cerebrospinal fluid communication pathway or by axon transport; thus, they may excite extra-synaptic receptors located at sites distant from synthesis which in turn influence multiple nerve cell aggregates organized to orchestrate specific complex behavioural or physiological processes (Barker, 1977). De Wied and colleagues were among the first to demonstrate a behavioural effect of one of these central nervous system (CNS) hormones by showing that vasopressin administration restores defective memory consolidation in vasopressin-deficient rats, and improves memory function in normal rats (de Wied and Gispen, 1977). These findings stimulated our group to investigate vasopressin function in disorders of human behaviour, particularly primary affective disorder. This paper summarizes our preliminary findings concerning the relationship between vasopressin function and the symptom complex of affective illness, and suggests some future studies.

METHODS

The patients were hospitalized in the clinical research unit of the National Institute of Mental Health (NIMH), Bethesda, USA, and met standard Research Diagnostic Criteria for major affective disorder (Spitzer et al., 1978). Volunteer subjects were studied in the same clinical research units. During each hospital day, patients were rated twice daily under double-blind conditions by a trained nursing research team using the revised NIMH scale for global items of depression, anxiety, psychosis, mania and anger (Kotin and Goodwin, 1972). Both patients and volunteers adhered to a controlled monoamine diet and received no active medication for three weeks prior to participating in only vasopressin function studies or the clinical trial of the vasopressin analogue, 1-deamino-D-arginine (DDAVP)˙ In three patients the plasma arginine vasopressin (AVP) response to sustained hypertonic saline infusion was monitored longitudinally during both the depressed and manic states. Lumbar punctures for cerebrospinal fluid arginine vasopressin (CSF AVP) were performed in 15 bipolar patients during the depressed phase and 13 patients during the manic phase. CSF AVP was also obtained by lumbar puncture from 33 control subjects (age range 19–64). Four depressed subjects received intranasal DDAVP in doses of 40–160 µg/day for 3–7 weeks. Plasma vasopressin responses were studied following the infusion of $0.05 \, ml \, kg^{-1} min^{-1}$ of 5% hypertonic saline for 2 h according to the method of Robertson et al. (1973). At this rate of infusion, plasma osmolality rises approximately 2%/h giving a linear rate of vasopressin secretion commensurate with the increase in plasma osmolality. When subjects are tested repeatedly with this hypertonic saline administration paradigm, a given individual's threshold for AVP secretion and the rate of AVP release which changes is osmolality shows a variance of less than 10%. Such reproducibility makes this paradigm particularly useful for following plasma AVP responses longitudinally in clinical populations. All infusions were conducted after an overnight fast, and patients were at bedrest for at least 2 h before the first of two baseline AVP samples. After the start of the infusion, blood was drawn for AVP and osmolality every 15 min for 2 h. Because of the sensitivity of AVP levels to change in blood pressure, this parameter was monitored every 5 min throughout the procedure.

Cerebrospinal fluid was obtained at 9 a.m. and analysed for both vaso-pressin and osmolality. Plasma and CSF AVP were analysed by radio-immunoassay as previously described using the highly specific and sensitive Glick-1 AVP antibody (Robertson et al., 1973).

In patients receiving DDAVP, cognitive functions were assessed by admin-istering a different but equivalent word list at the same time of day at least 10 times before, during, and after treatment. First, patients were asked to listen to and remember standardized lists of 32 random words made up of categories of structurally balanced or related items. The number of items recalled and the strategies used to remember, e.g. whether words from the same category are clustered at the time of recall, were measured. This task provides measures of the amount of organization imposed on information by the subject, and how organization is used to facilitate the laying down of memory traces. This is summarized by a measure of the number of related words correctly recalled

Table 1   Cognitive effects of 1-deamino-D-arginine vasopressin (DDAVP) in depressed patients

Patient No.	Total recall		Percent consistency of recall	
	Placebo	DDAVP	Placebo	DDAVP
1	12.0 ± 0.4 (4)	18.5 ± 0.5 (7)	58 ± 2.0 (4)	93 ± 1.0 (7)
2	6.33 ± 0.3 (3)	13.8 ± 0.9 (7)	16.7 ± 6.7 (3)	43.4 ± 4.2 (7)
3	7.67 ± 1.4 (3)	13.3 ± 1.4 (7)	18 ± 4.0 (3)	53 ± 1.0 (7)
4	7.3 ± 0.8 (3)	9.3 ± 0.7 (7)	32 ± 8.0 (3)	60 ± 10 (7)

Data expressed as Mean + SEM; number of trials in parentheses
Placebo significantly different from DDAVP ($p < 0.01$; ANOVA with repeated measures)

('total recall') (Table 1). A second procedure required subjects to listen to a list of 14 random words and remember them. Words are presented on subsequent recall trials that were not successfully remembered on the previous trial. Subjects would again try to remember all the words, those remembered on the previous trial, as well as those 'missed' or forgotten. The first recall trial can be seen as a measure of short-term or immediate memory. Performance on the subsequent 'prompted' trials indicates how much information had been learned, how much has been shifted from short- to long-term memory, and how much information can be consistently accessed from long-term memory.

This latter measure is particularly useful to evaluate the strength and organization of information in memory and is reported as 'percent consistency of recall' (see Table 1).

RESULTS

CSF AVP was significantly lower in drug-free bipolar patients in the depressed compared with the manic phase ($p < 0.01$, see Figure 1). CSF AVP levels tended to be lower in bipolar depressed patients compared with normals ($p < 0.1$). but there was no difference between manic patients and the controls (see Figure 1).

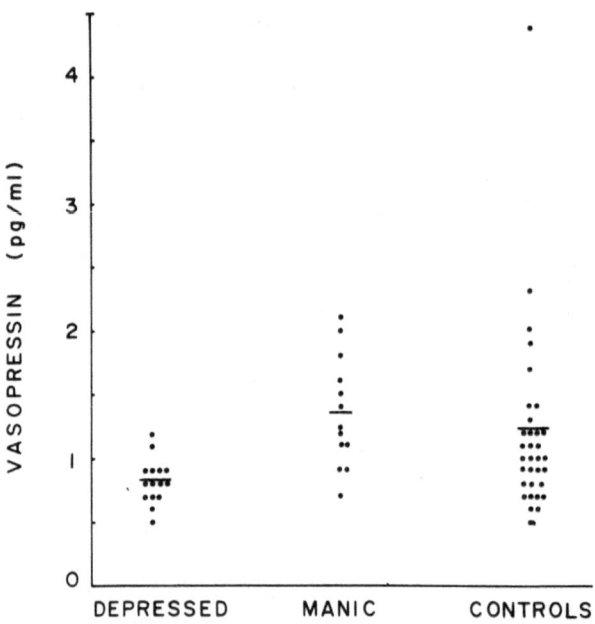

Figure 1   Cerebrospinal fluid vasopressin in patients with affective illness and in controls

In the three patients studied longitudinally with hypertonic saline infusion during depression and mania, the threshold and sensitivity (slope of the regression line relating AVP to osmolality) were substantially lower in depression compared with mania (see Figure 2).

Prior to DDAVP treatment each of the depressed patients studied demonstrated the moderate and stable impairments in cognitive performance usually associated with major depressive illness. Specifically, they showed difficulty in accessing and maintaining information in memory. and using organization to process and recall information. On the other hand, immediate recall of information. initial learning performance and attention appeared unimpaired.

Following DDAVP treatment, three of the four patients demonstrated significant enhancement in learning and memory, particularly in the formation of well-learned organized information that could be consistently recalled. For the group, the overall 'total recall' (see Table 1), and the overall 'mean percent consistency' (see Table 1) were significantly greater during DDAVP treatment compared with the placebo period (analysis of variance with repeated measures).

Each of the patients who showed enhancements on DDAVP was tested at intervals after discontinuation of the drug, and each showed considerable

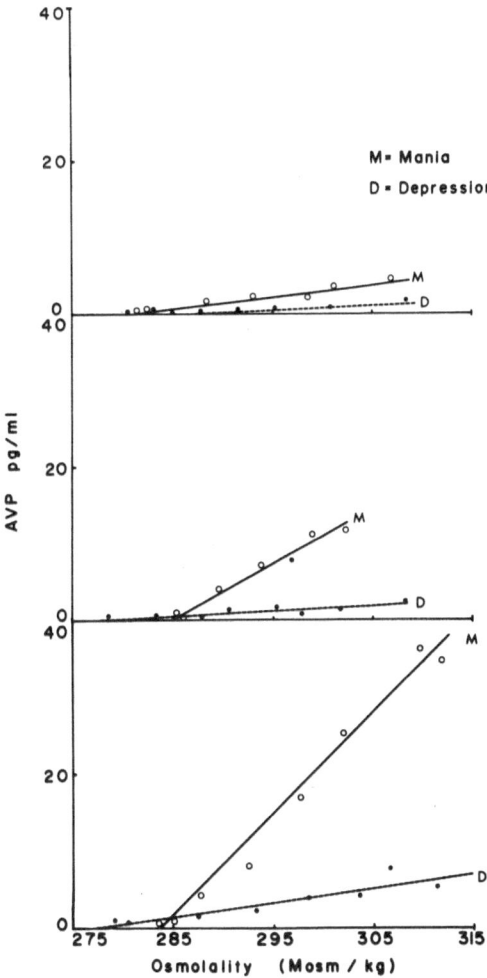

Figure 2 Vasopressin response to hypertonic saline in drug-free patients with bipolar affective illness

decline in cognitive enhancements attributable to DDAVP at varying times during the post-DDAVP period. In two subjects, the decline occurred about 14 days after DDAVP was discontinued; one subject did not show loss of cognitive enhancements until several weeks after DDAVP was stopped.

Two of four patients showed statistically significant amelioration of depressive and psychotic symptomatology during the trial. For patient 1, the amelioration lasted throughout the trial, and when DDAVP was discontinued, severe depressive and psychotic symptoms recurred. Patient 2 showed clear-cut, but transient, improvement in depressive symptoms during the second week of DDAVP treatment that lasted about two weeks and returned essentially to pre-treatment levels before DDAVP was discontinued. Patient 3, with rapidly cycling depressions and manias, showed no change in depressive symptoms, but some improvement during the manic phase of her illness. In addition, the length of the manic phase seemed lengthened by DDAVP treatment. Patient 4's severe depression was unaffected by DDAVP treatment. The clinical and cognitive responses of patient 1 are summarized in Figure 3.

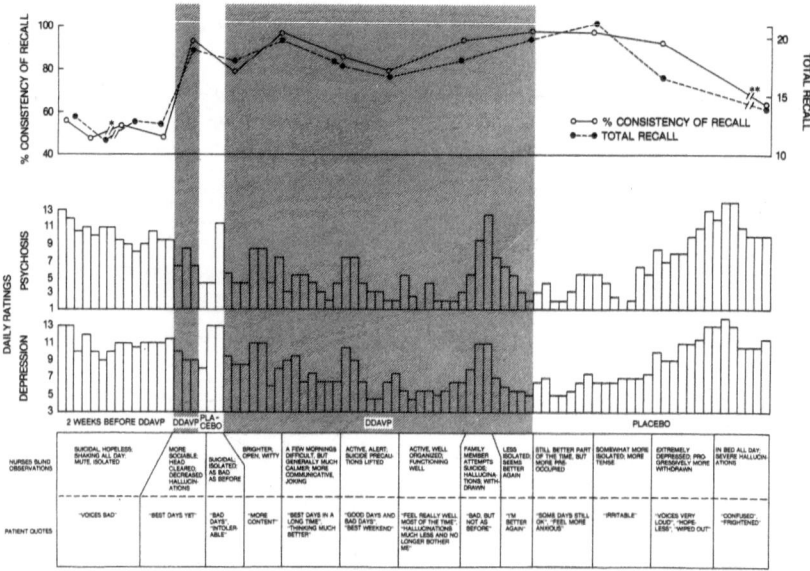

Figure 3 Cognitive and behavioural responses of one patient to 1-deamino-D-arginine vaso-pressin (DDAVP) treatment

DISCUSSION

In bipolar patients CSF levels of AVP and the plasma AVP response to hypertonic saline are lower in the depressed phase than in the manic phase. In addition, vasopressin analogue administration to depressed patients results in cognitive enhancements, and in some instances, in anti-depressant responses. These data suggest that vasopressin exerts specific behavioural and cognitive effects in man in addition to its established role as the anti-diuretic hormone.

Vasopressin is synthesized in the magnacellular system of the hypothalamus in clusters of cells that form several hypothalamic nuclei. Three pathways have been identified for vasopressin secretion. The major pathway is the supraoptico-hypophysial tract to the posterior pituitary for secretion into the blood. The second is to the external zone of the median eminence for secretion into the hypophysial portal blood. The third pathway is to the third ventricle for secretion into the cerebrospinal fluid. Vasopressin in CSF is derived largely from neurons other than those that secrete into the blood (Leurssen and Robertson, 1979); although originating in different neurons, the secretion of AVP into CSF and plasma seems to be influenced by many of the same stimuli, the most important of which seems to be the osmolality of body water. Whether the osmoreceptors regulating plasma and CSF AVP are functionally and/or anatomically different is unknown. Non-osmotic stimuli, such as haemorrhage, nausea, and glucopenia, also have a significant influence on the secretion of AVP into both CSF and plasma. In addition, neuropeptides such as angiotensin and the opiates, the biogenic amine neurotransmitters, and pharmacological agents such as ethanol, can influence both plasma and CSF AVP levels (Leurssen and Robertson, 1979).

The results of our CSF and plasma vasopressin studies do not seem to reflect non-specific factors such as changes in body osmolality, since baseline plasma and CSF osmolalities were similar in all groups tested. Certain non-osmolar stimuli, such as volume depletion, glucopenia, nausea, or prior drug ingestion can also be excluded as discriminating factors in the results of these studies. Thus, alterations in CSF vasopressin and the plasma response to hypertonic saline in patients with affective illness would seem to result from alterations in the synthesis, storage, release, or action of one or more of the neuropeptides or neurotransmitters that modulate AVP secretion. Alterations in CSF vasopressin or plasma responses to osmotic stimuli could also reflect changes in the permeability of the osmoreceptor cell membrane to either water or solute. The parallel findings of diminished CSF AVP and reduced plasma sensitivity to an osmolar stimulus in depression compared with mania suggest overlap in the regulatory apparatus that modulates both CSF and plasma AVP secretion.

The preliminary findings of cognitive and behavioural responses to DDAVP in depressed patients, although consistent with the alterations in vasopressin reported here, require replication in a larger series. These preliminary data show that DDAVP treatment preferentially influences those components of cognitive functioning that seem impaired in depression. Thus, the formation of long-term, relatively permanent trace events in memory and their effect on encoding and organization are altered more than those processes that are either attentional or are measures of immediate or short-term memory. It is of interest that this pattern of enhancement resembles that noted following amphetamine administration, although quantitatively, greater improvement is seen after DDAVP administration.

The fact that CSF and plasma AVP levels and responses differ between depressed and manic patients does not necessarily implicate AVP function in the pathophysiology of primary affective disorder. However, these data, in association with the clinical and cognitive responses to DDAVP in depression, are compatible with our previously stated hypothesis that central AVP function may be diminished in depression compared with mania (Gold et al., 1978). This hypothesis was based on a review of existing experimental and pharmacological data that indicated that vasopressin influences several behavioural and physiological processes of relevance to the symptom complex of affective illness, including alterations in memory function, pain sensitivity, sleep, the synchronization of biological rhythms, and the regulation of fluid and electrolyte balance. Here we shall briefly review the data that support this hypothesis and attempt to relate it to any biochemical and behavioural findings reported.

De Wied and his co-workers demonstrated that AVP facilitates memory processes in both vasopressin-deficient and normal experimental animals (de Wied and Gispen, 1977). We postulate that the well-documented impairments in memory function noted in depressed patients could partially relate to diminished central AVP function reflected by low CSF AVP. Of interest is our finding in normal subjects that CSF AVP is significantly and positively correlated with performance on standardized tests of memory (Ballenger et al., 1979). The preliminary study in which DDAVP augmented memory function and produced anti-depressant responses in patients with affective illness also supports the idea that diminished vasopressin function in depressed patients could be related to the memory deficits reported in these subjects. It has been previously reported that vasopressin administration augments memory function in subjects with dementia or post-traumatic amnesia (Legros et al., 1978; Oliveros et al., 1978).

Whether or not increases in central vasopressin function are related to the cognitive changes seen in mania is conjectural; however, there has been one case report that cites the occurrence of hypomania in a subject receiving exogenous vasopressin for the treatment of amnesia (Oliveros et al., 1978). In one of our patients with a pattern of rapid cycles of manic and depressed episodes, the manic phase seemed lengthened by DDAVP treatment.

The major pharmacological agents used in the treatment of affective illness exert important effects on vasopressin function in experimental animals. Certain tricyclic anti-depressants have been reported to augment vasopressin function, while lithium, the drug of choice in the treatment of mania, is well-known to antagonize vasopressin-stimulated production of adenyl cyclase, and thus, diminish vasopressin's functional activity. These data are compatible with the hypothesis that vasopressin function may be reduced in depression and relatively augmented in mania. This pharmacologically generated 'rheostatic' model of vasopressin function in affective illness requires some qualification, however, in light of clinical evidence that lithium exerts some anti-depressant effects in addition to its classic anti-manic properties. A recent report suggests that one tricyclic anti-depressant drug (carbamazepine), also may have both anti-manic and anti-depressant effects (Ballenger *et al.*, 1979). Thus, if both the anti-manic and the anti-depressant properties of lithium and carbamazepine are related to their effects on vasopressin, these agents may not simply act by augmenting or diminishing central vasopressin functional activity, but may act to prevent sudden perturbations that could trigger an active clinical episode.

To elucidate further the effects of lithium and carbamazepine on AVP function in man, we administered hypertonic saline infusions to a number of subjects with affective illness during a placebo period and after at least three weeks' treatment with either lithium or carbamazepine. The results of these studies (unpublished) show that while lithium seems to function as a vasopressin receptor antagonist, it also induces an augmentation (perhaps compensatory) in vasopressin secretion to an osmotic stimulus, and significantly increases the sensitivity of the AVP response to hypertonic saline. Conversely, although carbamazepine is known to augment vasopressin function, and has been used to treat partial central diabetes insipidus in man, this drug nevertheless induces a significant reduction in the sensitivity of the vasopressin response to hypertonic saline (Gold *et al.*, unpublished observation). Carbamazepine seems to be acting as a vasopressin receptor agonist, since lower levels of vasopressin are necessary to promote anti-diuresis and maintain plasma osmolality when hypertonic saline is administered during the carbamazepine treatment period compared with the drug-free state. Lithium and carbamazepine may exert therapeutic effects in bipolar affective illness by the initiation of compensatory changes in vasopressin secretion in a direction opposite to their effects on the putative central vasopressin receptor; possibly these drugs function by circumscribing the range of central vasopressin action analogous to their established effects on other regulated systems. This formulation represents a somewhat different concept of psychotrophic drug action, in which drug efficacy is related to the stabilization of the functional activity of a central peptide.

Vasopressin may also be involved in the modulation of the periodicity of circadian rhythms, that are thought to be slowed in depression and accelerated in mania (Wehr *et al.*, 1979). Pharmacological agents reported to slow circadian periodicity, such as ethanol, deuterium, and lithium, all antagonize AVP function, while tricyclic anti-depressants, reported to accelerate circadian rhythms, seem to augment AVP activity. One of the hypothalamic sites of AVP synthesis is the suprachiasmatic nucleus, thought to be the locus of the endogenous biological clock (Gold *et al.*, 1978).

Considerable interest is centred on interactions between vasopressin and endogenous opiate activity. It has been suggested that vasopressin and the endogenous opiates participate in a mutual regulatory loop, in which each modulates the other's release. Vasopressin was reported to influence the rate of development of tolerance to morphine administration, and to alter self-stimulation behaviour in rats. Thus, vasopressin function may be involved in the postulated role of endogenous opiates in phenomena relating to pleasure, pain, and reward that seem altered in both depression and mania (reviewed in Gold et al., 1978).

Vasopressin as the anti-diuretic hormone acting to regulate free water reabsorption at the level of the renal tubular epithelium has been established. This central peptide may also play a role in the fluid and electrolyte alterations reported in patients with affective illness, an effect yet to be fully investigated (Gold and Robertson, 1979).

In summary, in patients with bipolar affective illness, the level of CSF AVP and plasma responses to osmotic stimuli are lower in depression than in mania. While there is no firm evidence that these differences in CSF vasopressin responses are relevant to the aetiology and/or symptom complex of affective illness, the results are suggestive, particularly in association with the cognitive and behavioural responses to vasopressin analogue administration in depressed patients and in light of the experimental data linking vasopressin to important components of the overall symptom complex of affective illness.

FUTURE DIRECTIONS

The availability of the Brattleboro rat, unable to synthesize vasopressin, offers a unique opportunity for the study of a variety of important questions concerning central vasopressin function in affective illness. For instance, studies of circadian and long-term rhythms in the Brattleboro rat may help determine whether or not vasopressin plays a role in the modulation of biological rhythms that seem deranged in depression and mania. In addition, various other physiological parameters in Brattleboro rats that may be of relevance to the pathogenesis of affective disorder should also be examined, such as the phenomenon of neuronal 'kindling' after repeated pharmacological or electrical stimulation. Post and Kopanda (1976) have postulated that 'kindling' may represent a form of cellular memory and play an important role in the development of manic symptomatology. The elucidation or clarification of other possible physiological derangements in Brattleboro rats that may be an outgrowth of vasopressin deficiency, such as alterations in central oxytocin, angiotensin, or endorphin function, may also shed light on possible pathophysiological alterations in patients with affective illness.

A variety of further clinical studies are warranted in patients with affective illness, such as further trials with the newer AVP analogues, as well as investigations of the clinical effects of specific vasopressin antagonists and endogenous peptides with actions antagonistic to vasopressin. The role of central AVP function in neuroendocrine abnormalities already described in affective illness also deserves further exploration. One of the most enduring psychoneuroendocrine findings in affective illness is that of altered hypothalamic–pituitary–adrenal function in depression, specifically elevated corticosteroid production and failure to suppress corticosteroid and/or adrenocorticotrophic hormone following exogenous dexamethasone administration. The role of vasopressin in these findings has not yet been systematically studied, though for years it has been thought that vasopressin is an important corticotrophin releasing factor. Thus, alterations in central vasopressin function would certainly be expected to alter the functional activity of the hypothalamic–pituitary axis. Vasopressin has also been reported to release growth hormone; thus, it might be involved in the blunted growth hormone responses reported in depressed patients.

The specificity of the behavioural and cognitive effects of vasopressin administration should receive close scrutiny in future studies. An important question is whether vasopressin will prove to reinforce differentially aversive behaviour vs. pleasurably charged experience in human subjects. If vasopressin is shown to differentially reinforce aversive phenomena, there may be a relationship between vasopressin function during a critical period of painful stress and the subsequent development of the persistent ruminative pessimism typical of depressed patients. Conversely, it may be possible to devise behavioural–pharmacological paradigms in which specific positive psychosocial reinforcers and/or specific pleasurable experiences will be combined with vasopressin administration to enhance their retention and retrievability. Such studies may not be too far off in the future as part of a comprehensive programme of examining the central roles of vasopressin and its analogues in man.

References

Ballenger, J. C., Post, R. M. and Bunney, Jr., W. E. (1979). Carbamazepine (Tegretol) in manic-depressive illness: a new treatment. *Am. J. Psychiat.* (In press)

Barker, J. L. (1977). Physiological roles of peptides in the nervous system. In H. Gainer (ed.). *Peptides in Neurobiology*, pp. 295–345. (New York: Plenum Press)

Gold, P. W., Reuss, V. I. and Goodwin, F. K. (1978). Hypothesis: vasopressin in affective illness. *Lancet*, **1**, 1233

Gold, P. W. and Robertson, G. L. (1979). Central peptide regulation of fluid and electrolyte balance: psychiatric implications. In P. Alexander (ed.). *Fluid and Electrolyte Disturbances in Psychiatry*. (New York: Spectrum). (In press)

Kotin, J. and Goodwin, F. K. (1972). Depression during mania: clinical observations and theoretical implications. *Am. J. Psychiat.*, **129**, 679

Legros, J. J., Gilot, P., Seron, X., Claessers, J., Adam, A., Moeglen, J. M., Audibert, A. and Benghier, P. (1978). Influence of vasopressin on learning and memory. *Lancet*, **1**, 41

Leurssen, J. G. and Robertson, G. L. (1979). Cerebrospinal fluid vasopressin and vasotocin in health and disease. In J. H. Wood (ed.). *Neurobiology of Cerebrospinal Fluid.* (New York: Plenum Press). (In press)

Oliveros, J. C., Jandol, M. K., Timsit-Berthier, M., Remy, R., Benghezala. A., Audibert, A. and Moeglen, J. M. (1978). Vasopressin in amnesia. *Lancet.* **1**, 42

Post, R. M. and Kopanda, R. (1976). Cocaine, kindling, and psychosis. *Am. J. Psychiat.*, **133**, 627

Robertson, G. L., Mahr, E. A., Athar, S. and Sinha, T. (1973). Development and clinical application of a new method for the radioimmunoassay of arginine vasopressin in human plasma. *J. Clin. Invest.*, **52**, 2340

Spitzer, R. L., Endicott, J. and Robins, E. (1978). Research diagnostic criteria: rationale and reliability. *Arch. Gen. Psychiat.*, **35**, 773

Wehr, T. A., Wirz-Justice, A., Duncan, W., Gillin, J. C. and Goodwin, F. K. (1979). Phase advance of the circadian sleep–wake cycle as an anti-depressant. *Science.* (In press)

Weingartner, H. (1979). The pharmacology of cognition in man: a review. *Am. J. Psychiat.* (In press)

de Wied, D. and Gispen, W. H. (1977). Behavioural effects of peptides. In H. Gainer (ed.). *Peptides in Neurobiology*, pp. 397–448. (New York: Plenum Press)

Address for correspondence

Dr F. K. Goodwin, National Institute of Mental Health, Clinical Psycho-biology Branch, 9000 Rockville Pike, Building 10, Room 4S239, Bethesda, MD 20205, USA

3.4
ECT, mood and hormones

M. FINK

ABSTRACT

From the experience of more than four decades, we find that the
repeated and spaced induction of seizures (convulsive therapy) relieves the symptoms of severe depressive mood disorders, particularly
those with vegetative symptoms. Bilateral seizures are evidence of
brain stem stimulation, reflecting the cerebral biochemical events
which are the basis for a therapeutic result. Two recent threads in
studies of depression provide the basis for a hypothesis of the action
of convulsive therapy. Patients with severe depression demonstrate
neuroendocrine abnormalities, particularly in tests of hypothalamic
function. These functions return to normal with ECT. Some peptides
which originate or are found in high concentrations in hypothalamic
structures have both behavioural (extra-endocrine) effects and diffuse
cerebral distributions. It is probable that the antidepressant efficacy
of convulsive therapy results from the increased release and more
widespread distribution of peptides with behavioural effects. Such a
hypothesis provides a basis for clinical trials of centrally active
peptides in cases of endogenous depression.

INTRODUCTION

Convulsive therapy is an effective empirical treatment for endogenous
depression. It has been extensively studies since its introduction in 1934,
and it has been found to be more effective than other available therapies,

particularly antidepressant drugs and psychotherapies.* Despite its demonstrated efficacy, its practice remains outside the main stream of clinical practice and receives little consideration in modern psychiatric research.

It has undergone many modifications in its 40-year history; so much so, that the present usage is hardly similar in its procedures to the original treatment, reflecting it mainly in its name and the antipathy that it arouses. Many modifications have been made to reduce the incidence of complications. In the course of this experience, we have learned much of what is essential for the therapeutic process.

Concurrently, studies of the brain as both a source of hormones and an object of their influence have provided additional information about human behaviour.

These two sets of data—the efficacy of convulsive therapy in modifying behaviour, and the developments in psychoneuroendocrinology—can be brought together for a hypothesis of the mode of action and as a basis for the search for a pharmacologic substitute for convulsive therapy.

CONVULSIVE THERAPY

In usage, convulsive therapy has changed from an indiscriminate symptomatic procedure with little specificity, to one of high specificity for patients with severe endogenous depression. Examinations of its clinical results find the treatment most effective in cases of psychotic depression, usually requiring 4 to 9 seizures (an average of 7 seizures) for prolonged antidepressant effects. In patients with depression, convulsive therapy is more effective than the available drug therapies, particularly in reducing the incidence of death.

While patients with mania also respond, they usually require more seizures. In patients with schizophrenia, favourable results are usually achieved with 12 to 20 seizures, often at daily intervals. Convulsive therapy is no longer a principal treatment of schizophrenia, being reserved for those patients for whom other regimens have clearly failed. In our present selection of suitable cases, it is the severity of depression, suicidal features, retardation, and the degree of vegetative symptoms that provide the principal indications.

In the diagnosis of depression, vegetative symptoms distinguish the endogenous form from other types of depression. The severity of anorexia, refusal of food, and weight loss, insomnia and early morning awakening, decreased libido, and decreased bodily secretions, with amenorrhea, constipation, and lack of crying are usually cited as the best criteria for a good clinical result with ECT. These symptoms are most often found among

---

* The citations for the references to efficacy, physiology, chemistry, neuroendocrine effects, and theories of ECT are to be found in Fink, M. (1979). *Convulsive Therapy: Theory and Practice* (New York: Raven Press). Only those of special relevance to psychoneuroendocrine research are cited in the present instance.

depressed patients with diagnoses of bipolar or unipolar affective disorder, involutional depression, depression in the elderly, and some types of postpartum psychoses.

In its history, both chemical and electrical inductions of seizures were examined. The comparisons of pentylenetetrazol (Metrazol) and of flurothyl (Indokolon) with ECT found the inductions to be equivalent in efficacy, although ECT was clearly safer and easier to administer. Some authors enquired whether subconvulsive currents were clinically as effective as convulsive, and reported that subconvulsive applications were not therapeutic. Others noted that longer seizures (more than 25 seconds) were more effective than shorter.

Some clinicians induced Jacksonian or unilateral motor seizures, and found that such incomplete seizures were clinically ineffective. Others induced bilateral grand mal seizures using electrical currents delivered through unilateral (one side of the scalp) electrodes to the non-dominant hemisphere. They found that improvement was equivalent to seizures induced through bilateral electrodes, although the amnesia and aphasia were significantly reduced. Today such inductions through unilateral electrodes are favoured.

Amnesia is a common sequel to seizures in man, varying in extent and duration. It may be reduced by increasing the time between seizures, by placing electrodes on the non-dominant side of the head, and by hyperoxygenation without reducing therapeutic efficacy. The incidence of fractures following convulsions may be lessened by inducing muscle paralysis with succinylcholine (Anectine). Apprehension and the fear of the treatments may be diminished by sedation and anaesthesia. While barbiturate or benzodiazepine sedation will raise the seizure threshold requiring greater amounts of electrical energy for a successful induction, their use does not impair clinical efficacy. Similarly, the changes in blood pressure and in cardiac rate occurring during a seizure can be lessened by atropine. These modifications (anaesthesia, oxygenation, type of induction, electrode placement) affect the safety and side effects of ECT, but contribute little to the antidepressant efficacy.

The factor of time must also be considered. While successful treatment in depressed patients requires 4 to 9 seizures, it was not always clear how frequently the seizures should be applied. Various spacings were tried, from multiple seizures (up to 8) within a few minutes, to seizures spaced from a few hours to a week. For example, the efficacy of 4 to 8 seizures at 2–5-minute intervals in one sitting was examined, but few patients responded, with most still requiring additional seizures in 6 to 14 days for a successful course. These experiences demonstrated that the shorter the interval, the greater the degree of amnesia. Present usage finds seizures at intervals of 48 to 72 hours to yield a favourable balance between amnesia and clinical efficacy.

These experiences identify repeated bilateral cerebral seizures at intervals of days as essential for a lasting behavioural response.

Other observations should be considered in understanding the convulsive therapy process. During convulsive therapy, plasma, cerebrospinal fluid (CSF) and urinary calcium levels fall, with a peak effect after 5 to 7 spaced seizures. The levels and turnover rates of brain catecholamines increase, achieving persistent measurable levels after 4 to 6 seizures. There is also a persistent increase in the permeability of the blood–brain barrier.

NEUROENDOCRINE CONSIDERATIONS

The greatest behavioural improvement after convulsive therapy occurs in patients with endogenous depression and severe vegetative symptoms. In such cases, neuroendocrine tests are often abnormal. The release of growth hormone (GH) by hypoglycaemia, l-dopa, and thyrotrophin (TSH) is either reduced or lacking (Gregoire et al., 1977; Kendler and Davis, 1977). Thyrotrophin releasing hormone (TRH) normally stimulates the liberation of pituitary TSH, and this response is blunted in severe depression (Loosen et al., 1978). The secretion of cortisol is elevated, its phasic rhythmicity lost, and dexamethasone fails to suppress its secretion (Carroll and Mendels, 1976; Carroll, Greden and Feinberg, 1980). Other studies have found the hypothalamic–pituitary–adrenal, hypothalamic–pituitary–thyroid, and hypothalamic–pituitary–gonadal axes deficient in severe depressive states (Brambilla et al., 1978).

Not only do patients with endogenous depression show these neuroendocrine dysfunctions, but the functions revert to normal with convulsive therapy. The abnormalities in GH release (Gregoire et al., 1977; Kendler and Davis, 1977), TSH response to TRH (Kirkegaard and Smith, 1978; Kirkegaard and Bjørum, 1980), and the levels of cortisol and response to dexamethasone (Sachar, 1976) all respond with resolution of the depressive syndrome (Dysken et al., 1979; Albala and Greden, 1980). These observations encourage the speculations that hypothalamic-pituitary dysfunction is a feature of the endogenous depressive syndrome, and that successful antidepressant therapy results in normalization of these functions.

While many seek to relate hormonal changes to behaviour in patients with schizophrenia, the greatest abnormalities in tests of neuroendocrine integrity are reported in cases of endogenous depression. Furthermore, these functions return to normal patterns after successful ECT. The predictive value of vegetative symptoms for a favourable outcome in ECT also points to a central role for diencephalic functions in the process.

A connection between biogenic amine theories of the mode of action of antidepressant drugs and neuroendocrine theories may be made by examining the modulation of the release of hypothalamic hormones by biogenic amines. Production of adrenocorticotrophic hormone (ACTH) increases with increased serotonin and acetylcholine activity. GH secretion increases with alpha-adrenergic or dopamine stimulation, and is reduced with beta-adrenergic stimulation (Ettigi and Brown, 1977). Acetylcholine, 5-hydroxytrypt-amine, and angiotensin II release corticotrophin releasing hormone from the isolated hypothalamus of the rat, while noradrenaline and glycine decrease its production. Dopamine, adrenaline, and histamine fail to alter its production (Buckingham and Hodges, 1977).

A NEUROENDOCRINE HYPOTHESIS

Can these diverse observations be accommodated into a testable hypothesis to explain the antidepressant efficacy of convulsive therapy? The evidence that hypothalamic dysfunction is a feature of an endogenous depressive psychosis is increasingly persuasive, and encourages the following speculation regarding the mode of action of convulsive therapy.

Hypothalamic dysfunction is central to endogenous depressive disease. Convulsive therapy increases the release and cerebral distribution of substances (most probably peptides) from the hypothalamus which modify the mood and behaviour associated with mood disturbances.

This speculation is consistent with the available physiological data. Generalized seizures with bilateral cerebral representation arise from basal centrencephalic nuclei. The slowing of EEG frequencies and increased amplitudes and burst patterns seen in the inter-seizure and seizure records are bilateral, reflecting biochemical changes in centrencephalic structures. This is true whether the seizures are induced chemically or electrically, through unilateral or bilateral electrodes. Biogenic amine activity increases transiently after one seizure, but persists after 4 to 6 seizures. Normally, hypothalamic and pituitary hormones are found largely outside intracerebral flow patterns; increasing the permeability of the blood–brain barrier, as occurs in ECT, increases their availability to brain tissues. And the intracellular movement of calcium, necessary for the discharge of hormones, is typical in the ECT process.

The measurement of the behavioural effects of hypothalamic peptides is a new thread in behavioural research. Much of the data is found in animal studies, but some substances have been examined in man with encouraging results (Table 1). While none has clear antidepressant activity, their behavioural effects are striking. Behavioural alerting, transient euphoria, and antidepressant efficacy have been reported for TRH (Prange *et al.*, 1978; Kastin *et al.*, 1976) and MIF-1 (Ehrensing and Kastin, 1978 and 1974). The mood altering effects of TRH are seen in cases of depression and not in those of schizophrenia (Prange, *et al.*, 1978; Kastin, *et al.*, 1976). The central effects of TRH and MIF-1 are reflected directly in quantitative EEG studies, which have found both compounds to elicit profiles similar to such psychostimulant compounds as dextroamphetamine (Itil, 1974). TRG is widely distributed in rat brain (Winokur and Utiger, 1974).

While far from compelling, recent reports have found β-endorphin (Kline *et*

Table 1   Peptides with possible behavioural effects in man

Peptide	Code	Citations
Thyrotrophin releasing factor	TRH	Kastin et al.. 1978 and 1976; Prange et al., 1978; Ehrensing et al.. 1974; Itil. 1974
Melanocyte stimulating hormone (MSH) release inhibiting factor	MIF-1	Ehrensing and Kastin. 1978 and 1974; Kastin et al.. 1978; Itil. 1974
Vasopressin		Legros et al.. 1978; Oliveros et al.. 1978
Adrenocorticotrophic hormone (ACTH)$_{4\ 10}$ (α-MSH)	OI-63	Miller et al.. 1977
β-endorphin		Catlin et al.. in press; Gerner et al.. 1980; Kline et al.. 1977
Des-Tyr-γ-endorphin	GK-78	Verhoeven et al.. 1979
Methionine-enkephalin analogue	FK33-824	Krebs and Roubicek. 1979; Nedophil and Rütter, 1979

al., 1977) and des-Tyr-γ-endorphin (Verhoeven et al., 1979) to be clinically active. The first reports of β-endorphin claimed both antidepressant and antipsychotic effects (Kline et al.. 1977). but a more recent study emphasizes its antidepressant activity (Catlin et al., in press; Gerner et al., 1980). ACTH, somatostatin, and the peptide fragments ACTH$_{4-10}$ and α-MSH stimulate measurable effects on learning and memory (Miller et al., 1977; de Wied, 1969).

Plasma peptide levels increase with ECT. CSF levels of β-endorphin-like immunoreactivity were not measurably increased pre-treatment in schizophrenic patients. but the plasma levels increased 10 minutes after ECT (Emrich et al., 1979). In another study. the plasma levels of arginine-vasopressin were elevated 5 and 15 minutes after a seizure (Raskind et al., 1979). Plasma prolactin levels increase immediately after a seizure. both in depressed and schizophrenic patients. with a return to baseline in 24 hours (Meco et al.. 1978; O'Dea et al., 1978; Öhman et al., 1976; Arato et al., 1980). While these changes in néurohormones may not be directly implicated in the therapeutic process. they demonstrate that peptide release is a feature of repeated seizures.

Further evidence of the persistent effects of ECT on hypothalamic–pituitary function is seen in a particularly instructive clinical case reported by Pitts and Patterson (1979). A severely depressed male patient. responsive to ECT, found that dexamethasone induced a euphoria which allowed him to function. He took dexamethasone chronically and developed hypothalamic–hypopituitarism (CRF-ACTH type). This syndrome persisted even after withdrawal from dexamethasone. Recurrent depression led to re-assessment and on endocrine tests he showed no response to metyrapone. indicating persistent suppression of hypothalmic–pituitary function. Another course of ECT (17 bilateral treatments) resulted in some relief of depression with a persistent return of responsivity to metyrapone (four- to five-fold increase in the serum cortisol and 24-hour urinary output of 17-hydroxysteroids). The response has remained normal for two years of the follow-up after treatment.

This hypothesis encourages our belief that the enthusiastic search for endogenous ligands with behavioural effects may yield substances specifically able to relieve the symptoms of endogenous depression. Present psychoneuro-endocrine research focuses on the effects of peptides in cases of schizophrenia. This interest is based on the thin threads that naloxone reduces hallucinations in schizophrenic patients, that β-endorphin produces cataplexy in mice, and that des-Try-γ-endorphin shows a pharmacological profile similar to that of haloperidol. In contrast, the threads for a relationship between neuroendo-crine change and endogenous depression seem more secure. We find convul-sive therapy to be a specific therapy for endogenous depression, a syndrome in which neuroendocrine abnormalities are commonly present and are reversed by successful treatment. A centrencephalic seizure increases the blood–brain barrier permeability as well as the intracellular movement of calcium ions, thereby increasing the release and distribution of hypothalamic peptides. Some peptides of hypothalamic origin have demonstrated cerebral effects, cerebral distributions, increase in CSF with ECT, and alter mood in psychi-atric patients. If these analyses resemble reality, it is probable that peptides will be found to reverse the pathophysiology of endogenous depression and to replace the present complex procedures of convulsive therapy (Fink and Ottosson. 1980).

References

Albala. A. A. and Greden. J. F. (1980). Serial dexamethasone suppression tests in affective disorders. *Am. J. Psychiat.*. **137**. 383

Arato. M.. Erdos. A.. Kurcz. M.. Vermes. I. and Fekete. M. (1980). Studies on the prolactin response induced by electro convulsive therapy in schizophrenics. *Acta Psychiat. Scand.* **61**. 239

Brambilla. F.. Smeraldi. E.. Sacchetti. E.. Negri. E.. Cocchi. D. and Müller. E. E. (1978). Deranged anterior pituitary responsiveness to hypothalmic hormones in depressed patients. *Arch. Gen. Psychiat.*. **35**. 1231

Buckingham. J. C. and Hodges. J. R. (1977). Production of corticotrophin releasing hormone by the isolated hypothalamus of the rat. *J. Physiol.*. **272**. 469

Carroll. B. J.. Greden. J. F. and Feinberg. M. (1980). Neuroendocrine disturbances and the diagnosis and aetiology of endogenous depression. *Lancet*. **1**. 321

Carroll. B. J. and Mendels. J. (1976). Neuroendocrine regulation in affective disorders. In E. J. Sachar (ed.). *Hormones. Behaviour and Psychopathology*. pp. 193–224. (New York: Raven Press)

Catlin. D. H.. Poland. R. E.. Gorelick. D. A.. Gerner. R. H.. Hui. K. K.. Rubin. R. T. and Li. C. H. (1981). Intravenous infusion of β-endorphin increases serum prolactin but not growth hormone on cortisol. in depressed subjects and withdrawing methadone addicts. *Arch. Gen. Psychiat.* (in press)

Dysken. M. W.. Pandey. G. N.. Chang. S. S.. Hicks. R.. and Davis. J. M. (1979). Serial post dexamethasone cortisol levels in a patient undergoing ECT. *Am. J. Psychiat.*. **136**. 1328

Ehrensing. R. H. and Kastin. A. J. (1978). Dose-related biphasic effect of prolyl-leucyl-glycinamide (MIF-1) in depression. *Am. J. Psychiat.*. **135**. 562

Ehrensing. R. H. and Kastin. A. J. (1974). Melanocyte-stimulating hormone-release inhibiting hormone as an anti-depressant: A pilot study. *Arch. Gen. Psychiat.*. **30**. 63

Ehrensing. R. H.. Kastin. A. J.. Schalch. D. S.. Friesen. H.. Vargas. R. and Schally. A. V. (1974).

Affective state and thyrotropin and prolactin response after repeated injections of thyrotropic releasing hormone in depressed patients. *Am. J. Psychiat.*, **161**, 714

Emrich, H. M., Höllt, V., Kissling, W., Fischler, M., Lapse, H., Heinemann, H., v. Zerssen, D. and Herz, A. (1979). β-Endorphin-like immunoreactivity in cerebrospinal fluid and plasma of patients with schizophrenia and other neuropsychiatric disorders. *Pharmakopsychiat. Neuro-Psychopharm.*, **12**, 269

Ettigi, P. G. and Brown, G. M. (1977). Psychoneuroendocrinology of affective disorder: An overview. *Am. J. Psychiat.*, **131**, 493–501

Fink. M. and Ottosson. J.-O. (1980). A theory of convulsive therapy in endogenous depression: Significance of hypothalamic functions. *Psychiatry Research*, **2**, 49

Gerner. R. H.. Catlin. D. H.. Gorelick. D. A.. Hui, K. K. and Li, C. H. (1980). β-Endorphin: Intravenous infusion causes behavioral change in psychiatric inpatients. *Arch. Gen. Psychiat.*, **37**. 642

Gregoire, F., Brauman, H., de Buck, R. and Corvilain, J. (1977). Hormone release in depressed patients before and after recovery. *Psychoneuroendocrinology.*, **2**, 303

Itil, T. M. (1974). The neurophysiological models in the development of psychotropic hormones. In *Psychotropic Action of Hormones*. pp. 53–77. (New York: Spectrum)

Kastin, A. J., Coy, D. H., Schally. A. V. and Miller, L. (1978). Peripheral administration of hypothalamic peptides results in CNS changes. *Pharmacol. Res. Commun.*. **10**. 293

Kastin, A. J., Schally, A. V., Gonzalez-Barcena, D., Zurate. A., Besser. M. and Hall, R. (1976). Clinical studies with hypothalamic peptides. In A. L. C. Salgado, R. Fernandez-Duragno and J. G. Lopez del Campo (eds). *Applications and Clinical Uses of Hypothalamic Hormones*. pp. 235–243. (New York: American Elsevier)

Kendler, K. S. and Davis, K. L. (1977). Elevated corticosteroids as a possible cause of abnormal neuroendocrine functions in depressive illness. *Commun. Psychopharmacol.*. **3**, 183

Kirkegaard. C. and Bjørum. N. (1980). TSH responses to TRH in endogenous depression. *Lancet*. **1**. 152

Kirkegaard, C. and Smith, E. (1978). Continuation therapy in endogenous depression controlled by changes in the TRH stimulation test. *Psychol. Med.*. **8**. 501

Kline, N. S., Li, C. H., Lehmann, H. E.. Lajtha. A.. Laski, E. and Cooper, T. (1977). β-endorphin-induced changes in schizophrenic and depressed patients. *Arch. Gen. Psychiat.*, **34**, 1111

Krebs, E. and Roubicek, J. (1979). EEG and clinical profile of a synthetic analogue of methionine-enkephalin FK 33–824. *Pharmakopsychiat. Neuro-Psychopharm.*, **12**. 86

Legros, J. J., Gilot, P., Seron, X., Claessens, J., Adam. A.. Moeglen, J. M., Audibert. A. and Berchier, P. (1978). Influence of vasopressin on learning and memory. *Lancet*. **1**, 41

Loosen, P. T., Prange, A. J. and Wilson, I. C. (1978). Influence of cortisol on TRH-induced TSH responses in depression. *Am. J. Psychiat.*, **135**. 244

Meco, G., Casacchia, M., Carchedi, F., Falaschi, P., Rocco, A. and Frajese, G. (1978). Prolactin response to repeated electroconvulsive therapy in acute schizophrenia. *Lancet*. **1**, 999

Miller, L. H., Sandman, C. A. and Kastin, A. J. (1977). Neuropeptide influences on the brain and behaviour. *Advances in Biochemical Psychopharmacology*. vol. 17, p. 298. (New York: Raven Press)

Nedophil, N. and Rütter, E. (1979). Effects of the synthetic analogue of methionine enkephalin FK 33-824 on psychotic symptoms. *Pharmakopsychiatr. Neuro-Psychopharm.*. **12**. 277

O'Dea, J. P. K., Gould, D., Hallberg, M. and Wieland, R. G. (1978). Prolactin changes during electroconvulsive therapy. *Am. J. Psychiat.*. **135**. 609

Öhman, R., Balldin, J., Walinder, J. and Wallin, L. (1976). Prolactin response to electroconvulsive therapy. *Lancet*. **1**, 936

Oliveros, J. C., Jandali, M. K., Timsit-Berthier, M.. Remy, R., Benghezel, A.. Audibert. A. and Moeglen, J. M. (1978). Vasopressin in amnesia. *Lancet*. **1**. 42

Pitts, F. N. and Patterson, C. W. (1979). Electroconvulsive therapy for iatrogenic hypothalamic-hypopituitarism (CRF-ACTH type). *Am. J. Psychiat.*. **136**. 1074

Prange, A. J., Nemeroff, C. B. and Lipton, M. A. (1978). Behavioural effects of peptides: Basic and clinical studies. In M. A. Lipton, A. DiMascio and K. F. Killam (eds), *Psychopharmacology: A Generation of Progress*, pp. 441–463. (New York: Raven Press)

Raskind, M., Orenstein, H. and Weitzmann, R. E. (1979). Vasopressin in depression. *Lancet*, 1, 164

Sachar. E. J. (1976). *Hormones, Behaviour and Psychopathology*. (New York: Raven Press)

Verhoeven. W. M., van Praag. H. A., van Ree, J. M. and de Wied, D. (1979). Improvement of schizophrenic patients treated with [Des-Tyr¹]-γ-endorpin (DTγE). *Arch. Gen. Psychiat.*, 36, 294

de Wied, D. (1969). Effects of peptide hormones on behaviour. In W. F. Ganong and L. Martini (eds.), *Frontiers in Neuroendocrinology*, pp. 97–140. (New York: Oxford Press)

Winokur, A. and Utiger, R. O. (1974). Thyrotropin-releasing hormone: Regional distribution in rat brain. *Science*, 185, 267

Address for correspondence

Professor M. Fink, State University of New York at Stony Brook, Health Sciences Center School of Medicine, Department of Psychiatry and Behavioral Science, Stony Brook, NY 11794, USA

3.5
Neurohypophysial peptides and ethanol

H. RIGTER and J. C. CRABBE

ABSTRACT

Ethanol was chronically administered to mice to induce tolerance and physical dependence. Ethanol treatment was stopped and withdrawal severity and residual tolerance was measured.

Vasopressin and its fragment des-Gly⁰-AVP (DGAVP) were found to enhance functional tolerance to ethanol, without changing responses of naive animals to acutely administered ethanol. The efficacy of vasopressin in modulating tolerance was not restricted to a particular effect of ethanol. The efficacy of DGAVP, a peptide with greatly reduced peripheral endocrine activity, suggests that the effect of vasopressin-like peptides on tolerance is mediated within the central nervous system. Since restricting peptide treatment to the period of tolerance was effective in increasing residual tolerance, DGAVP presumably influences the development of tolerance to ethanol. It is possible that vasopressin-like peptides also affect the decay of tolerance.

Continuous infusion of DGAVP throughout the induction of dependence and testing for withdrawal exacerbated withdrawal convulsions. This effect is not likely to be due to subconvulsive activity of the peptide by itself nor to changes in blood or brain levels of ethanol. The exacerbation of withdrawal may reflect modulation of physical dependence by DGAVP.

Vasopressin-like peptides have also been reported to enhance acquisition of ethanol drinking by rats. This finding suggests that these peptides may facilitate learning components involved in the development and decay of ethanol responses. It remains to be seen whether this explanation can account for the effects of vasopressin and DGAVP on tolerance and withdrawal.

INTRODUCTION

Ethanol affects the release of the neurohypophysial hormone vasopressin (cf. review by Crabbe and Rigter, 1980). It is not known whether changes in levels of endogenous vasopressin influence further actions of ethanol. This possibility is suggested by the results of studies reviewed in this chapter. These studies were inspired by the earlier work of Krivoy *et al.* (1974) and of van Ree and de Wied (1980) who found that vasopressin-like peptides modulate the development of tolerance to and physical dependence on morphine. It now appears that these peptides similarly affect the development of tolerance to and physical dependence on ethanol and, additionally, also affect the acquisition of ethanol drinking.

Before presenting the experimental data, the phenomena to be discussed will be briefly defined (cf. Rigter and Crabbe, 1980). Tolerance to ethanol is often conceptually divided into acute and protracted (chronic) tolerance. The studies reported here deal with the latter type. Repeated or prolonged exposure to ethanol leads to the development of tolerance, defined as the diminution of the initial effect of ethanol and best illustrated by a lateral shift in the dose–response curve. Prolonged exposure to ethanol can also lead to the development of physical dependence, as evidenced by the occurrence of characteristic withdrawal signs upon cessation of ethanol administration. In rodents, the most frequently studied withdrawal sign is handling-induced convulsions. Tolerance and physical dependence develop in parallel but are not necessarily expressions of the same process or processes. Another phenomenon featuring in this chapter is ethanol preference. Some strains of rodents may prefer ethanol over water, but generally animals do not drink sufficient amounts of ethanol for marked tolerance or physical dependence to occur. This ethanol preference, therefore, cannot be strictly equated with alcoholism. An adequate animal model of alcoholism would require the voluntary selection of intoxicating amounts of ethanol, leading to physical dependence in at least a substantial percentage of the animals (Lester and Freed, 1973). Unfortunately, such models are not yet available for routine use.

NEUROHYPOPHYSIAL PEPTIDES AND TOLERANCE TO ETHANOL

Hoffman *et al.* (1978) were the first to report effects of neurohypophysial hormones on tolerance to ethanol. These investigators rendered mice tolerant to and dependent on ethanol by forcing them to drink a 7% ethanol liquid diet for seven days. At the end of this period ethanol was abruptly withdrawn. Animals were reported to exhibit withdrawal signs. Each three days thereafter, residual tolerance to ethanol was assessed by administering an acute 3 g/kg intraperitoneal dose of ethanol and measuring the duration of the loss of the righting reflex (sleep time) and hypothermia. Six days after withdrawal the animals were no longer tolerant to the effects of ethanol when compared with controls which had not been chronically treated with ethanol.

Some mice were given daily subcutaneous injections of 10 μg [Arg^8]-vasopressin (AVP), oxytocin or saline during the drinking period and for nine days after withdrawal, excluding the day of withdrawal. Animals treated with AVP retained tolerance to ethanol for as long as the peptide was administered. When peptide administration was stopped, at nine days, tolerance gradually subsided over the following six days. Thus, vasopressin appeared to maintain tolerance during the period of its administration. Thereafter, it had no residual effect on the rate at which tolerance was lost. Oxytocin was ineffective in this study. Neither peptide had any effect on temperature in animals not chronically treated with ethanol.

The efficacy of AVP in delaying decay of tolerance could have been due to a peripheral effect rather than to an effect mediated by the central nervous system. One—preliminary—approach for the study of this issue is to examine des-Gly^9-AVP, a vasopressin fragment sharing behavioural effects with the parent hormone in spite of having reduced pressor, antidiuretic, oxytocin- and corticotrophin-releasing properties (de Wied, 1971). If this fragment could also affect ethanol tolerance in the same manner as AVP, it would suggest a central site of action, although more research would be required to definitely confirm this suggestion. Our studies with des-Gly^9-AVP citrate (DGAVP) yielded evidence that this peptide influences ethanol tolerance in a fashion similar to the parent hormone. Hoffman and Tabakoff have obtained comparable data with a similar vasopressin fragment (personal communication).

In our studies of tolerance (Rigter et al., 1980), we rendered mice physically dependent by forcing them to inhale ethanol vapour for three days and treating them daily with an inhibitor of ethanol metabolism, pyrazole. The inhalation technique has the advantage of offering excellent control over blood levels of ethanol, although the results may be confounded by the fact that pyrazole may have effects on the central nervous system. However, when used with appropriate controls, the effects of pyrazole may be discounted. One or more days after withdrawal of dependent mice from ethanol, we injected the animals with an acute intraperitoneal challenge dose of 3 g/kg ethanol and measured the resulting drop in body temperature 45 minutes after injection. Naive mice which had not been made dependent were used as controls to assess initial sensitivity to the challenge dose of ethanol. It was shown that one day after withdrawal marked residual tolerance to the hypothermic effect of ethanol remained, but that tolerance had dissipated two days after with-drawal. The tolerance measured was probably functional since we did not find evidence of faster metabolism of ethanol one day after withdrawal.

We explored the efficacy of DGAVP in modulating tolerance by administer-ing this peptide via Alzet® osmotic minipumps. Subcutaneously implanted minipumps deliver fluid at a constant rate for approximately 8–9 days. In the first study, minipumps were implanted on Day 1, before the induction of dependence, and left in the mice throughout testing for withdrawal and tolerance. Minipumps contained either saline or a solution of DGAVP (release rate: 0.8 μg/hour). The results of this experiment indicate that con-tinuous infusion of DGAVP enhanced residual tolerance to the hypothermic effect of ethanol measured one day after withdrawal, i.e. all dependent-withdrawn mice exhibited tolerance compared with naive control animals, but

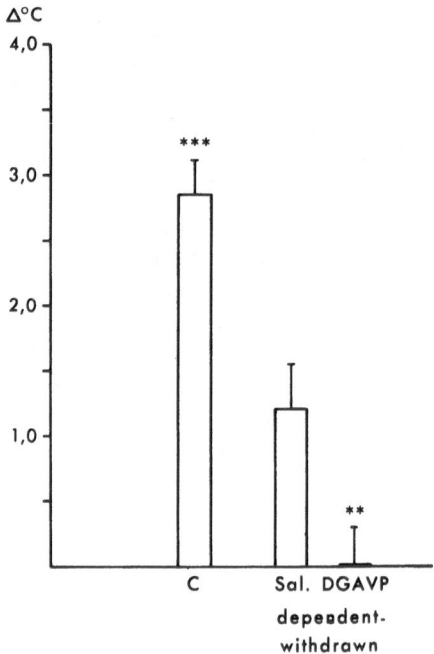

Figure 1   Enhancement of residual tolerance to the hypothermic effect of a challenge dose (3 g/kg i.p.) of ethanol produced by continuous infusion of DGAVP (0.8 μg/hour). Δ°C represents the difference (mean ± SEM) between base line rectal temperature, recorded 5 min before acute administration of ethanol, and temperature measured 45 min after acute treatment with ethanol. C: non-dependent naive control group (20 mice). Sal. and DGAVP: dependent-withdrawn mice bearing minipumps with saline ($n = 28$) or DGAVP ($n = 7$). respectively. Minipumps were implanted prior to induction of physical dependence. Tolerance was assessed one day after withdrawal from ethanol. $**p < 0.01$, $***p < 0.001$. relative to Sal. group. (Reproduced from H. Rigter and J. C. Crabbe, Jr (1980). In Sandler. M. (ed.) *The Psychopharmacology of Alcohol.* Courtesy of Raven Press, New York.)

the degree of tolerance was more marked in the peptide-treated mice. In fact, in this particular study, DGAVP-treated mice showed virtually no hypothermia in response to the challenge dose of ethanol (Figure 1). In the next experiment this effect of DGAVP was confirmed. However, this study also demonstrated that the effect of DGAVP was lost when testing for tolerance was delayed two days following withdrawal (Figure 2). The latter finding seems to be inconsistent with the protracted activity of AVP reported by Hoffman *et al.* One apparent difference between our results and those of Hoffman and co-workers is the rapid loss of residual tolerance observed for our placebo-treated mice, and perhaps this may account for the difference in time course of efficacy of DGAVP in the two investigations.

In subsequent studies we administered DGAVP during restricted portions of the experiment in order to try to distinguish peptide effects on development from those on decay of tolerance. First, we examined the effect of treatment with DGAVP during dependence induction. Minipumps were removed at the time of withdrawal and tolerance was assessed one day later. Several doses of

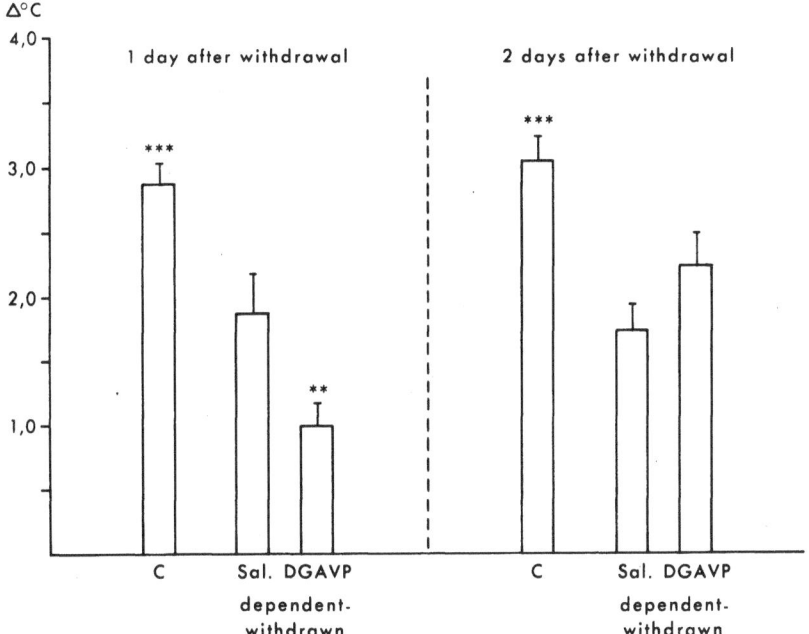

Figure 2 Time course of the effect of continuously infused DGAVP on residual tolerance to the hypothermic effect of 3 g/kg i.p. ethanol. Tolerance was assessed 1 day (left panel) or 2 days (right panel) after withdrawal. Minipumps containing saline or DGAVP (release rate: 0.8 μg/hour) were implanted prior to induction of physical dependence. C: control group ($n = 20$); Sal.: saline group ($n = 24$–25); DGAVP: peptide groups ($n = 14$ each). **$p < 0.01$. ***$p < 0.001$. relative to Sal. group. (Reproduced from H. Rigter and J. C. Crabbe. Jr (1980). In Sandler. M. (ed.) *The Psychopharmacology of Alcohol.* Courtesy of Raven Press. New York)

peptide were used. The results showed increased tolerance in mice which had been treated with 0.08 or 0.8 µg/hour (Figure 3). In a second study, restriction of DGAVP treatment to the period of testing for withdrawal and tolerance tended to enhance tolerance, but none of the differences was statistically significant (Figure 3). It should be noted, however, that in a recent series of experiments Hoffman *et al.* (1979) found AVP to be effective in enhancing residual tolerance when peptide treatment was restricted to the period of testing for tolerance. Taken together these results suggest that DGAVP facilitates development (or 'acquisition') of tolerance, but that evidence that it inhibits decay of tolerance is as yet weak.

Control experiments demonstrated that the enhancement of tolerance by DGAVP was probably not due to an interaction with pyrazole or to changes in blood levels of ethanol. Treatment with pyrazole for three days did not affect ethanol-induced hypothermia in non-dependent mice. Moreover, continuous infusion of DGAVP had no effect on body temperature, either before or after

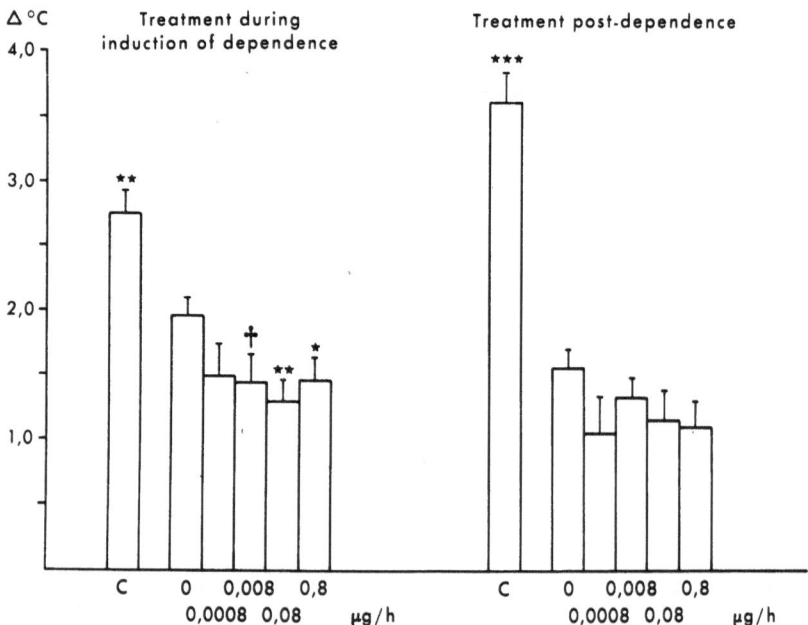

Figure 3 Enhancement of residual tolerance to the hypothermic effect of ethanol: effect of treatment with DGAVP during restricted portions of the experiment. Left panel: groups of 17–20 mice were implanted with minipumps containing saline (0) or different concentrations of DGAVP (release rates: 0.0008–0.8 µg/hour). Minipumps were implanted prior to induction of dependence and removed at the time of withdrawal from ethanol. Right panel: groups of 14–16 mice were implanted with minipumps at the time of withdrawal. In both studies testing for tolerance was performed one day after withdrawal. $\dagger p < 0.01$, $*p < 0.05$, $**p < 0.01$, $***p < 0.001$, relative to saline group (0). (Reproduced from Rigter *et al.* (1980). Courtesy of Elsevier/North Holland Biomedical Press, Amsterdam)

acute administration of ethanol, either in pyrazole-treated or in placebo-treated non-dependent animals. Finally, continuous infusion with the peptide did not change blood ethanol levels measured in dependent-withdrawn mice after an acute challenge dose of ethanol.

These data raise a number of questions which should be considered in future studies. More time course studies are needed to distinguish between the effects of DGAVP on the development of tolerance and those influencing its decay. Also, the effect of the peptide on ethanol tolerance should be further characterized by assessing whether parallel shifts in ethanol dose–response curves occur. The generality of the peptide effect could be tested by determining a possible action of DGAVP on the development and/or maintenance of ethanol-barbiturate cross tolerance. Future experiments should also determine the possible involvement of the central nervous system in the effects of DGAVP and localize the site or sites of action of this peptide. Finally, one obvious goal of future research should be the determination of the structural requirements of vasopressin and related peptides necessary for the expression of the effect on tolerance.

NEUROHYPOPHYSIAL PEPTIDES AND PHYSICAL DEPENDENCE ON ETHANOL

Hoffman *et al.* (1978) did not find evidence of an effect of AVP or oxytocin on withdrawal symptoms in mice but their study was not designed to test this notion explicitly. We have undertaken an investigation of the ability of DGAVP to modulate the development and decay of physical dependence in mice as measured by changes in severity or incidence of withdrawal convulsions. The results from this investigation show that the vasopressin fragment exacerbates withdrawal convulsions (Rigter *et al.*, 1980).

The methods used to induce dependence were identical to those described in the section on tolerance. In fact, many of the mice used for assessment of tolerance were also employed to obtain measures of physical dependence. Thus, mice were rendered dependent on ethanol by application of the inhalation-pyrazole technique for 3 days and were abruptly withdrawn from ethanol on the fourth day. The severity of withdrawal was assessed by hourly checking of the severity of convulsions caused by picking the animal up by its tail or twirling it gently through 180 degrees. The severity of such convulsions increased gradually for several hours after withdrawal, peaking between 6 and 10 hours, and then gradually subsided. There was virtually no residual hyperexcitability 24 hours after withdrawal.

The development of physical dependence requires the prolonged presence of ethanol in the organism. We reasoned that in order to influence the development of physical dependence on ethanol DGAVP should be given both chronically and continuously. We therefore administered DGAVP

using minipumps. The rate of release of peptide was 0.8 µg/hour. Treatment
was started at the beginning of the induction of dependence and continued
throughout testing for withdrawal. Continuous administration of DGAVP
produced exacerbated convulsions throughout the course of the withdrawal
syndrome (Figure 4). The peptide enhanced the maximum intensity of withdrawal convulsions, as well as the cumulative score of withdrawal convulsions.

In order to distinguish between effects on the development of physical
dependence and those on its decay, we administered DGAVP during the
period of induction of physical dependence or during testing for withdrawal.
For the former purpose, minipumps containing saline or one of several
concentrations of DGAVP were implanted immediately prior to exposing the
animals to ethanol vapour and removed before withdrawal testing. Groups of
peptide-treated mice and the placebo group did not differ significantly with
respect to peak intensity of withdrawal convulsions nor to the cumulative
convulsion score across the testing period, although animals treated with a
dose of 0.08 µg peptide/hour tended to display higher convulsion scores. To
evaluate a possible effect of DGAVP on decay of physical dependence,
DGAVP was administered hourly by means of subcutaneous injections
throughout portions of the period of testing for withdrawal. A dose of

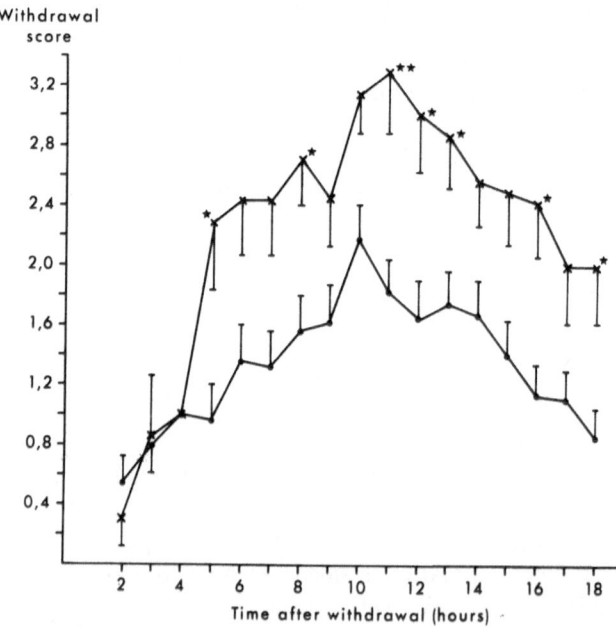

Figure 4   Graded withdrawal convulsions in dependent-withdrawn mice continuously infused
with saline ($n = 28$; bottom curve) or DGAVP (0.8 µg/hour; $n = 7$; top curve). Scores are
means $\pm$ SEM. *$p < 0.05$; **$p < 0.01$. relative to Sal. group. (Reproduced from Rigter *et al.*
(1980). Courtesy of Elsevier/North Holland Biomedical Press, Amsterdam)

10 μg per injection per mouse delayed the dissipation of the withdrawal syndrome. The effect became evident after the peak withdrawal score in placebo animals had been reached.

The data suggest that DGAVP facilitates the development and/or decay of physical dependence as evidenced by exacerbated withdrawal convulsions. Control studies demonstrated that this effect of the peptide probably cannot be attributed to changes in blood or brain levels of ethanol, nor to an interaction between the peptide and pyrazole. Continuous infusion with DGAVP (0.08 or 0.8 μg/hour) did not alter ethanol levels in the blood measured at the end of the period of dependence induction. Similarly, repeated subcutaneous injections of 10 μg DGAVP did not influence elimination of ethanol from blood or brain in mice withdrawn from ethanol. Pyrazole by itself sometimes produced weak convulsions in non-dependent mice but their frequency and intensity was far less than in dependent-withdrawn animals. Continuous infusion with DGAVP was ineffective in changing convulsion scores in non-dependent saline- or pyrazole-treated mice.

We also wondered if the efficacy of DGAVP could be due to covert neural excitatory properties of the peptide. In order to investigate this we administered the convulsive agent pentylenetetrazol to mice bearing minipumps with saline or DGAVP (0.8 μg/hour). The two groups did not differ with respect to the dose of pentylenetetrazol needed to produce clonic convulsions. Therefore, we did not find evidence of an interaction between the peptide and the convulsive agent. The fact that our usual DGAVP treatment regimens did not affect the behaviour of mice in an open field test also indicates that the peptide has no general stimulant action on the central nervous system under our experimental conditions.

It would thus appear that the effect of DGAVP is due to a direct action on some component of physical dependence. This tentative conclusion needs to be substantiated by future experiments. Further examination is also required of the relationship between the effects of DGAVP on physical dependence and those on tolerance. Another important question is whether the peptide affects some adaptive process underlying the development and/or decay of both physical dependence on and tolerance to ethanol, or whether these effects are independent. Structure-activity studies may aid in answering this question. We are presently investigating the effects of a number of vasopressin congeners on ethanol withdrawal convulsions. This investigation is not yet complete but preliminary findings suggest that oxytocin may also exacerbate withdrawal convulsions when repeatedly injected during testing for withdrawal.

Vasopressin-like peptides may be useful in providing insight into the acute development of tolerance and physical dependence in naive animals, and this would obviously be of great theoretical importance. However, we are also interested in the question of whether there is a way to affect the re-acquisition of physical dependence in organisms previously dependent on ethanol. To this end, we have subjected dependent-withdrawn mice to a second cycle of dependence induction and implanted minipumps before the start of this second cycle. Again DGAVP (0.8 µg/hour) exacerbated withdrawal con vulsions, but only in those mice which displayed low withdrawal scores in the first cycle (Rigter, unpublished data). Therefore, DGAVP appears also to facilitate the re-acquisition of physical dependence though perhaps in a smaller percentage of animals than initially.

ROLE OF LEARNING IN ETHANOL TOLERANCE AND PHYSICAL DEPENDENCE

The importance of hormones in the consolidation of newly learned experience and subsequent retrieval from memory is well documented (Rigter and Crabbe, 1979; van Ree et al., 1978; de Wied, 1971). In particular, vasopressin and related peptides enhance memory consolidation and retrieval whereas oxytocin exerts opposite effects (Bohus et al., 1978; van Ree et al., 1978; de Wied, 1971). Deficits in acquisition of new responses due to hypophysectomy, inherited vasopressin deficiency or the administration of amnesia-inducing treatments can be corrected by vasopressin and peptides such as DGAVP (Rigter and Crabbe, 1979; van Ree et al., 1978; de Wied, 1971). Moreover, the administration of vasopressin-like peptides shortly after a learning experience has frequently been found to improve retention in animals. Such post-trial efficacy probably reflects a specific effect on consolidation processes.

Given the evidence that vasopressin modulates memory, the question arises of whether the effects of DGAVP on ethanol tolerance and withdrawal are based on the same mechanism of action. There are indeed data suggesting that, among other factors, there may be a learning component in the development of drug tolerance and physical dependence. Most of the evidence is indirect (Crabbe and Rigter, 1979); the sorts of neurobiological manipulations that are known to alter learning ability and memory strength have also been reported to affect acquisition and retention of drug tolerance. More direct evidence stems from the demonstration that animals can learn to compensate for ethanol-induced behavioural impairments and that this learning contributes to the development of tolerance (LeBlanc et al., 1978). Tolerance to ethanol may also depend partly on the organism's learning to associate ethanol-induced cues with environmental cues (Hinson and Siegel, 1980). Evidence regarding a role of learning in the development of physical dependence is more equivocal, though the existence of a learning component is suggested by reports that in alcoholics the presence of environmental cues associated with prior alcohol use, or the taste of alcohol itself, can elicit withdrawal distress (Hinson and Siegel, 1980).

It thus seems possible that DGAVP and other vasopressin-like peptides affect tolerance to and physical dependence on ethanol by modulating some aspect of these processes which involve learning. Such an interpretation was made by van Ree and de Wied (1980) to account for the facilitatory effects of these peptides on tolerance to and physical dependence on morphine. However, one feature of our experiments may prove to be inconsistent with this possibility. Conceivably, learning may play a clear role in the development of tolerance to and physical dependence on ethanol if the ethanol is administered at spaced intervals so that animals are able to learn discrete stimulus–response associations. However, ethanol was administered continuously in our studies and, therefore, it seems more difficult, though not necessarily impossible, to specify discrete stimulus–response relations.

There is another argument against the unqualified acceptance of the view that the interaction of vasopressin-like peptides with ethanol responses reflects an effect on learning. One theory attempts to specify this learning component by assuming that during learning environmental cues are associated with the administration of ethanol (Hinson and Siegel, 1980). These cues then elicit compensatory responses that result in a weakening of (or 'tolerance' to) the consequences of ethanol administration. For instance, environmental cues may produce hyperthermia as a compensation for anticipated ethanol-induced hypothermia. We have obtained data suggesting that the development of this conditioned hyperthermia is not facilitated by DGAVP (Crabbe et al., 1980); surprisingly, DGAVP seems to block conditioned hyperthermia in mice repeatedly challenged with ethanol. Similarly, Niesink et al. (cited in van Ree and de Wied, 1980) found that DGAVP inhibited the development of a possibly different learning component of ethanol tolerance, 'behavioural augmentation'. However, it remains possible that other forms of learning also play a role in the development of tolerance and physical dependence (Le Blanc et al., 1978) and that these are the substrate of the facilitatory effects of vasopressin-like peptides.

In conclusion, there is a striking parallel between the effects of DGAVP and related peptides on development and decay of ethanol tolerance and withdrawal, on one hand, and the effects of these peptides on acquisition and extinction of conditioned behaviour, on the other. There is good evidence that the latter effects reflect modulation of memory. It is tempting to speculate that the effects on tolerance and withdrawal are based on the same mechanism of action. However, this working hypothesis remains to be specified before it can be adequately tested. At any rate, the fact that vasopressin-like peptides modulate tolerance to and physical dependence on both morphine and ethanol strongly suggests that these peptides influence some general process of adaptation in the face of chronic exposure to (addictive) compounds.

ALCOHOLISM

In view of the complexity of the clinical picture, it is not surprising that no completely satisfactory animal model of alcoholism is available (Lester and

Freed, 1973). Some inbred strains of mice and genetically selected lines of rats will drink alcohol by choice but they do not become intoxicated. Experimental manipulations may enhance the intake of alcohol but this excessive intake is usually not maintained on subsequent removal of these manipulations. Even the induction of physical dependence does not generally lead animals to persistently or episodically select intoxicating amounts of alcohol. Some of these issues are elegantly illustrated in the studies of Kalant and co-workers (Mucha and Kalant. 1979).

These investigators examined the effects of des-Gly^9-[Lys^8]-vasopressin (DGLVP) on the acquisition of an alcohol-drinking habit in rats. Sham-operated or hypophysectomized animals were forced to drink increasing concentrations of alcohol in water. Sham-operated rats treated with DGLVP accepted higher concentrations of alcohol during the training period and consequently showed higher amounts of daily alcohol intake (although probably not high enough to produce substantial tolerance or physical dependence). Hypophysectomized rats initially accepted alcohol, but within six days began to reject all but the lowest alcohol concentrations. DGLVP did not affect this pattern. On termination of training, animals were given the choice to drink either water or alcohol. Alcohol intake of sham-operated animals declined under free-choice conditions to about half their forced intake levels but relative group positions remained about the same. These findings indicate that DGLVP might have enhanced acquisition of (forced) alcohol drinking and, additionally, might have delayed the rate of extinction during the choice conditions. In a subsequent study (Mucha and Kalant. 1979), DGLVP, LVP and the tail amino acid sequence of oxytocin, Pro-Leu-Gly-amide (PLG), were examined. Both DGLVP and PLG enhanced alcohol acceptance when given during training, whereas LVP was ineffective at the doses used. DGLVP did not affect intake of alcohol after a final level of acceptance had been reached, supporting the view that the peptide facilitated initial acquisition of alcohol drinking rather than asymptotic acceptance levels.

The facilitated acquisition of alcohol drinking is consistent with the facilitatory effect of vasopressin-like peptides on acquisition (and extinction) of conditioned behaviour. However, it must be re-emphasized that this finding cannot be taken to predict an activity of vasopressin-like peptides in alcoholism. Van Ree and de Wied (1980) distinguish between two separate effects of vasopressin-like peptides on opiate-related responses. For example, DGAVP facilitated the development of tolerance to and physical dependence on morphine in their studies but, in contrast, impaired acquisition of *voluntary* self-administration of heroin in rats. The latter finding, of course, is of great clinical relevance. However, whether there are any clinical prospects for the use of DGAVP in alcoholism cannot be predicted from animal studies before appropriate models become available.

References

Bohus, B., Kovács, G. L. and de Wied, D. (1978). Oxytocin, vasopressin and memory: opposite effects on consolidation and retrieval processes. *Brain Res.*, **157**, 414

Crabbe, J. C. and Rigter, H. (1980). Hormones and ethanol. In H. Rigter and J. C. Crabbe (eds). *Alcohol: Studies on Tolerance and Dependence*, (Amsterdam: Elsevier/North-Holland Biomedical Press), pp. 291–313

Crabbe, J. C. and Rigter, H. (1979). Learning and the development of tolerance to and dependence on alcohol: the role of vasopressin-like peptides. *Trends Neurosci.*, **3**, 20

Crabbe, J. C., Rigter, H. and Kerbusch, S. (1980). Genetic analysis of tolerance to ethanol hypothermia in recombinant inbred mice: effect of des-glycinamide-arginine^8-vasopressin. *Behav. Genet.*, **10**, 139

Hinson, R. E. and Siegel, S. (1980). The contribution of Pavlovian conditioning to ethanol tolerance and dependence. In H. Rigter and J. C. Crabbe (eds). *Alcohol: Studies on Tolerance and Dependence*. (Amsterdam: Elsevier/North-Holland Biomedical Press)

Hoffman, P. L., Ritzmann, R. and Tabakoff. B. (1979). The influence of arginine vasopressin and oxytocin on ethanol dependence and tolerance. In M. Galanter (ed.). *Currents in Alcoholism*. vol. 5, pp. 5–16. (New York: Grune and Stratton)

Hoffman, P. L., Ritzmann, R. F., Walter, R. and Tabakoff, B. (1978). Arginine vasopressin maintains ethanol tolerance. *Nature*. **276**, 614

Krivoy, W. A., Zimmermann, E. and Lande, S. (1974). Facilitation of development of resistance to morphine analgesia by desglycinamide^9-lysine vasopressin. *Proc. Natl. Acad. Sci. (Wash.)*, **71**, 1852

LeBlanc, A. E., Poulos, C. X. and Cappell. H. D. (1978). Tolerance as a behavioural phenomenon: evidence from two experimental paradigms. In N. A. Krasnegor (ed.). *Behavioural Tolerance: Research and Treatment Implications*, pp. 72–89. (Rockwell: U.S. Government Printing Office, NIDA Research Monograph 18)

Lester, D. and Freed, E. X. (1973). Criteria for an animal model of alcoholism. *Pharmacol. Biochem. Behav.*, **1**, 103

Mucha, R. F. and Kalant, H. (1979). Effects of desglycinamide^9-lysine^8-vasopressin and prolyl-leucyl-glycinamide on oral ethanol intake in the rat. *Pharmacol. Biochem. Behav.*. **10**, 229

van Ree, J. M., Bohus, B., Versteeg, D. H. G. and de Wied, D. (1978). Neurohypophyseal principles and memory processes. *Biochem. Pharmacol.*. **27**, 1793

van Ree, J. M. and de Wied, D. (1980). Brain peptides and psychoactive drug effects. In Y. H. Israel *et al.* (eds). *Research Advances in Alcohol and Drug Problems*, vol. 6. (New York: Plenum Press). (In press)

Rigter, H. and Crabbe, J. C. (eds) (1980). *Alcohol: Studies on Tolerance and Dependence*. (Amsterdam: Elsevier/North-Holland Biomedical Press)

Rigter, H. and Crabbe. J. C. (1979). Modulation of memory by pituitary hormones and related peptides. *Vitam. Horm.*. **37**, 153

Rigter, H., Rijk, H. and Crabbe, J. C. (1980). Enhancement of tolerance to ethanol and severity of withdrawal in mice by a vasopressin fragment. *Eur. J. Pharmacol.*. **64**. 53

de Wied, D. (1971). Long-term effect of vasopressin on the maintenance of a conditioned avoidance response in rats. *Nature*, **232**, 58

Address for correspondence

Dr H. Rigter, Organon International BV, Scientific Development Group, CNS Pharmacology Department. PO Box 20, 5340 BH Oss, The Netherlands

Section 4
Hormonal Changes in Psychopathology

4.1
Circadian changes in pituitary hormone levels in manic-depressive illness

J. MENDLEWICZ

ABSTRACT

Manic-depressive disorder can be conceptualized as a biological clock disorder with periodic oscillations in mood, energy level and such physiological factors as sleep, appetite, sex and drive. Hypothalamic pituitary disturbances have been described in the pathogenesis of affective disorder but very few studies have been reported on circadian alterations of hypothalamic and pituitary hormones in affective illness. This paper reviews some of the neuroendocrine abnormalities described in primary depression and provides preliminary data on circadian alterations in the levels of the pituitary hormones prolactin, thyroid-stimulating hormone, growth hormone, and melatonin during the depressive phase of manic-depression. The findings are discussed in the light of the biogenic amine hypothesis of major affective illness, and with reference to recent advances in neuropeptide research.

INTRODUCTION

It is now clear that the pituitary gland is not merely a vestigial organ, but that it constitutes a major link in the neuroendocrine axis in man. Central neurotransmitters regulate the secretion of hypothalamic neurohormones which, in turn, may affect brain monoamine metabolism. These neuroendocrine parameters are subjected to circadian variations both in animal and in man, and may be implicated in the pathogenesis of cyclical manic-depressive syndromes. Some affective disorders are characterized by alternating depressive and manic episodes and by periodic disturbances in mood and biological functions such as sleep, appetite and sex. Furthermore, experimental studies have shown jet day and night shifts (desynchronization phenomenon) to modify energy levels and concentration abilities, while sleep deprivation has been reported to temporarily alleviate depression. The study of circadian and ultradian rhythms of biological functions is thus of great importance in psychopathology, in particular in manic-depression.

Over several centuries, observations of remarkably predictable recurrences of periodic psychoses have stimulated interest and raised hopes that the study of such cases might help us understand important aspects of the pathophysiology of affective psychoses (Jenner, 1968; Gjessing, 1960). Despite the fact that precise periodicities of psychosis are rare, there is a marked statistical tendency towards a specific timetable in a large number of patients. Such phenomena are highly relevant to the structural changes in mood observed in affectively ill patients.

A minority of manic-depressive patients, called 'rapid cyclers', show an unusually rapid shift from depression to mania and vice versa. This rapid switching offers a unique opportunity for the monitoring of biological variables in relation to sudden mood changes. Phase shifts in biochemical circadian rhythms in manic-depressive patients have also been suggested for steroids, electrolyte rhythms and neurochemical metabolites. While these studies based on brief observations suggest that there are circadian disturbances in manic-depressives, longitudinal observations are essential in order to demonstrate consistent circadian patterns in affectively ill patients.

The existence of circadian variations in the release in man of several pituitary and adrenal hormones is well-documented. Moreover, it has been shown that for certain of these hormones—adrenocorticotrophic hormone (ACTH), thyroid-stimulating hormone (TSH), cortisol, and melatonin—more frequent, non-periodic oscillations, corresponding to secretory episodes, are super-imposed on the basal circadian rhythms. As a consequence of this hormonal variability, studies of hormonal secretion necessitate repeated blood sampling over long periods of time, i.e. 24 h periods. This approach was used by Sachar and his colleagues who found that the normal 24 h pattern of cortisol secretion is disrupted in some depressed patients. These workers found an increase in the number of secretory episodes, with active secretion during the normal non-secretory episodes, and with elevation of all peaks of plasma cortisol throughout the 24 h period (Sachar et al., 1970). The pattern returned to normal when the patient recovered. Other workers had previously shown that the effects of dexamethasone and of insulin-induced hypoglycaemia on cortisol secretion are reduced in depressed patients (Carroll, 1969). They postulated an 'abnormal drive from limbic areas', a concept similar to Sachar's of 'central limbic dysfunction in depression'. Other studies have suggested that such disturbances cannot be explained entirely as a simple stress response, since (a) they are also present in unanxious patients during sleep, and (b) they are not corrected by the administration of large doses of sedative medication (Stokes, 1972).

METHOD

We have investigated pituitary activity in patients suffering from primary affective disorders. In this paper we report preliminary results on the diurnal variations of four pituitary hormones—prolactin (PRL), thyroid-stimulating hormone (TSH), growth hormone (GH), and melatonin—during the depressed phase of manic-depressive illness in subjects diagnosed as bipolar manic-depressives, i.e. patients experiencing both manic and depressive episodes, and in unipolar depressives, suffering from depression only. Plasma dopamine-β-hydroxylase (DBH) (an enzyme which catalyses the terminal step in the biosynthesis of norepinephrine) activity was also measured.

Serum concentrations of PRL, TSH, GH and melatonin were determined by radioimmunoassay. DBH activity in plasma was assayed by a modification of the spectrophotometric method described by Nagatsu and Udenfriend (1972). Estimated amplitudes and phases (day and night) of PRL, TSH, GH, melatonin and DBH patterns observed in depressed patients were compared to the control patterns recorded in healthy volunteers. All patients studied were free of medications for at least one week prior to the investigation, and were hospitalized for a primary depressive episode severe enough to warrant hospitalization. Our diagnostic criteria for diagnosing bipolar and unipolar depression have been described previously (Mendlewicz and Fleiss, 1974). The severity of the depressive illness was assessed by means of the Hamilton Rating Scale. Blood samples were drawn for 24 h through a plastic indwelling catheter; samples were collected every hour during the day time and every thirty minutes during the night. All patients were confined to bed, had normal breakfast, lunch and supper, and their nocturnal sleep was not interrupted.

RESULTS

The PRL patterns of all depressive patients as a group ($n = 18$) showed significant differences from those observed in healthy subjects ($n = 6$ males). The mean PRL level over 24 h was significantly lower in bipolar patients than in unipolars and controls. This was mainly due to the absence of sleep-related elevations of PRL in 6 out of 8 bipolar patients in whom maximum PRL secretion occurred during wakefulness; maximum PRL concentrations were observed during sleep in all unipolar patients, as in normal controls, but basal PRL levels were more elevated in unipolars because of increased secretion during wakefulness.

The diurnal patterns of TSH levels in the depressed patients ($n = 15$) differed greatly from those exhibited by normal subjects previously investigated ($n = 6$ males, 7 females). The mean 24 h TSH level was lower in all depressed patients than in the controls. In these patients the rhythm appeared to be desynchronized, no early morning peak being evidenced. In some cases a maximum occurred before midnight. Higher frequency variations were also present in most affectively ill patients. Differences in circadian variation of plasma TSH could also be observed between unipolar and bipolar patients. Thyroid function was found to be normal in all patients and in all controls.

The elevation of GH associated with the onset of sleep (during the first non-REM phase) is consistently observed in most normal controls. However, some depressed patients do not show such an elevation of GH with the onset of sleep, and there is thus an absence or delay of sleep-related secretory peaks of GH in some depressed patients. More important peaks of GH are seen during wakefulness. In this investigation, afternoon peaks were observed in all unipolar patients and 4 of the 7 bipolar patients. The mean GH level and standard deviation (index of variability) was twice as high in affectively ill patients as in normal controls.

Preliminary data on 24 h plasma melatonin concentrations are available for 4 depressed patients before and after treatment and 5 normal controls (males). Secretory episodes were observed during wakefulness in all subjects, but they were of higher magnitude in depressed patients and seemed to appear at abnormal times (late afternoon or evening before onset of sleep). The circadian rhythm of melatonin was less apparent in the depressed patients than in the controls. The night/day ratio for melatonin was 1.38 in depressed patients and 2.8 in the controls. A nocturnal rise of melatonin was almost absent in 3 of 4 depressed patients who showed an elevation during the day time. Finally, no significant changes in 24 h melatonin patterns were seen in depressed patients after anti-depressant treatment and following remission.

We have previously demonstrated striking alterations in 24 h plasma DBH activity in depressed patients, with more episodic variations during day time and the absence of circadian rhythms in some cases (van Cauter and Mendlewicz, 1978). These observations may provide an objective and quantitative biological indicator of the alteration of circadian peripheral dopaminergic activity in affective illness.

DISCUSSION

It is tempting to speculate from the above data that alterations in the circadian rhythms of plasma pituitary hormones in some depressed patients are somehow related to primary modifications in the circadian rhythms of central catecholaminergic and serotonergic activity in affective illness. It is also possible that cholinergic–adrenergic interactions are of significance. There is, however, no reason to assume that groups of patients labelled 'depressive' are necessarily similar genetically or biochemically. We have previously shown that it is possible to differentiate between several genetic sub-groups in depressive illness (Mendlewicz, 1974). At the same time it is conceivable that some forms of depressive illness are associated with abnormalities in, for example, serotonin metabolism, and that others are associated with catecholaminergic deficiencies; it seems likely, however, that in all cases there is a complex imbalance between several neurotransmitters. It is also becoming increasingly clear that neuropeptides play an important role in the modulation of normal and of abnormal behaviour. This imbalance is consistent with the concept of an internal desynchronization of biological rhythms in some manic-depressive patients. Circadian clock frequencies may be transmitted on an X-chromosome gene, as has been shown in animal studies (Konopka and Benzer, 1971), and may increase with age; this has been indicated by Kripke et al. (1978) in their work with manic-depressives.

The brain distribution of other releasing factors and peptides has not yet been sufficiently reported upon. It is likely that when more is known about the brain effects of hypothalamic hormones and peptides, depressive illnesses will be better understood. Meanwhile, the studies outlined above, the evaluation of enzymatic and endocrine levels over 24 h during abnormal behaviour and after remission, are most promising and may enable us to investigate alterations of hypothalamic and pituitary functions in man in psychopathological conditions. It is, however, premature at the present time to draw firm conclusions from neuroendocrine abnormalities as to the specific nature of underlying neurotransmitter or neuropeptide disturbances in psychopathology.

Acknowledgements

Acknowledgements are due to E. van Cauter, P. Linkowski, C. Robyn, M. L'Hermite, J. Golstein, G. Copinschi, L. van Haelst, U. Weinberg and E. Weissman for their collaboration in this study. Support was also provided by the Association for Mental Health Research.

References

Carroll, B. J. (1969). Hypothalamic–pituitary function in depressive illness: insensitivity to hypoglycemia. Br. Med. J., 3, 27
van Cauter, E. and Mendlewicz, J. (1978). 24-hour dopamine-bêta-hydroxylase pattern: a possible biological index of manic-depression. Life Sci., 22, 147
Gjessing, R. (1960). Beiträge zur kenntnis der pathophysiologie des katatonen stupors. Arch. Psychiat. Nervenkr., 200, 350

Jenner, F. A. (1968). Periodic psychoses in the light of biological rhythm research. *Int. Rev. Neurobiol.*, **11**, 129

Konopka, R. J. and Benzer, S. (1971). Clock mutants of drosophila melanogaster. *Proc. Natl. Acad. Sci. (Wash.)*, **68**, 21

Kripke, D. F., Mullancy, D. J., Hatkinson, M. and Wolf. S. (1978). Circadian rhythm disorders in manic-depressives. *Biol. Psychiat.*, **13**, 335

Mendlewicz, J. (1974). Le concept d'hétérogénéité dans la psychose maniaco-dépressive. *Inform. Psychiat.*, **2**, 1044

Mendlewicz, J. and Fleiss, J. L. (1974). Linkage studies with X-chromosome markers in bipolar (manic-depressive) and unipolar (depressive) illness. *Biol. Psychiat.*, **9**, 261

Nagatsu, R. and Udenfriend, S. (1972). Photometric assay of dopamine-bêta-hydroxylase activity in human blood. *Clin. Chem.*, **18**, 980

Sachar, E. J., Hellman, L. and Fukushima, D. K. (1970). Cortisol production in depressive illness. *Acta. Gen. Psychiat.*, **23**, 289

Stokes, P. E. (1972). Studies on the control of adrenocortical function in depression. In Williams, Katz and shiled (eds.). *Recent Advances in the Psychobiology of Depressive Illnesses*, pp. 199–220. (Washington, D.C.: U.S. DEHW pub. 70-9053)

Address for correspondence

Professor J. Mendlewicz, Université Libre de Bruxelles, Hôpital Erasme, Route de Lennick 808, 1070 Bruxelles, Belgium

4.2
Hormonal changes as a consequence of jet lag: corticotrophic axis

G. COPINSCHI, D. DÉSIR, V. S. FANG, J. GOLSTEIN,
E. MARTINO, C. JADOT, S. REFETOFF and E. van CAUTER

ABSTRACT

Five normal male volunteers were subjected to seven consecutive studies at 10-day intervals over a total period of 10 weeks. The investigation comprised a basal study in Brussels, a westward 7-hour time shift to Chicago, three studies in Chicago, an eastward flight back to Brussels, and three studies in Brussels. During each study, blood was drawn at 15 min intervals for 25 hours. Plasma adreno-corticotrophic hormone (ACTH) and cortisol were measured in each sample. No quantitative alterations of the adrenocortical secretion were caused by jet lag. In all subjects the temporal organization of ACTH and cortisol secretion was disrupted by the time shifts for at least 11 days after the flights. A dissociation in the rapidity of the adaptation of the time of maximal secretion and of the quiescent period was observed. This suggests that the maximal and minimal secretory periods may be controlled by different mechanisms.

INTRODUCTION

Long-distance transmeridian flights are frequently followed for several days by sleep disturbances, fatigue and a general feeling of physical and psychological discomfort. This 'jet lag' syndrome is most likely due to a disruption

285

and desynchronization of bodily rhythms (MacFarland, 1974; Siegel *et al.*, 1969), especially of the endocrine system since hormones are known to play a major role in the adaptation to environmental changes. Little is known, however, about the characteristics of nyctohemeral hormonal variations after time zone shifts. Several previous investigations have attempted to analyse the adaptation of the pituitary–adrenal activity, but these were based on low frequency sampling of plasma or urine corticosteroids and provided only rough descriptions of the nyctohemeral patterns (Sekigushi *et al.*, 1976; Elliott *et al.*, 1972; Wegmann *et al.*, 1970; Haus *et al.*, 1968; Lafontaine *et al.*, 1967; Flink and Doe, 1959). Other hormones had not been studied.

The effects of real westward and eastward time zone shifts on circadian and ultradian variations of several hormones have been the subject of recent studies undertaken by us. In this paper we make a preliminary report on the results obtained for adrenocorticotrophic hormone (ACTH) and for cortisol.

SUBJECTS AND METHODS

Five normal male volunteers aged 21–29, originating in Belgium, were carefully selected. The selection procedure included physical and psychological examination, routine laboratory tests, electrocardiogram, electroencephalogram, X-ray films of the skull, plasma and urinary corticosteroids estimations, thyroxine and tri-iodothyronin measurements, and a combined thyroliberin–gonadoliberin stimulation test. Subjects with endocrine, metabolic or psychiatric history were rejected. None of the volunteers had experienced shift work or transmeridian flight for at least one year before the investigation. All of them had regular sleep, feeding and professional schedules.

The investigation was carried out between 17th October, 1977 and 1st January, 1978. Prior to the first study each subject spent four nights in the sleep study room of the Metabolic Unit at the St Pierre hospital in Brussels in order to foster habituation to the experimental procedure and particularly to polygraphic sleep recording which was performed every night. During the entire investigation period the subjects complied with standardized sleep (23.00 h–07.00 h) and meal (08.00 h, 12.30 h and 19.00 h) schedules. Snacks between meals, naps and bed-rest during day-time were prohibited.

Seven successive studies were performed at 10-day intervals. Each study included blood sampling at 15 min. intervals for 25 hours and nocturnal polygraphic sleep recording; the latter was also performed the night before. Particular attention was paid to the technical design of blood sampling and of sleep recording in order to avoid arousal due to the procedure. Anaemia was successfully prevented by oral iron supplementation. Total plasma proteins were measured in each plasma sample in order to detect any plasma dilution resulting from the sampling procedure. A significant dilution was detected in 36 samples (out of a total of 3264) which were discarded.

The basal study S_1 was performed in Brussels. The subjects were then flown to Chicago in K.L.M. jets. Studies S_2 to S_4 were carried out in Chicago, blood sampling for these studies starting 25 hours, 11 and 21 days after arrival. All subjects remained in Chicago for 30 days, then returned to Brussels by the same route as on the onward journey. Studies S_5 to S_7 were performed in Brussels, blood sampling starting 32 hours, 11 and 21 days after the return. The time shift resulting from the flights was of 7 hours in both directions.

Plasma cortisol was estimated by a competitive protein binding technique (Rosenfield et al., 1969) derived from Murphy (1967). Plasma ACTH was determined radioimmunologically (Virasoro et al., 1974).

Each individual hormonal profile was submitted to statistical analysis. Low frequency variations were analysed using the periodogram method, which has been described in detail by van Cauter (1979). In brief, the significant components are determined using repeated periodogram calculations and are summed up to build a 'best fit' pattern. Only components of periods of 8 hours or more are considered for inclusion in this best fit pattern, which may be unimodal, bimodal or trimodal. A circadian rhythm is considered to be present if a significant 23–24 hours component is detected. Acrophases and nadirs are, respectively, the times of occurrence of maxima and minima of the best fit pattern; the amplitude of the best fit pattern corresponds to half the difference between its global maximum (i.e. major acrophase) and its global minimum (i.e. major nadir). Confidence intervals at the 90% level are estimated for acrophases, nadirs and amplitudes. Bimodal and trimodal best fit patterns may have two or three major acrophases (nadirs) if similar values are found at two or three acrophases (nadirs).

In each cortisol pattern, the 'period of minimal secretion' (PMS) was also determined; this period was considered to begin when plasma concentrations lower than half the 24-hour mean level were present for at least 30 min and to end when concentrations higher than half this mean level were observed for at least 30 min.

The number of secretory peaks of each cortisol profile was estimated according to Weitzman et al. (1971); similar criteria were used to calculate the number of ACTH secretory peaks taking into consideration a rise of 10 pg/ml and a fall of 5 pg/ml.

RESULTS

All grouped data shown in this section are expressed as means $\pm$ SD.

The 24-hour mean ACTH and cortisol levels, the number of ACTH and of cortisol secretory peaks and the amplitudes of the best fit patterns (Table 1) were not significantly modified by the time shifts.

Classical cortisol (Figure 1) and ACTH profiles were obtained in all subjects but one in the basal study S_1: asymmetric patterns with short-lasting

Table 1 ACTH and cortisol: 24-hour mean levels, number of secretory episodes, amplitudes of circadian variations (mean ± SD)

Study	24-hour mean levels		Number of secretory episodes		Amplitude (% of the 24-hour mean level)	
	ACTH (pg/ml)	Cortisol (μg/dl)	ACTH	Cortisol	ACTH	Cortisol
S_1	36 ± 10	5.3 ± 1.2	8 ± 1	7 ± 2	76 ± 31	87 ± 22
S_2	36 ± 12	6.2 ± 0.9	9 ± 4	7 ± 2	64 ± 55	64 ± 15
S_3	34 ± 17	5.4 ± 1.0	8 ± 2	6 ± 2	77 ± 34	82 ± 18
S_4	31 ± 12	5.3 ± 1.3	9 ± 2	5 ± 2	69 ± 39	99 ± 20
S_5	37 ± 8	5.8 ± 1.3	8 ± 3	7 ± 2	65 ± 54	77 ± 25
S_6	30 ± 8	5.4 ± 0.8	8 ± 2	7 ± 2	91 ± 44	93 ± 16
S_7	38 ± 16	5.0 ± 0.8	7 ± 2	6 ± 2	87 ± 48	91 ± 13

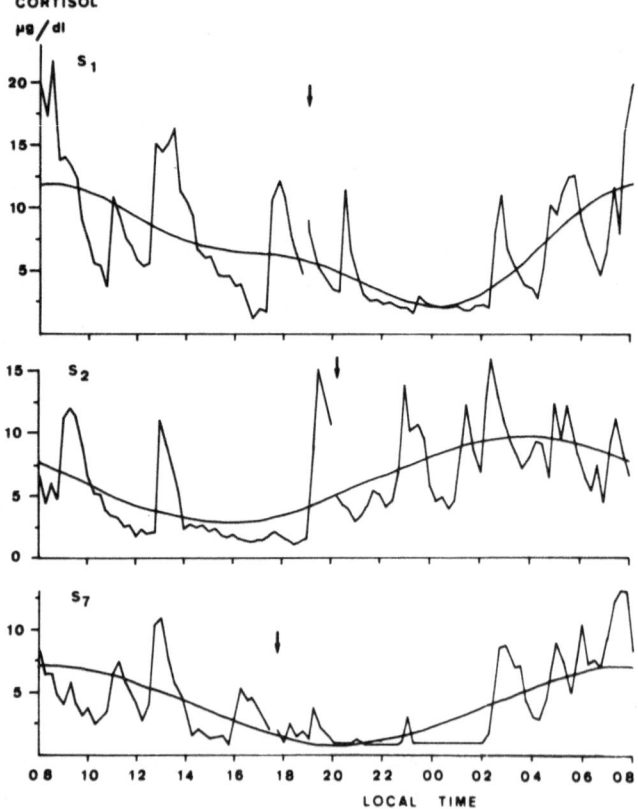

Figure 1 Twenty-four-hour profiles of plasma cortisol in a representative subject during the basal study (S_1), 25 hours after arrival in Chicago (S_2), and 21 days after return to Brussels (S_7). Experimental data and best fit patterns are shown. All profiles are plotted according to local time. Arrows denote the first samples

maximal values around 07.30 h, intermittent secretory activity of decreasing magnitude during day-time, prolonged quiescent period around midnight followed by secretory episodes of increasing magnitude (one subject had maximal secretory activity in the afternoon and minimal secretion in the morning but subsequent patterns of this subject were similar to those of the other volunteers; this single altered basal profile was not included in the statistical analysis).

The 24-hour cortisol profiles in studies S_1, S_2 and S_7 in one representative subject are shown in Figure 1.

In all subjects, the classical patterns were markedly disorganized after the flights. A number of bimodal profiles, with split acrophases and/or nadirs were observed for both hormones in studies S_2 to S_6 (Figure 2, Table 2). The rapidity of adaptation to the new clocktime was similar for ACTH and cortisol, but different for periods of maximal and minimal hormonal secretion (Figure 2). Thus most acrophases were partially or fully adapted to the Chicago local time (CLT) one day after arrival and all but one were fully synchronized with CLT 11 days after arrival. Important inter-individual variation in acrophases adaptation was observed in study S_5, one day after return to Brussels; acrophases were fully synchronized with Brussels local time (BLT) 11 days after return, except splitting of ACTH in two subjects; no splitting persisted 21 days after return.

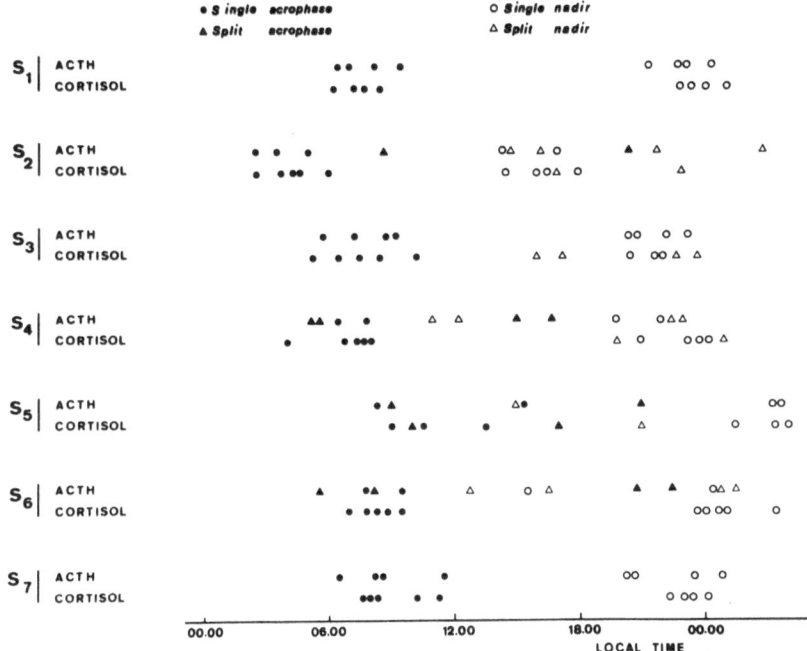

Figure 2   Individual acrophases and nadirs. Note absence of splitting in S_1 and in S_7

Table 2   Characteristics of best fit patterns

Study	Hormone	Total number of patterns	Number of split acrophases	Number of split nadirs
S₁	ACTH	4	0	0
	Cortisol	5	0	0
S₂	ACTH	4	1	2
	Cortisol	5	0	1
S₃	ACTH	4	0	0
	Cortisol	5	0	2
S₄	ACTH	4	2	2
	Cortisol	5	0	1
S₅	ACTH	3	1	1
	Cortisol	4	1	1
S₆	ACTH	4	2	2
	Cortisol	5	0	0
S₇	ACTH	4	0	0
	Cortisol	5	0	0

In contrast, all ACTH and cortisol profiles had a nadir still synchronized with BLT one day after arrival in Chicago, but a second major nadir, already synchronized with CLT, appeared in some profiles. Eleven days after arrival, most patterns exhibited split nadirs and/or partial adaptation of nadirs; even 21 days after arrival, similar phenomena were observed in a number of profiles. One day after return to Brussels, cortisol nadir was completely synchronized with BLT in only one subject; split ACTH nadirs were still

Table 3   Structure of the period of minimal secretion (PMS)

Study	Major uninterrupted period of minimal secretion expressed as a percentage of the total PMS duration (Mean ± SD)
S₁	93 ± 8
S₂	81 ± 12
S₃	63 ± 14
S₄	89 ± 7
S₅	74 ± 26
S₆	95 ± 6
S₇	92 ± 8

observed in two subjects 11 days after return, while all but one cortisol nadirs were synchronized with BLT; complete synchronization of nadirs without any splitting was achieved in all patterns 21 days after return.

The normal structure of the period of minimal secretion (PMS) was disrupted by time shifts. In studies S_1, S_4, S_6 and S_7, the PMS mainly consisted of one major uninterrupted episode (MPMS), centred around midnight (local time). This pattern was slightly altered in study S_2. In studies S_3 and S_5, the PMS was split into two or three episodes scattered around midnight for both BLT and CLT. The duration of the MPMS represented a significantly smaller percentage ($p < 0.005$) of the total duration of the PMS in study S_3, than in studies S_1, S_4, S_6 and S_7 (Table 3).

DISCUSSION

The present data indicate that ACTH and cortisol secretions were not quantitatively altered by transmeridian flights. On the other hand, the temporal organization was markedly disrupted. The period of maximal secretion was already partially adapted one day after arrival on both continents and almost fully synchronized to the new clocktime after 11 days. In contrast, the adaptation of the quiescent period to CLT was still not completely achieved three weeks after the westward flight, and it took 11 and 21 days, respectively, for cortisol and ACTH quiescent periods to be fully synchronized with BLT after the eastward flight. Thus, the adaptation occurred more rapidly for the secretory than for the quiescent period. This dissociation suggests that maximal and minimal secretory periods may be controlled by different mechanisms. Multiple control of the overt circadian rhythm has previously been postulated by others in animal studies to explain split phenomena (Krieger and Aschoff, 1979).

The synchronization of the new clocktime appeared to occur more rapidly after the eastward than after the westward flight. This finding contrasts with previous data (Sekigushi et al., 1976; Wegmann et al., 1970), probably because the previous data included only—inadequate—statistical analyses of acrophase evolution.

The dissociation in the rapidity of adaptation of the various components of the adrenocortical circadian periodicity and the split phenomenon resulted in a profound disorganization of the normal temporal structure of ACTH and cortisol secretions. This disorganization is very likely a major cause of the jet lag syndrome, which every year affects thousands of transatlantic travellers. The elucidation of this disorganization will, hopefully, be the first step towards the successful prevention of this syndrome.

Acknowledgements

This work was supported by the Belgian F.R.S.M., the A.P.M.O. Foundation, the International Health Foundation, K.L.M., T.A.P., the Belgian divisions of Pfizer, Hoechst, Ciba-Geigy and Upjohn Laboratories, and U.S. Public Health Service grants AM 15.070 and RR 55. It was performed, in part, under contract of the Ministère Belge de la Politique Scientifique within the framework of the Association Euratom-Universities of Pisa and Brussels.

We wish to thank Jacques E. Dumont for his active support. We are also grateful to Drs Ruska Ristannovic, Nicole Hermanus, Anne Segers, Morris Brown, Colleen Carey and Didier Gervy for their skilful assistance, and to Drs Jean-Paul Spire and Pierre Noel for supervising the sleep studies. Finally, we are indebted to the subjects who volunteered for this investigation, and to the staffs of the Hôpital Universitaire St Pierre in Brussels and of Billings Hospital in Chicago for their consistent co-operation.

References

van Cauter, E. (1979). Method for the characterization of 24-hour temporal variations of blood components. Am. J. Physiol., 6, E255

Elliott, A. L., Mills, J. N., Minors, D. S. and Waterhouse, J. M. (1972). The effect of real and simulated time-zone shifts upon the circadian rhythms of body temperature, plasma 11-hydroxy-corticosteroids, and renal excretion in human subjects. J. Physiol (Lond.)., 221, 227

Flink, E. D. and Doe, R. P. (1959). Effect of sudden time displacement by air travel on synchronization of adrenal function. Proc. Soc. Exp. Biol. (N.Y.), 100, 498

Haus, E., Halberg, F., Nelson, W. and Hillman, D. (1968). Shifts and drifts in phase of human circadian system following intercontinental flights and in isolation. Fed. Proc., 27. 224

Krieger, D. T. and Aschoff, J. (1979). Endocrine and other biological rhythms. In L. J. de Groot (ed.). Endocrinology, Vol. II, p. 2079. (New York: Grune and Stratton)

Lafontaine, E., Lavernhe, J., Courillon, J., Medvedeff, M. and Ghata, J. (1967). Influence of air travel east–west and vice versa on circadian rhythms of urinary elimination of potassium and 17-hydroxycorticosteroids. Aerospace Med., 38, 944

MacFarland, R. A. (1974). Influence of changing time zones on air crews and passengers. Aerospace Med., 45, 648

Murphy, B. E. P. (1967). Some studies of the protein-binding of steroids and their application to the routine micro- and ultramicro-measurement of various steroids in body fluids by competitive protein-binding radio-assay. J. Clin. Endocrinol., 27. 973

Rosenfield, R. L., Eberlein, W. R. and Bongiovanni, A. M. (1969). Measurement of plasma testosterone by means of competitive protein-binding analysis. J. Clin. Endocrinol.. 29, 854

Sekigushi, C., Yamagushi, O., Kitajima, T. and Ueda, Y. (1976). Effects of rapid round trips against time displacement on adrenal cortical-medullary circadian rhythms. Aviation Space Environ. Med., 47, 1101

Siegel, P. V., Gerathewohl, S. J. and Mohler, S. R. (1969). Time-zone effects. Science, 164, 1249

Virasoro, E., Copinschi, G. and Bruno, O. D. (1974). Degradation of labelled hormone in radioimmunoassay of ACTH. In Radioimmunoassay and Related Procedures in Medicine, Vol. I, pp. 323–335. (Vienna: International Atomic Energy Agency)

Wegmann, H. M., Brüner, H., Jovy, D., Klein, K. E., Marbarger, J. P. and Rimpler, A. (1970). Effects of transmeridian flights on the diurnal excretion pattern of 17-hydroxycorticosteroids. Aerospace Med., 41, 1003

Weitzman, E. D., Fukushima, D., Nogeire, C., Roffwarg, H., Gallagher, T. F. and Hellman, L. (1971). Twenty-four-hour pattern of the episodic secretion of cortisol in normal subjects. J. Clin. Endocrinol., 33. 14

Address for correspondence

Dr G. Copinschi, Clinique Médicale et Laboratoire de Médecine Expérimentale, Département d'Endocrinologie, Hôpital Universitaire St Pierre, Rue Evers 2, 1000 Bruxelles, Belgium

4.3
Aspects of brain development in children and adolescents with pituitary growth hormone deficiency

Z. LARON and A. GALATZER

ABSTRACT

Head circumference was measured in children with isolated growth hormone deficiency (IGHD) before and during growth hormone therapy. It was found that children below five years of age when therapy began showed a marked catch-up growth in head circumference, whereas older children did not. Secondly, intellectual function, school achievement and social adjustment of children with Laron-type dwarfism (LTD) were compared with those of children with IGHD, before and during therapy. It was found that the children receiving human growth hormone (HGH) therapy had a tendency for higher IQ and better scholastic performance and social adjustment. It is concluded that, as in hypothyroidism, there may be a critical age at which HGH affects brain development and maturation. This should be an additional stimulus for early diagnosis and treatment of growth hormone deficiency.

INTRODUCTION

The aetiology of hypothalamic pituitary dysfunctions in childhood is variable (Laron, 1980 and 1969; Costin, 1979), though several classifications have been proposed (Laron, 1980). Until now almost no systematic studies have been made of brain development and brain function in these diseases. This is due partly to the fact that the distinction between the various entities has been made possible only recently by the introduction of specific radioimmuno-assays for each pituitary hormone, and partly to the lack of communication between the medical and behavioural professions. The introduction of a multi-disciplinary approach at our institute in Israel (Laron et al., 1970), first in the treatment of juvenile diabetics and then in the treatment of all chronic endocrine disorders including dwarfism, has enabled us in the last ten years to carry out a series of investigations related to brain function and behaviour in hypothalamic pituitary diseases in childhood (Laron, 1975; Shurka and Laron, 1975b; Frankel and Laron, 1968). The present paper reports on our recent studies in this field.

HEAD CIRCUMFERENCE AS AN INDEX OF BRAIN GROWTH

Although it is difficult to obtain direct measurements of brain growth in children with hypothalamic pituitary disease, an indirect index may be derived from changes in head circumference, assuming that cranial growth is mainly determined by pressure exerted from within by the growing brain. Studies in children with different types of growth hormone deficiency have shown that in those with isolated growth hormone deficiency (IGHD) the head circumference is subnormal for age though the deficit is less than that of height (Table 1)

Table 1 The effect of HGH therapy on head circumference in cases of isolated growth hormone deficiency

	Chronological age (years)		Bone age (years)		Head circumference (cm, SD)			
	Before therapy	After therapy	Before therapy	After therapy	Before therapy		After therapy	
(a) Younger than 5 years at initiation of therapy $(n=8)$								
Mean	$2\frac{10}{12}$	$7\frac{4}{12}$	$1\frac{2}{12}$	$5\frac{11}{12}$	45.6	−2.6	49.5	−1.4
±SD	$1\frac{6}{12}$	$4\frac{5}{12}$	$0\frac{11}{12}$	$4\frac{8}{12}$	1.2	1.4	2.5	1.3
(b) Older than 9 years at initiation of therapy $(n=6)$								
Mean	$12\frac{2}{12}$	$15\frac{4}{12}$	$8\frac{11}{12}$	$12\frac{5}{12}$	49.7	−2.7	51.5	−2.9
±SD	$2\frac{8}{12}$	$3\frac{5}{12}$	$3\frac{5}{12}$	$3\frac{5}{12}$	2.7	1.8	1.5	1.8

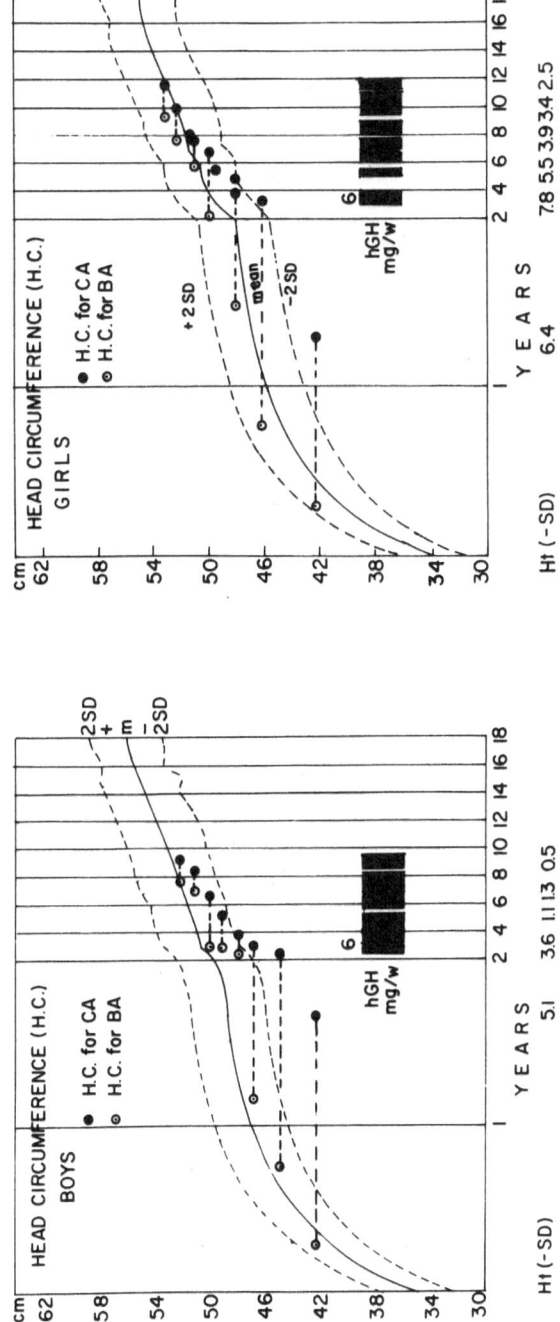

Figure 1 Effect of HGH treatment on the head circumference of (a) a boy and (b) a girl suffering from isolated growth hormone deficiency. CA = chronological age, BA = bone age. (Laron *et al.*, 1979. Reproduced with permission)

(Laron *et al.*, 1979). Subdivision of these patients according to age reveals that patients younger than five years of age at the start of therapy show marked catch-up growth of head circumference in response to human growth hormone (HGH) therapy. This is illustrated in Figure 1. It is speculated that the rapid increase in head circumference, with achievement of normal head size, represents actual brain growth. In three adult patients with IGHD who had received no treatment the head circumference was small, ranging from -2.3 to 4.4 SD below the normal means. It was of interest to find that in children with a deficiency of multiple pituitary hormones (MPHD), including that of HGH, the deficit in head circumference was less than that in the children with IGHD. The reason for this is not clear, but it is suspected that it may be due to the existence of hypothalamic pituitary growth inhibiting hormones.

PSYCHO-SOCIAL FUNCTIONING

Laron-type dwarfism (LTD)

Patients with Laron-type dwarfism (LTD) syndrome, first described in 1966 (Laron *et al.*), resemble those with IGHD (Laron, 1977) both clinically and in many of the laboratory findings, but have high levels of plasma immunoreactive growth hormone (IR-HGH) in the presence of low levels of serum somatomedin (Laron *et al.*, 1971). They represent an extreme model of hereditary deficiency of growth hormone and somatomedin activity. Of the 33 patients with this syndrome originally followed in our clinic, 21 were evaluated for psycho-social functioning. (Of the remaining 12, some are infants, one has died, and several live abroad and so were unavailable for this study.)

The distribution of the IQ scores of this group of 21 LTD patients, in comparison with normal distribution, is shown in Table 2. It is evident that the IQ scores of the LTD patients are strongly skewed towards the lower part of the curve. None of the patients scored above 108. The mean total IQ score at the last examination was 82.1 ± 17.4 (SD). The mean verbal IQ score was

Table 2 Distribution of IQ scores of 21 patients with Laron-type dwarfism

IQ	Expected	Verbal	Performance	Total
	%	%	%	%
>130	2.2	0	0	0
120–129	6.7	0	0	0
110–119	16.1	0	5.4	4.8
90–109	50.0	31.6	31.6	28.6
80–89	16.1	31.6	21.0	33.3
70–79	6.7	21.0	21.0	9.5
<69	2.2	15.8	21.0	23.8

80.8 ± 16.5 and the performance IQ score was 82.6 ± 17.3. Twelve of these LTD patients were tested repeatedly (2–4 tests) but no learning effect was evident.

It must be noted that approximately half of these patients belong to a low socio-economic class. When the achievements of the lower and higher socio-economic groups were compared it was seen that the patients from the higher socio-economic group had a higher IQ score than those of the lower socio-economic group, 96.0 ± 10.6 cf. 71.8 ± 13.9; $t = 4.53$, $p < 0.001$).

The Bender-Gestalt test (Bender, 1938), which evaluates visuo-motor co-ordination, was performed in 18 patients, and the results of the younger children were assessed using the scoring system of Koppitz (1964). The mean score number of errors of the 9 patients below the age of 12 was −2 SD below the average. The older children could not be similarly assessed as the Koppitz scoring system is designed only for children up to the age of 12, but the drawings of 8 of the 9 children over this age were regarded as 'very poor'.

The psycho-social problems of the families of these patients, studied by means of interviews in the clinic, at home, and in school, as well as by means of personality questionnaires (Fitts, 1965), are presented below along with those of the families of patients with IGHD.

Isolated growth hormone deficiency (IGHD)

Of 49 patients with total isolated growth hormone deficiency (IGHD) followed in our clinic, 21 were subjected to tests of intellectual and psycho-social functioning. In another 7 patients we have information only on the psycho-social aspects. Table 3 gives the distribution of IQ scores at the last examinations made. Included in this table are patients who received therapy with exogenous HGH for various lengths of time and those who received no therapy (Laron and Pertzelan, 1976). The overall mean IQ score was 91.8 ± 21.8 (SD) (n = 21), the mean verbal IQ was 97.1 ± 16.7 (SD) (n = 19) and the mean performance IQ was 95.8 ± 21.8 (n = 19). When the patients

Table 3 Distribution of IQ scores of 21 patients with isolated growth hormone deficiency

IQ	Expected	Verbal	Performance	Total
	%	%	%	%
> 130	2.2	0	5.3	4.8
120–129	6.7	10.5	10.5	4.8
110–119	16.1	10.5	10.5	9.5
90–109	50.0	42.1	42.1	38.1
80–89	16.1	31.6	5.3	23.8
70–79	6.7	0	15.8	4.8
<69	2.2	5.3	10.5	14.2

Table 4   Comparison of distribution of IQ scores of 21 patients with Laron-type dwarfism and 21 patients with isolated growth hormone deficiency)

IQ	Expected %	Verbal		Performance		Total	
		LTD %	IGHD %	LTD %	IGHD %	LTD %	IGHD %
>110	25	0	20.1	5.4	26.3	4.8	19.1
90–109	50	31.6	42.1	31.6	42.1	28.6	38.1
<89	25	68.4	36.9	63.0	31.6	66.6	42.8

with IGHD were compared with those with LTD the mean IQ score of the former group was found to be higher (Table 4), probably due to the HGH treatment received. The distribution of socio-economic class did not differ in these two groups. When the IQ score of the IGHD patients was analysed according to socio-economic class, the patients from the higher socio-economic class were again found to score better, but the difference was not as striking as in the LTD group (102.2 ± 14.7 cf. 74.6 ± 24.0; $t = 2.94$, difference N.S.).

In four patients tests were performed both before and during HGH therapy (Table 5). The two patients who received HGH before the chronological age of 5 and bone age of 2 had a greater catch-up in IQ than the two in whom therapy was started after the chronological age of 5 and a bone age of $4\frac{6}{12}$. It is noteworthy that this increase in IQ paralleled a catch-up growth in head circumference, thought to represent brain growth.

The mean Bender-Gestalt score in 10 IGHD patients aged below 12 was -1.1 SD. In 3 of the 8 patients above that age the quality of the drawings was poor.

School achievements, graded by the teachers at our request, show a good or fair achievement by 76% of the IGHD children but by only 52% of the LTD children. (It is of note, however, that one female patient with LTD has obtained a Master's Degree in microbiology.)

Social adjustment was evaluated on the basis of interviews and question-naires completed by the parents, school personnel, and, in the case of older individuals, by the patients themselves. The results show most of the Laron-type dwarfs to be badly adjusted, mainly because of their very short stature and grotesque appearance (Shurka and Laron, 1975a). Among the IGHD patients there was a high percentage of good adjustment in the younger patients who had received HGH treatment, but the older ones, who had missed the benefits of early treatment, were poorly adjusted, like the LTD patients. The dwarfed patient is apt to have many sexual problems, par-ticularly the male, who has a stronger sexual drive than the female. One of the female LTD patients is married and has two children but reported physical difficulties during intercourse because of her body build.

Table 5 IQ scores before and after HGH therapy of 4 patients with isolated growth hormone deficiency

Sex	Before therapy							After therapy						
			IQ score			Head circumf.				IQ score			Head circumf.	
	CA	BA	Verbal	Perform.	Total	cm	SD	CA	BA	Verbal	Perform.	Total	cm	SD
F	3,3	0,9	—	—	80	46.2	−2.3	8,2	6,0	95	107	101	51.4	−0.2
M	4,5	1,6	—	—	100	47.6	−2.5	13,7	11,0	103	106	105	55.0	+0.8
F	9,1	4,6	87	111	99	47.8	−3.0	8,7	6,6	125	121	125	50.3	−1.6
M	13,5	15,6	86	76	80	48.0	−4.0	14,3	11,0	92	132	112	50.0	−3.0
								14,10	15,9	89	78	82	49.2	−3.9

CA = chronological age, years and months
BA = bone age, years and months

Evaluation of personality in these patients showed a damaged body image in both types of patients, with self-concept being particularly poor in the LTD patients. In some of the IGHD patients who had had the benefit of HGH treatment and who approached the lower limits of normal height the extent of the damage was less severe.

From the interviews and questionnaires it was evident that the parents of children with LTD, a condition for which at present there is no treatment, showed the greatest degree of despair. The parents of children with IGHD, in contrast, had high expectations for their children and manifested a high degree of anxiety as to the availability of drugs for treatment.

Multiple pituitary hormone deficiencies (MPHD)

This is a very variable group of patients and it is difficult to draw any definite conclusions about them as a group. A recent review of 16 juvenile patients with craniopharyngioma led to the conclusion that the physical and mental changes observed before operation are due to the presence of the tumour itself but that surgery and the consequent hormone deficiencies are responsible for the changes in behaviour and achievement seen later (Galatzer, unpublished observations).

DISCUSSION AND CONCLUSIONS

In order to test the influence of changes in pituitary hormone secretion on brain dysfunction we chose to study the model of isolated lack of growth hormone activity. The patients with IGHD were found to score more highly than those with LTD. In each group the patients coming from a lower socio-economic class scored less than those from a higher class, a phenomenon described previously (Gil, 1974; Kennet and Cropley, 1970), but since there was a similar distribution between the two classes in both groups this factor cannot account for the difference in IQ scores. The fact that most of the patients with IGHD received treatment with exogenous HGH may well account for the better performance of these patients. Direct evidence for this assumption is the finding that in four patients studied before and during HGH therapy the hormone clearly induced brain growth and an improvement in intellectual functioning. Furthermore, this effect was found to be greater when treatment was instituted early in life.

Also of interest is the finding that in the IGHD patients HGH therapy induces a catch-up in visuo-motor function towards puberty. The lack of this phenomenon in the treatment-deprived LTD patients may explain some of the difficulties which these latter patients have in adjusting to the manual professions to which most of them are compelled to turn due to their low level of intellectual achievement.

The difference between our results and those of Steinhausen and Stahnke (1977), who found that GH had no effect on psychological variables, may be due to the small number of IGHD patients examined by those authors (only 7), the wide range in age, and the methods of investigation used.

In conclusion, it is proposed that, as in hypothyroidism, there may be a critical age at which GH can affect brain development and maturation, either directly or via somatomedin, and that late initiation of therapy may not be effective in influencing the maturational processes of the brain. Thus we might hope that early diagnosis and treatment would not only lead to a normalization of stature, and with it an improvement in body image and self-concept, but that it would also result in a higher level of intellectual functioning and social achievement.

Acknowledgements

The authors thank Ms N. Beit-Halachmi and Ms O. Aran of the Rehabilitation Unit for Growth Problems, Beilinson Medical Center, for their valuable assistance in the preparation of this manuscript.

References

Bender, L. (1938). *A Visual Motor Gestalt Test and its Clinical Use.* (New York: The American Orthopsychiatric Association)

Costin, G. (1979). Endocrine disorders associated with tumours of the pituitary and hypothalamus. *Pediatr. Clin. N. Am.*, **26**, 15

Fitts, W. H. (1965). *Manual for the Tennessee Self Concept Scale.* (Nashville: Counsellor Recordings and Tests)

Frankel, J. J. and Laron, Z. (1968). Psychological aspects of pituitary insufficiency in children and adolescents with special reference to growth hormone. *Israel J. Med. Sci.*, **4**, 953

Gil, R. (1974). Wechsler verbal intelligence and Bender Gestalt performance of children of Western and Oriental origins from the upper and lower socio-economic levels. M.A. Thesis, Bar Ilan University, Israel

Kennet, K. F. and Cropley, A. J. (1970). Intelligence, family size and socio-economic status. *J. Biosoc. Sci.*, **2**, 3

Koppitz, E. M. (1964). *The Bender Gestalt Test for Young Children.* (New York: Grune and Stratton)

Laron, Z. (1980). The etiology of pituitary dwarfism. In D. W. Daughaday (ed.), *Comprehensive Endocrinology—Endocrine Control of Growth.* (New York: Elsevier/North Holland). (In press)

Laron, Z. (1977). Syndrome of familial dwarfism and high plasma immunoreactive growth hormone (IR-hGH)—Laron type dwarfism. *Paediatrician*, **6**, 106

Laron, Z. (1975). Hypopituitarism and mental functions (Abstract). In *Hormones and Behaviour.* European Training Programme in Brain and Behaviour Research. Zuoz, Switzerland.

Laron, Z. (1969). The hypothalamus and the pituitary gland (Hypophysis). In D. W. Hubble (ed.), *Paediatric Endocrinology*, pp. 35–111. (Oxford: Blackwell)

Laron, Z., Karp, M., Greenberg, D., Averbuch, Z. and Nitzan, D. (1970). Intensive and comprehensive care of the juvenile diabetic in his surroundings. In Z. Laron (ed.), *Habilitation and Rehabilitation of Juvenile Diabetics*, pp. 154–158. (Leiden: H. E. Stenfert Kroese)

Laron, Z. and Pertzelan, A. (1976). Intermittent versus continuous hGH treatment of hypo-oituitary dwarfism. In A. Pecile and E. E. Muller (eds.), *Growth Hormone and Related Peptides*, pp. 297–311. (New York: American Elsevier)

Laron, Z., Pertzelan, A., Karp, M., Kowadlo-Silbergeld, A. and Daughaday, W. H. (1971). Administration of growth hormone to patients with familial dwarfism with high plasma immunoreactive growth hormone. Measurement of sulfation factor, metabolic and linear growth responses. *J. Clin. Endocrinol.*, **33**, 332

Laron, Z., Pertzelan, A. and Mannheimer, S. (1966). Genetic pituitary dwarfism with high serum concentration of growth hormone. A new inborn error of metabolism? *Israel J. Med. Sci.*, **2**, 152

Laron, Z., Roitman, A. and Kauli, R. (1979). Effect of hGH therapy on the head circumference in children with hypopituitarism. *Clin. Endocrinol.*, **10**, 393

Shurka, E. and Laron, Z. (1975a). Rehabilitation of children and adolescents with growth retardation. *Harefuah*, **89**, 112

Shurka, E. and Laron, Z. (1975b), Adjustment and rehabilitation problems of children and adolescents with growth retardation. I. Familial dwarfism with high plasma immunoreactive human growth hormone. *Israel J. Med. Sci.*, **11**, 352

Steinhausen, H. C. and Stahnke, N. (1977). Negative impact of growth hormone deficiency on psychological functioning in dwarfed children and adolescents. *Eur. J. Pediat.*, **126**, 263

Address for correspondence

Professor Z. Laron, Director, Institute of Pediatric and Adolescent Endocrinology, Beilinson Medical Center, Petah Tiqva, Israel

4.4
Hormonal effects of neuroleptics and dopamine: relationship with change in psychopathology

G. LANGER

ABSTRACT

The longitudinal studies in five schizophrenic patients summarized in this paper were conducted in order to investigate the relationship between neuroleptic (NL) treatment, plasma prolactin (PRL) response, suppression of NL-induced PRL elevation by dopamine (DA) infusion, and psychopathological change. In the course of treatment with a potent NL, haloperidol or droperidol, a given patient showed several levels of plasma PRL concentration rather than one sustained maximal level. Frequently, PRL levels were not further elevated by the NL, although PRL levels were submaximal at the time of NL infusion. DA infusions in relatively low doses, comparable in strength with the hypothalamic DA drip, suppressed NL-induced elevated PRL concentration regardless of the dose of NL pre-treatment. Rapid though transient psychopathological improvement was induced by most of the droperidol infusions. In line with the results of culture studies on pituitary prolactin-secreting cells, our data in man suggest a mixed DA-antagonist–agonist action of haloperidol. This may explain some 'paradoxical' phenomena in clinical practice. The data appear to open up new vistas for the

validity of the 'prolactin-model' in studying the pharmacodynamics
of NLs in man.

INTRODUCTION

The secretion of prolactin (PRL) by the prolactin-secreting cells of the
pituitary gland is regulated by inhibitory and by stimulatory influences from
the hypothalamus (Macleod, 1976). The major influence is a tonic inhibition
mediated primarily by hypothalamic dopamine (DA) (Langer et al., 1978a;
Macleod, 1976; Lu and Meites, 1972). A variety of conditions, physiological
and pharmacological, stimulate the secretion of PRL. 'Stimulation' is to be
distinguished from 'disinhibition', the effect exerted by neuroleptic drugs
(NL); both mechanisms result in the secretion of PRL, but stimulation results
in a higher maximal PRL secretion (Langer et al., 1977).

PRL concentration in human plasma may be reliably increased by the
administration of a NL. The increase is dose-related and highly reproducible
within a subject (Langer et al., 1977). A relatively small dose of a NL can
significantly elevate PRL levels, and a single dose well below the regimen
ordinarily given to treat schizophrenic patients can induce maximal PRL
response (Langer et al., 1977). The pituitary's prolactin-secreting cells have
been identified as the locus of action of NLs in releasing PRL in stalk-
sectioned monkeys (Langer et al., 1978a) and in normal men (Langer et al.,
1978b).

NLs have been shown to block dopaminergic transmission (Snyder et al.,
1974); by this mechanism they increase the secretion of PRL. DA in doses
required to suppress plasma PRL concentration (agonistic effects to endogenous hypothalamic DA) may be safely administered to man (Leblanc et al.,
1976). Hence it was intriguing for us to study, in man, dopaminergic–
antidopaminergic interactions as evidenced by fluctuations in plasma PRL
concentration.

The longitudinal studies in five schizophrenic patients summarized in this
paper were conducted in order to investigate the relationship between NL
treatment, plasma PRL response, suppression of NL-induced PRL elevation
by DA infusion, and psychopathological change. Some of the data have
already been published (Langer and Pühringer, 1979; Langer et al., 1979). In
the course of treatment with a potent NL, haloperidol or droperidol, a given
patient showed several levels of plasma PRL concentration rather than one
sustained maximal level. Frequently, PRL levels were not elevated by the NL,
although PRL levels were submaximal at the time of NL infusion. DA
infusions in a relatively low dose, comparable in strength to the hypothalamic
DA drip (the 'exogenous DA-equivalence' of half-maximal hypothalamic

human PRL inhibition) (Langer *et al.*, 1979), suppressed NL-induced elevated PRL concentration regardless of the dose of NL pre-treatment. Haloperidol-induced PRL levels and their suppression by exogenous DA were not related to psychopathological change. In contrast, most droperidol infusions induced a rapid, though transient, improvement in psychopathological factors.

It has been shown in culture studies of pituitary prolactin-secreting cells that PRL secretion may be reduced by increasing the dose of haloperidol (Macleod and Lamberts, 1978). Our data in man also suggest a mixed DA-antagonist–agonist action of haloperidol, which may be of clinical relevance.

MATERIAL AND METHODS

Data are presented of five schizophrenic in-patients who have been studied longitudinally. All patients met research diagnostic criteria for schizophrenia (Endicott and Spitzer, 1978). The schizophrenic woman (patient A), 35 years old, had not received neuroleptic medication for several weeks prior to admission to hospital. On day 2 of hospitalization she was given three dosages of dopamine hydrochloride (Dopamine Giulini®): 15 μg/min, 45 μg/min, and 90 μg/min; each dose was infused over 20 min and the doses were separated by pauses of 20 min. The dopamine was dissolved in normal saline immediately prior to administration and was infused at the rate of 1 ml/min. The patient was then treated with haloperidol, 25 mg/day intramuscularly, for 7 days, and the dopamine tests were then repeated. Following this the patient's intramuscular haloperidol regimen was gradually reduced as psychotic symptoms vanished. Upon psychopathological normalization the patient was given oral haloperidol 5 mg/day for 7 days, and the dopamine tests were then repeated on two consecutive days, days 22 and 23 of treatment.

Patient B, a young schizophrenic man, had never previously been treated with NLs. Upon admission to hospital he was treated with oral haloperidol 8 mg/day for 10 days, followed by 16 mg/day for 8 days. On day 18 of treatment, dopamine hydrochloride was infused in incremental doses of 15 μg/min, 60 μg/min, and 300 μg/min; each dose was infused over 45 min.

Patients C, D and E were, similarly, young schizophrenic men who had never previously been treated with NLs. In all three cases treatment was started shortly after admission to hospital. The NL used in these patients was droperidol (Dehydrobenzperidol®), a very potent butyrophenone NL (Cocito *et al.*, 1970), which is reported to have a rapid onset of action but a relatively short biological half-life. It was infused intravenously over 20 min in dosages of 75 mg (patient C) and 100 mg (patients D and E), and was used whenever psychopathology deteriorated to the point at which pharmacological treatment was warranted. Blood samples for analysis of PRL were drawn at intervals of one or three hours. PRL was analysed by radioimmunoassay. Depth of sleep and intensity of psychopathological signs and symptoms

(psychomotor activity, affect, thought, delusions and hallucinations) were
rated by the same psychiatrist throughout the study.

RESULTS

Effects of DA infusions on haloperidol-induced PRL elevation: relationship with change in psychopathology

Figure 1 shows four different PRL response patterns to DA infusions in a
schizophrenic woman. Curve A, the results when the patient had been free of
NLs for several weeks, shows that PRL levels remained suppressed, without
rebound, when DA was discontinued. (The elevated PRL level at time 0 is
'incidental', and certainly not due to NL medication. This may be concluded
from the fact that 8 hours after the DA test, before NL medication was
initiated, the PRL level was within the normal range [data not shown].) The
patient was then treated with haloperidol intramuscularly, 25 mg/day for 7
days. On day 7 the DA tests were given again (curve B). The PRL suppressive
effects of DA at this time do not appear to be attenuated by NL pre-treatment,

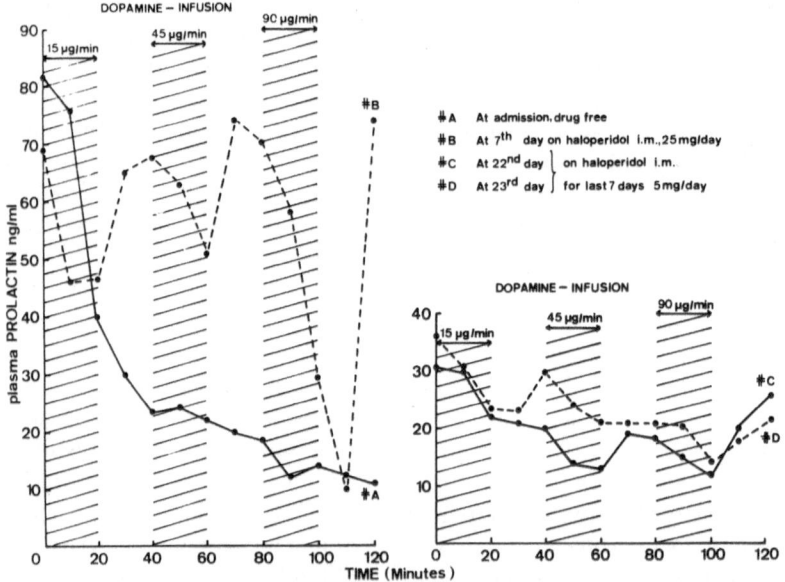

Figure 1   Four prolactin response patterns to intravenous infusions of dopamine hydrochloride
in a female schizophrenic aged 35. Curve A shows the results of tests performed when the patient
had been free from neuroleptic treatment for several weeks. Curve B shows the results after 7 days'
treatment with 25 mg/day i.m. haloperidol. The treatment was then gradually reduced, and curve
C shows the results on day 22 of treatment when the patient had been receiving 5 mg/day oral
haloperidol for 7 days. Curve D shows the results on day 23. (Langer and Pühringer, 1979.
Reproduced with permission)

PRL responses being comparable with those obtained a week earlier when no NLs had been given. The patient's haloperidol regimen was then progressively reduced and the tests were re-performed on two consecutive days (days 22 and 23 of treatment) after the patient had been receiving 5 mg/day oral haloperidol for 7 days. The high test–retest reproducibility of DA's suppressive effect on NL-induced elevated PRL levels is seen in the results obtained on these occasions, Figure 1, curves C and D.

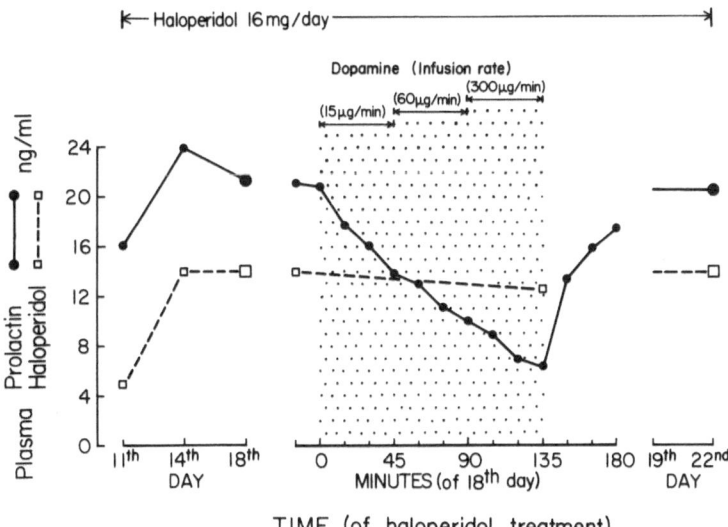

Figure 2 Plasma concentrations of prolactin (solid dots) and haloperidol (open squares) in a young male schizophrenic (patient B). Haloperidol was given orally in doses of 8 mg/day on days 1–10, and 16 mg/day on days 11–18. On day 18 (shaded area) dopamine hydrochloride was intravenously infused in doses of 15 µg/min. 60 µg/min and 300 µg/min. (Langer and Pühringer. 1979. Reproduced with permission)

Figure 2 demonstrates PRL suppression by DA infusion in a young schizophrenic man (patient B). Upon admission to hospital this patient was given oral haloperidol 8 mg/day for 10 days followed by 16 mg/day for a further 8 days. On the 18th day of hospitalization he was tested with DA infusions of 15 µg/min, 60 µg/min, and 300 µg/min. As was seen in the former patient, in this patient NL (haloperidol) pre-treatment did not prevent PRL suppression by DA. Upon discontinuation of DA a rapid PRL rise to the previous level was seen. The haloperidol plasma level appeared unaltered by DA.

Psychotic symptoms (delusions, auditory hallucinations) did not occur in either of these haloperidol-treated patients during DA infusion. While PRL levels were suppressed by DA, psychopathology was, as expected, not influenced, as DA does not penetrate the blood–brain barrier.

Relationship between droperidol treatment, PRL levels, dyskinesia, and change in psychopathology

Figures 3–5 demonstrate the relationship between droperidol administration, PRL response, and changes in psychopathology in three young schizophrenic men (patients C, D and E). These patients were investigated continuously for four or five days. Unexpectedly, droperidol did not invariably raise plasma PRL levels in these patients. It failed to do so on two occasions in two of the

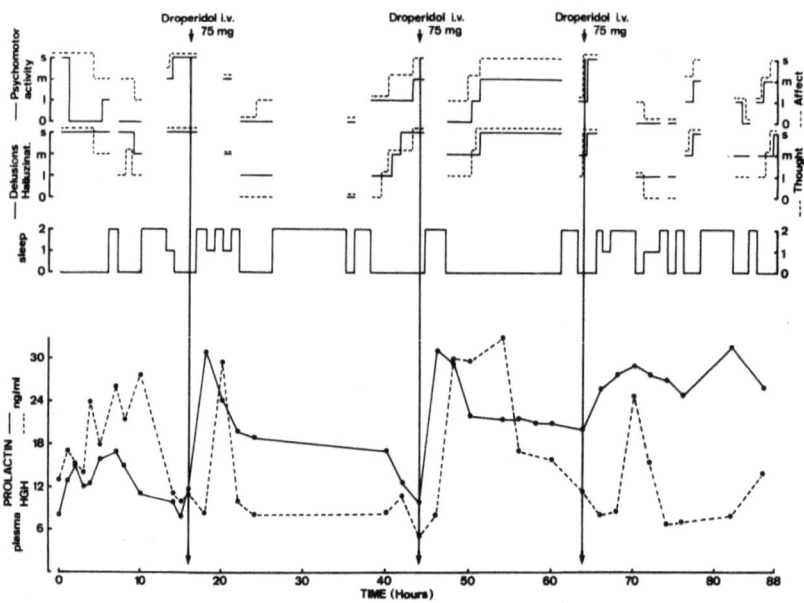

Figure 3   Patient C. a young schizophrenic man. The lower panel shows plasma prolactin (solid line) and growth hormone (broken line) responses to intravenous infusions of 75 mg droperidol at the times indicated by the arrows. The upper panels show ratings of sleep and psychopathology. Sleep: 0 = awake. 1 = light sleep, 2 = deep sleep. Psychopathology: 0 = normal. 1 = lightly disturbed. m = mediumly disturbed, s = severely disturbed. The uppermost panel shows psychomotor activity (solid line) and affect (broken line). The second panel shows delusions and hallucinations (solid line) and thought (broken line). (Langer and Pühringer. 1979. Reproduced with permission)

patients (4 occasions out of 12), even though PRL levels at the time of the droperidol administration were sub-maximal. Plasma PRL concentrations declined within a few hours of droperidol administration, presumably due to the short biological half-life of this drug. In every instance the patients fell asleep, to various degrees, shortly after the infusion had been given. Transient oral dyskinesia occurred at irregular intervals (Figures 4 and 5); no relationship was seen between these occurrences and droperidol administration. In one instance (Figure 5) dyskinesia occurred during the administration of

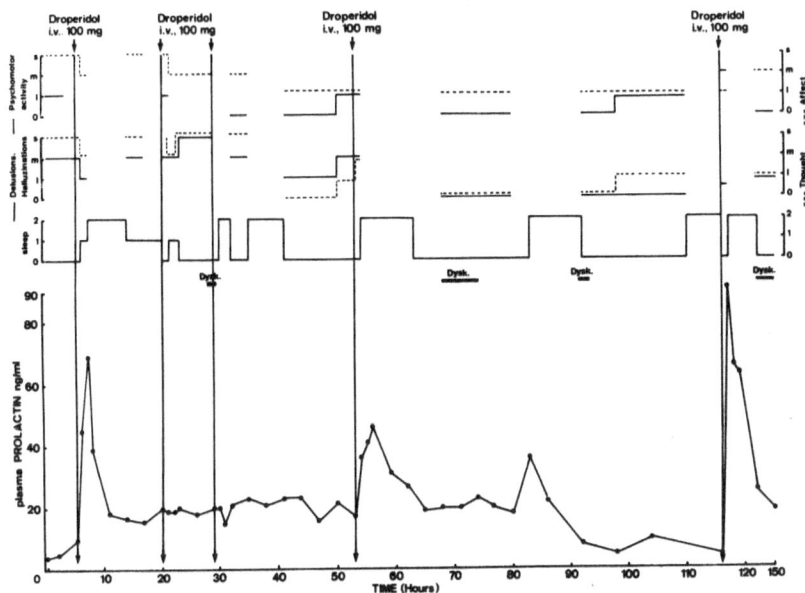

Figure 4 Patient D, a young schizophrenic man. 100 mg droperidol was administered intra-venously at the times indicated by the arrows. For further explanation see the legend of Figure 3. (Langer and Pühringer, 1979. Reproduced with permission)

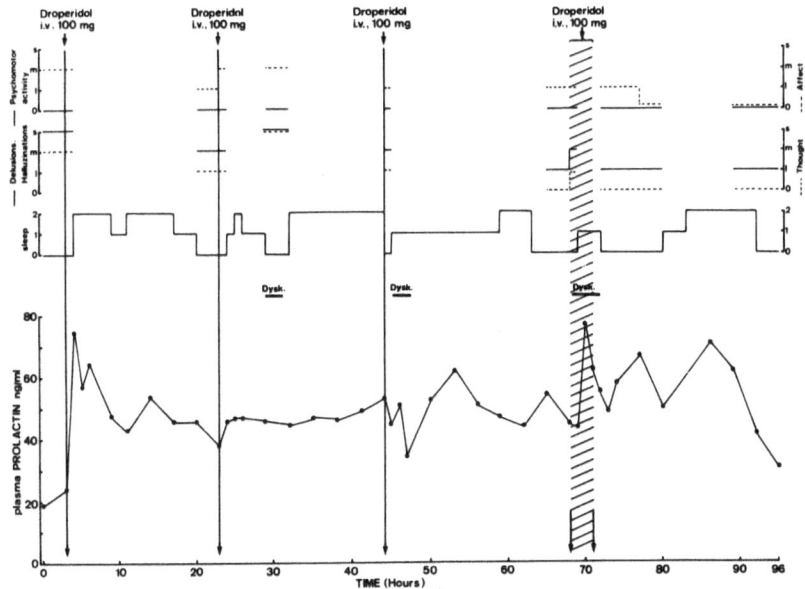

Figure 5 Patient E, a young schizophrenic man. 100 mg droperidol was administered intra-venously at the times indicated by the arrows. For further explanation see the legend of Figure 3

droperidol, which on that occasion was infused over 3 h. Likewise, no temporal relationship was seen between droperidol administration and transient improvement in schizophrenic affect and thought disorder, delusions and hallucinations.

There might, however, be a positive relationship between a transient therapeutic response to droperidol and a droperidol-induced PRL response. As illustrated, a total of twelve droperidol infusions was given to these three schizophrenics. If one considers change of psychopathology during the first 6 hours after droperidol infusion, improvement of thought, delusions and hallucinations occurred in five instances, while essentially no improvement was seen in three instances; in four instances the patients did not awake during this period so psychopathology could not be evaluated. PRL response to droperidol appeared to be blunted on the occasions when psychopathology remained unimproved, and a clear PRL response to droperidol was seen in those instances when psychotic psychopathology improved or was almost normal at the time of infusion.

DISCUSSION

The finding of the high test–retest reproducibility of DA's suppressive effects on NL-induced elevations of PRL (Figure 1) complements our previous data on the reliability of the 'prolactin model' (Langer et al., 1977). As has also been published recently (Langer and Pühringer, 1979; Langer et al., 1979), the small dose of 15 µg/min DA was enough to suppress PRL levels regardless of whether the patient was free of NLs or on high-dose treatment (Figures 1 and 2). It has recently been determined that in normal men this dose of exogenous DA is equivalent to the 'loss' of endogenous hypothalamic dopaminergic inhibition resulting from the administration of a NL in a dose half-maximal for PRL release (Langer et al., 1979). Of note is the fact that a five-fold difference in haloperidol regimen at the time of DA infusion did not affect the degree of DA's PRL suppression (Figure 1). This may raise the question of whether higher doses of NLs partially exert DA-agonistic effects. If replicated, these findings in man would be in line with in vitro studies on prolactin-secreting cells showing a suppression of PRL secretion with higher concentrations of haloperidol (Macleod and Lamberts, 1978). Whether this partial DA-agonistic effect of NLs could 'explain' treatment failures in some patients, and the occasionally seen agitating effects of high doses of NLs, cannot yet be decided. These data appear to question the simple hypothesis that NLs invariably block DA receptors (Snyder et al., 1974), and that this effect is sufficient to ensure their anti-psychotic effects. This statement may be corroborated by the longitudinal studies illustrated in Figures 3–5. Despite the very high neuroleptic potency of 100 mg droperidol given intravenously, which is equivalent in potency to the same dose of haloperidol, not every infusion ameliorated schizophrenic psychopathology. The fact that when amelioration did occur it was of relatively short duration may be partly explained by the relatively short biological half-life of droperidol.

The question of the relationship between treatment response and PRL response to NLs is clearly open. It cannot be settled by a simple statistical correlation of single morning PRL levels with psychopathology, as within a given patient several levels of NL-induced PRL elevation may be found which do not correspond linearly to the NL dose. Furthermore, not every infusion of NLs elevated PRL levels, even though PRL levels at the time of infusion were far below maximal level. It appears to be true, however, as shown by earlier studies in normal controls (Langer *et al.*, 1977), that each individual has his own maximal PRL response to a NL, and that this is quickly reached, even after a small dose, though obviously not maintained upon continued medication. The data in Figures 3–5, suggesting a relationship between a PRL response and a therapeutic response to a NL, and between a blunted PRL response and no therapeutic effect, should be confirmed before the interesting speculations to which they give rise are considered further.

We believe that the data presented here open up new vistas for the use of the 'prolactin model' as a means of investigating further the pharmacodynamics of NLs in the treatment of schizophrenic patients.

References

Cocito, E., Ambrosini, G., Arata, A., Bevilacqua, P. and Tortora, E. (1970). Clinical evaluation in 112 psychiatric patients of a butyrophenone neuroleptic, dehydrobenzperidol (R 4749). *Arzneimittel-Forsch.*, **20**, 1119

Endicott, J. and Spitzer, R. L. (1978). A diagnostic interview: The schedule for affective disorders and schizophrenia. *Arch. Gen. Psychiat.*, **35**, 837

Langer, G. and Pühringer, W. (1979). Haloperidol and droperidol treatment in schizophrenics: clinical application of the 'prolactin-model'. *Acta Psychiat. Belg.* (In press)

Langer, G., Ferin, M. and Sachar, E. J. (1978a). Effect of haloperidol and L-dopa on plasma prolactin in stalk-sectioned and intact monkeys. *Endocrinology*, **102**, 367

Langer, G., Sachar, E. J. and Halpern, F. S. (1978b). Effect of dopamine and neuroleptics on plasma growth hormone and prolactin in normal men. *Psychoneuroendocrinology*, **3**, 165

Langer, G., Sachar, E. J., Halpern, F. S., Gruen, P. H. and Solomon, M. (1977). The prolactin response to neuroleptic drugs—a test of dopaminergic blockade: Neuroendocrine studies in normal men. *J. Clin. Endocrinol.*, **45**, 996

Langer, G., Sachar, E. J., Nathan, R. S., Tabrizi, M. A., Perel, J. M. and Halpern, F. S. (1979). Dopaminergic factors in human prolactin regulation: A pituitary model for the study of a neuroendocrine system in man. *Psychopharmacology*. (In press)

Leblanc, H., Lachelin, G. C. L., Abu-Fadil, S. and Yen, S. S. C. (1976). Effects of dopamine infusion on pituitary hormone secretion in humans. *J. Clin. Endocrinol.*, **43**, 668

Lu, K. H. and Meites, J. (1972). Effects of L-dopa on serum prolactin and PIF in intact and hypophysectomized, pituitary-grafted rats. *Endocrinology*, **91**, 868

Macleod, R. M. (1976). Regulation of prolactin secretion. In L. Martini and W. F. Ganong (eds), *Frontiers in Neuroendocrinology*, pp. 169–195. (New York: Raven Press)

Macleod, R. M. and Lamberts. S. W. J. (1978). The biphasic regulation of prolactin secretion by dopamine agonist-antagonists. *Endocrinology*, **103**. 200

Snyder, S. H., Banerjee, S. P., Yamamura, H. I. and Greenberg, D. (1974). Drugs, neurotransmitters, and schizophrenia. *Science*, **184**. 1243

Address for correspondence

Dr G. Langer, Psychiatrische Universitätsklinik, Lazarettgasse 14, A-1097 Wien, Austria

4.5
Hormonal changes in addiction

F. BRAMBILLA

ABSTRACT

A study of the endocrine patterns of 119 male heroin addicts shows (a) a low basal secretion of follicle-stimulating hormone, luteinizing hormone and testosterone, with a blunted response to luteinizing hormone releasing hormone (LHRH) stimulation, (b) elevated basal prolactin levels in 41% of addicts, with blunted responses to thyrotrophin releasing hormone (TRH) and to sulpiride in some of them, (c) normal basal growth hormone levels, with a blunted response to glucose and an abnormal hypersecretion after TRH and LHRH stimulation, (d) normal basal tri-iodothyronine, thyroxine, and thyroid-stimulating hormone levels, with a blunted response to TRH stimulation in 50% of the cases, and (e) normal basal glucose and insulin levels, but with increased hyperinsulinaemia after a glucose load. The data suggest the possibility of a hypothalamic catecholamine deficiency as a result of heroin addiction. A parallel is proposed between the findings in heroin addicts and those observed in patients suffering from primary affective disorders.

INTRODUCTION

Drug abuse has become an increasing occurrence all over the world, representing a socio-economic, medical and psychological problem. Certain drugs, such as cannabis derivatives, can be used occasionally and in small

quantities for transitory hedonistic purposes, but morphine and its derivatives, in particular heroin, are different in that their use, once started, is
generally continuous with a minimal possibility for spontaneous or induced
diminution.

In the past five years we have had the opportunity to study the hormonal
profiles of a number of heroin addicts. This neuroendocrine investigation has
been undertaken in an attempt to clarify the mechanism of action of the drug
on the central nervous system (CNS). It is well known that neurotransmitters
act at the level of the hypothalamus, regulating the secretion of neurohormones and, therefore, the peripheral gland function. The study of basal
hormonal levels and of their capacity to respond to different stimuli may be
an easy way of investigating the steady state levels and turnover of neurotransmitters and their receptors, at least in the hypothalamus. For this purpose we have investigated pituitary–gonadal and pituitary–thyroid functions,
prolactin (PRL) and growth hormone (GH) secretions and their responses to
stimuli, and insulin-glucose metabolism in our heroin addict patients.

MATERIAL

Data are presented from 119 male heroin addicts. We chose to study only male
subjects in order to avoid hormonal fluctuations related to the menstrual
cycle. The patients were aged 18–40 years, and had histories of addiction to
heroin alone lasting from 6 months to 7 years. The daily intravenous intake
ranged from 200 to 3000 mg of the street preparations (containing c. 18% pure
heroin). The time lapse between the last heroin intake and the beginning of our
experiments was from 4 to 18 hours. All the patients had histories of intake of
other drugs of abuse, such as amphetamines, LSD, morphine, and cannabis,
but their drug use since they started to use heroin had been restricted to heroin
alone. All were hospitalized during the investigation. No medications were
given. During the experiments none appeared to suffer symptoms of the
abstinence syndrome when assessed on the Blackly Scale (Blackly, 1966).
Physical examination of the patients showed all to be of normal body build,
with no specific abnormalities, and no signs of malnutrition. No neurological
disorders were found.

Sixty-six normal male subjects from the hospital staff were used as controls.
These were matched for age with the patients, but they had never practised
any type of drug abuse and were taking no medications at the time of the
investigation.

METHODS

1. FSH (follicle stimulating hormone), LH (luteinizing hormone) and testosterone levels of 46 patients were measured at the moment of hospitalization

during maximal heroin intake. and then 48 hours and 10 days later during abstinence from the drug and in the absence of any medication. A similar test. performed once only. was also made in 14 controls. Ten patients and 10 controls then received a LHRH (luteinizing hormone releasing hormone) stimulation test. 150 µg being injected i.v. as a bolus. Blood was drawn at the time of stimulation and 30. 60. 90 and 120 min later. Plasma FSH and LH were assayed by the double antibody radioimmunological methods of Midgley (1967 and 1966). and testosterone was assayed by the method of Ismail *et al.* (1972).

2. PRL levels and responses to stimulation with TRH (thyrotrophin releasing hormone) or with sulpiride were examined in 17 patients during maximal heroin intake. and in 10 controls. TRH. 500 µg i.v.. was administered as a bolus to 9 patients and to 5 controls. and sulpiride. 100 mg i.m.. was administered to 8 patients and to 5 controls. Blood was drawn 30 min before the administration of TRH or sulpiride. at the time of administration. and 15. 30. 45. 60. 90 and 120 min later. Plasma PRL was assayed by the double antibody homologous radioimmunological method of Frantz *et al.* (1972).

3. GH (growth hormone) levels were analysed in 30 patients at the time of hospitalization during maximal heroin intake. and in 29 controls. Ten patients and 9 controls were then given a glucose load (100 g orally) and GH levels were assayed 30. 60. 90 and 120 min later. Eight other patients and 10 controls were given a TRH stimulation test (500 µg i.v. as a bolus) and 10 patients and 10 controls a LHRH stimulation test (150 µg i.v. as a bolus). with blood drawn at the moment of the stimulation and 15. 30. 60. 90 and 120 min later. Plasma GH levels were analysed by the double antibody radioimmunological method of Schalch and Parker (1964). Plasma GH responses to TRH and LHRH stimulations were defined as positive when there was both an increase to at least twice the baseline value and an increase greater than 5 ng/ml.

4. Levels of TSH (thyroid stimulating hormone). T_4 (thyroxine) and T_3 (triiodothyronine) were examined in 10 patients at the time of hospitalization during maximal heroin intake and in 9 controls. TRH. 500 µg i.v. as a bolus. was then administered and blood was drawn 15. 30. 60. 90 and 120 min later. Plasma TSH was assayed by the double antibody radioimmunoassay method of Odell *et al.* (1967) and plasma T_4 and T_3 were assayed by the double antibody radioimmunoassay method of Mitsuma *et al.* (1972).

5. Glucose and insulin levels were analysed in 16 patients at the time of hospitalization during maximal heroin intake and in 9 controls. Thirty minutes later the patients and controls were given an oral glucose tolerance test (OGTT) (100 g of glucose) and blood was drawn 30. 60. 90 and 120 min later. The OGTT was repeated in the patients 48 hours and 5 days later. when they were not taking heroin. The blood glucose was analysed by the

glucose-oxidase method. The plasma insulin was analysed by the double antibody radioimmunoassay method of Hales and Randle (1974).
6. Urinary heroin levels of each patient were analysed by the method of Spector and Parker (1970), using a double antibody radioimmunoassay.

In all the above-mentioned experiments patients fasted and rested in bed for 4 to 12 hours before each of the experiments. Blood was drawn through an indwelling catheter in a forearm vein, kept patent by saline infusion. The blood was immediately centrifuged and plasma frozen at $-20\,°C$. All data were subjected to the analysis of variance.

RESULTS

1. Basal levels of FSH and LH were low in all patients with the only change 10 days later being a modest increase in LH (Figure 1). The differences between the levels in the addicts and those in the controls were statistically

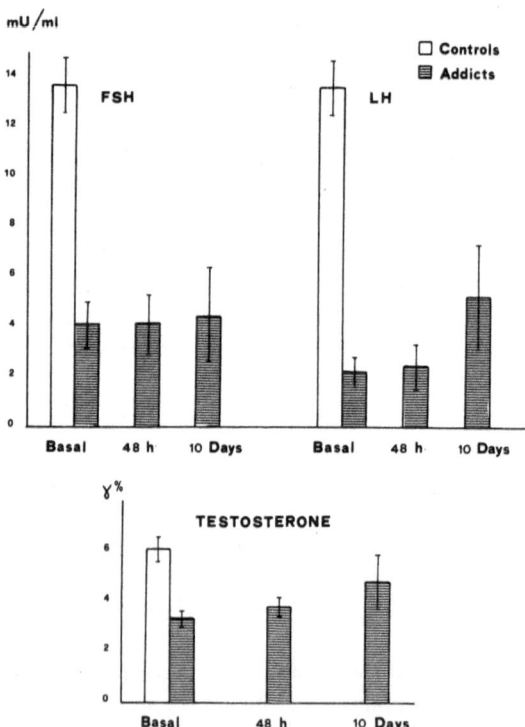

Figure 1 FSH, LH and testosterone levels in 46 heroin addicts during maximal heroin intake (basal) and 48 hours and 10 days later after withdrawal from the drug, and in 14 controls. Means ± S.E.

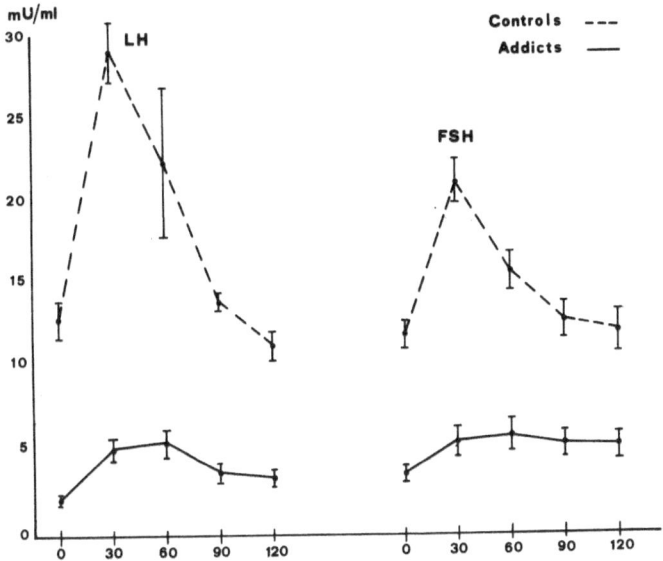

Figure 2 LH and FSH responses to LHRH stimulation (150 μg i.v.) in 10 heroin addicts and 10 controls. Means ± S.E.

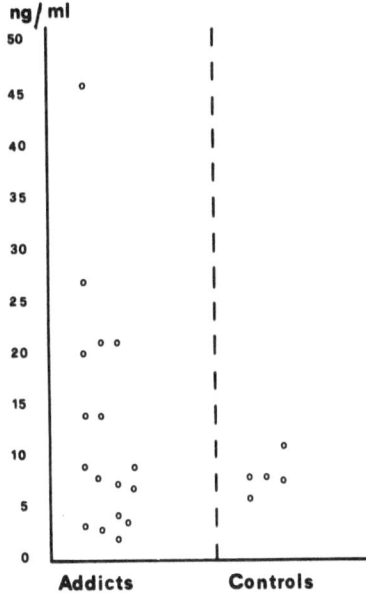

Figure 3 Basal prolactin levels in 17 heroin addicts during maximal heroin intake and in 5 controls

significant in all three studies ($p < 0.01$). Basal testosterone levels were low in all patients in all three studies (Figure 1). Ten days after withdrawal from heroin the levels tended to increase, though not significantly. The differences between the levels in the addicts and those in the controls were again statistically significant in all three studies ($p < 0.01$). LHRH stimulation (Figure 2) induced a smaller rise of FSH and of LH in the addicts than in the controls, and again the difference between the two groups was statistically significant ($p < 0.01$).

2. Basal PRL levels were elevated in 41% (7 of 17) of the patients tested (Figure 3), but the difference between the addicts as a group and the controls was not statistically significant. Stimulation with TRH induced a blunted response in 3 of the 9 patients examined (Figure 4). These 3 patients had basal hyperprolactinaemia. No statistically significant difference was observed between the addicts as a group and the controls. Stimulation with sulpiride (Figure 5) induced a blunted response in 1 of the 8 patients, again

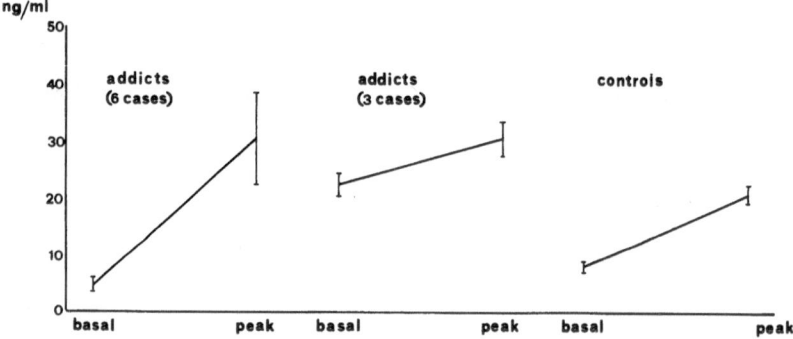

Figure 4 Prolactin response to TRH stimulation (500 µg i.v.) in 9 heroin addicts and in 5 controls. Means ± S.E.

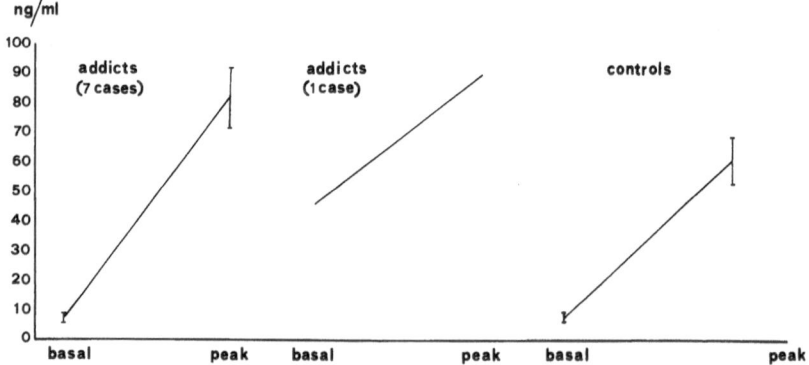

Figure 5 Prolactin response to sulpiride stimulation (100 mg i.m.) in 8 heroin addicts and 5 controls. Means ± S.E.

in a subject with basal hyperprolactinaemia. No statistically significant difference was observed between the addicts and the controls.

3. Basal GH levels were normal in all the patients (Figures 6 and 7). After a glucose load the addicts showed no decrease in GH levels (Figure 6). The difference between the addicts and the controls in this respect was statistically significant ($p < 0.05$). TRH stimulation (Figure 7, upper graph) induced a substantial rise in GH levels in half of the patients, with peak times occurring between 15 and 120 min after stimulation. LHRH stimulation (Figure 7, lower graph) induced a substantial rise in GH levels in 4 of the 10 patients involved, with peaks occurring between 60 and 90 min after stimulation. The overall means of GH values after TRH or LHRH stimulation were significantly higher in the addicts than in the controls ($p < 0.05$ and $p < 0.01$ respectively).

4. Basal T_4, T_3 and TSH levels were normal in all patients (Figure 8). Stimulation with TRH induced a blunted rise of TSH in half the addicts tested. There was no statistically significant difference between the addicts and the controls, either in basal values or in response to the stimulus when the addicts were considered as a group. However, when the addicts were divided into responders and non-responders to TRH, the post-stimulation levels of the non-responders were statistically different from those of the responders and the controls ($p < 0.01$).

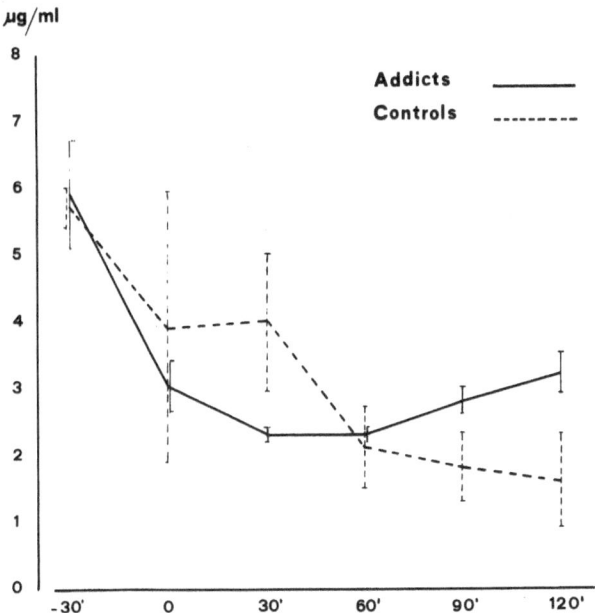

Figure 6 Growth hormone response to glucose load (100 g orally) in 10 heroin addicts and 9 controls. Means ± S.E.

5. Basal glucose and insulin levels were normal in all patients (Figures 9 and 10). The glucose load induced the same increase in blood glucose in addicts as in controls, but in addicts the peaks were delayed to 60 min (Figure 9). Insulin peaks were higher in the addicts in all three examinations than in the controls (Figure 10), and the differences were statistically significant ($p < 0.01$). In the addicts the peaks were delayed to 60–120 min and the hyperinsulinaemia was still present in all patients at 120 min; this was a statistically significant difference from the controls ($p < 0.01$).
6. Analysis of heroin in the urine revealed large quantities of the drug (from 150 to 800 ng/ml) in all cases. No heroin was found 48 hours, 5 days or 10 days after withdrawal from the drug.

DISCUSSION AND CONCLUSIONS

Our data indicate there to be very substantial impairments in heroin addicts of all the neuroendocrine axes studied. It is, however, rather difficult to arrive at a common interpretation for all the pathological data gathered.

Studies in animals suggest that acute morphine administration in rats

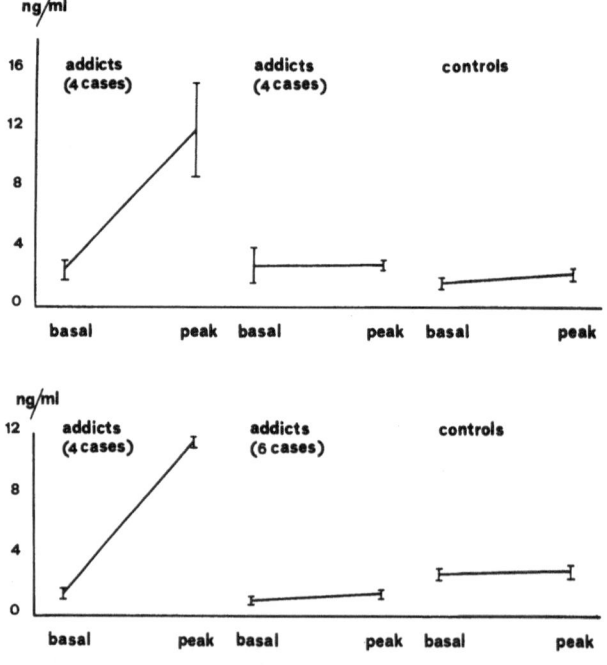

Figure 7   Upper graph: Growth hormone response to TRH stimulation (500 μg i.v.) in 8 heroin addicts and 10 controls. Lower graph: Growth hormone response to LHRH stimulation (150 μg i.v.) in 10 heroin addicts and 10 controls. Means ± S.E.

inhibits central dopaminergic activity and that chronic administration of this drug causes a decline in dopamine levels, resulting in a latent dopamine receptor super-sensitivity similar to that associated with neuroleptic drugs (Puri *et al.*, 1976; Ho *et al.*, 1975; Lal *et al.*, 1975; Simon *et al.*, 1975). Basal levels of adenylate cyclase have been reported to be increased in the striatum, thalamus, substantia nigra and cortex of morphine-dependent rats, one reason for which might be an increase in dopamine receptor sensitivity. However, dopamine stimulation of morphine-dependent rats induces a lower adenylate cyclase response, suggesting that the dopamine receptor sensitivity is not increased (Puri *et al.*, 1976). Conflicting results have been reported with regard to noradrenaline levels in the CNS, which have been seen at different times to be unaltered, increased and decreased (Simon *et al.*, 1975; de Wied *et al.*, 1974). Serotonin levels seem to be generally decreased in the CNS of morphine-dependent rats (Simon *et al.*, 1975).

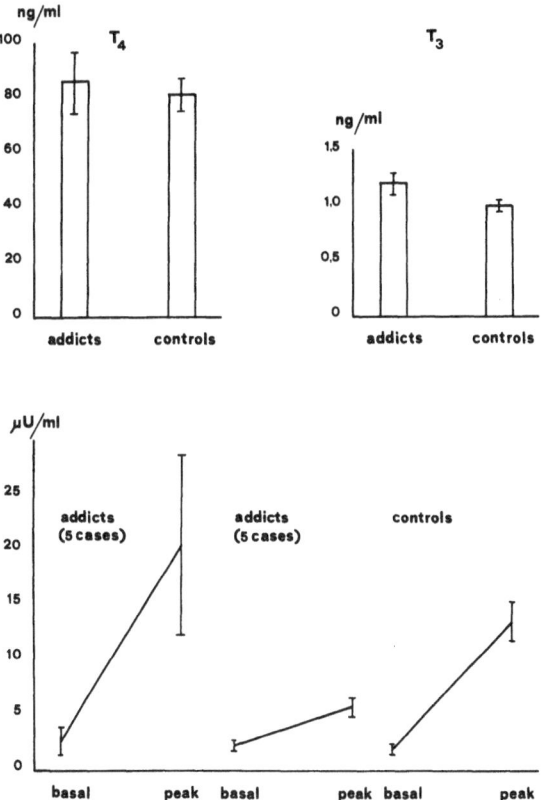

Figure 8 Upper graphs: Basal thyroxine (T_4) and tri-iodothyronine (T_3) levels in 10 heroin addicts and 9 controls. Lower graph: TSH response to TRH stimulation (500 µg i.v.) in 10 heroin addicts and 9 controls. Means ± S.E.

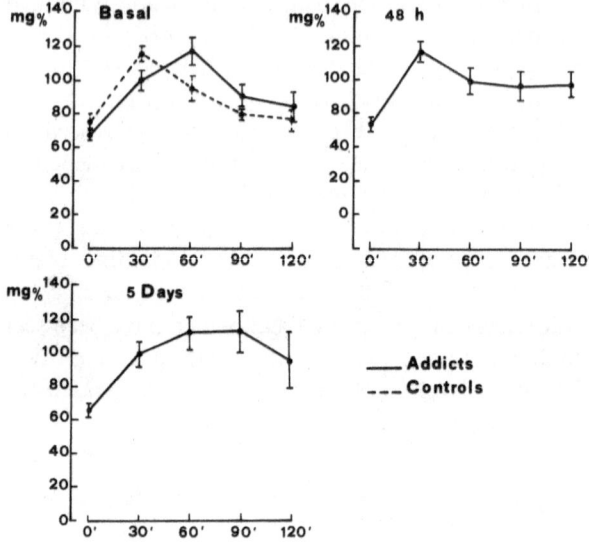

Figure 9   Glycaemic response to glucose load (100 g orally) in 16 heroin addicts during maximal heroin intake (basal) and 48 hours and 5 days later after withdrawal from the drug, and in 9 controls. Means ± S.E.

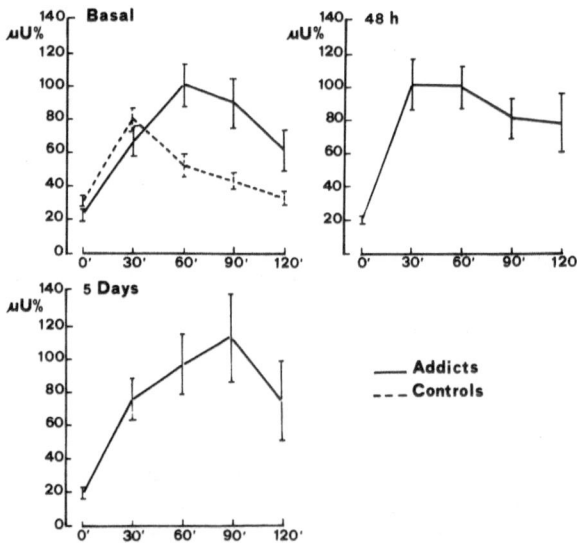

Figure 10   Insulinaemic response to glucose load (100 g orally) in 16 heroin addicts during maximal heroin intake (basal) and 48 hours and 5 days later after withdrawal from the drug, and in 9 controls. Means ± S.E.

Whilst it seems clear that opiate addiction results in a profound derangement of brain biochemistry, present knowledge does not permit us to conclude that opiate addiction induces or is connected with the impairment of any one specific neurotransmitter. It is even difficult, at this point in time, to establish which of the neurotransmitter alterations could be responsible for the neuroendocrine disorders observed in heroin addiction.

The hormonal profiles reported in the present paper tend to suggest a catecholaminergic deficiency induced by heroin addiction. The hormones studied are certainly affected by dopamine or by noradrenalin: GH, TSH and possibly FSH and LH being stimulated by them, PRL and insulin being inhibited (Müller *et al.*, 1977). There is a similarity between the neuroendocrine impairments seen in heroin addiction and those observed in primary affective disorders, and findings very similar to the present ones—low basal FSH, LH and testosterone levels and response to stimuli, reduced GH response to glucose inhibition, blunted TSH response to TRH stimulation, high basal PRL levels with blunted response to stimuli, and high insulin levels after glucose load—have also been previously reported in depressed patients (Brambilla *et al.*, 1978; Prange *et al.*, 1977; Sachar, 1976). It has been suggested that primary affective disorders and their related neuroendocrine impairments are associated with catecholamine deficiency (Schildkraut, 1974). It seems possible, therefore, and is tentatively suggested, that heroin addiction also induces a catecholamine deficiency, and that it is this which is responsible for the endocrine imbalances observed in addicts.

Another theory is that heroin addiction induces a disruption not only of the catecholaminergic system but also of the normal connections between neurotransmitters and neurohormones, and thus induces a complex impairment of pituitary–target gland function. The abnormal response of GH to stimulation with TRH and LHRH in our investigation supports this hypothesis. In physiological conditions each releasing factor would impede the responsiveness of a specific pituitary cell to non-specific stimuli; suppression or diminution of the specific neurohormonal influences would facilitate the interaction between non-specific receptors of the pituitary cells and other hypophysiotropic factors. Support for this view is found in experiments in rats: when the connections between the CNS and the pituitary are anatomically interrupted, TRH, LHRH and melanocyte-inhibiting hormone are all capable of releasing GH (Müller *et al.*, 1977; Panerai *et al.*, 1976; Udeschini *et al.*, 1976). It is tempting to speculate, therefore, that a 'functional disconnection' between the CNS and the anterior pituitary is present in our patients, and that this is responsible for the impairments observed.

Three lines of study are indicated for the future:

(1) Since our data seem to indicate that heroin addicts have a catecholaminergic deficiency, the effects of treatment with catecholamine precursors and agonists should be determined. Clonidine, a noradrenalin agonist, has

been used during withdrawal from heroin with good results on the symptoms of abstinence (Gold *et al.*, 1978). The use of agonists during heroin intake, in that they modify noradrenalin levels in the CNS and the receptor sensitivity, may reduce tolerance to the drug, and thus lower the need for increasing doses of heroin.

(2) The catecholamine receptor sensitivity should be determined during addiction and abstinence, as further proof of a drug-induced catecholamine deficiency in the CNS. Changes in secretion of GH and PRL could be used as indicators of the phenomenon of super-sensitivity.

(3) An attempt should be made to see whether or not there are any relationships between endogenous opioids, heroin, and the catecholaminergic system in the brain, both in basal situations and under various pharmacological treatments.

References

Blackly, P. H. (1966). Management of the opiate abstinence syndrome. *Am. J. Psychiat.*, **122**, 742

Brambilla, F., Smeraldi, E., Sacchetti, E., Cocchi, D. and Müller, E. E. (1978). Deranged anterior pituitary responsiveness to hypothalamic hormones in depressed patients. *Arch. Gen. Psychiat.*, **35**, 1231

Frantz, A. D., Kleinberg, D. and Noel, G. (1972). Studies on prolactin in man. *Recent Progr. Hormone Res.*, **28**, 527

Gold, M. S., Redmond, D. E., Jr. and Kleeber, H. D. (1978). Clonidine blocks acute opiate-withdrawal symptoms. *Lancet*, **2**, 599

Hales, C. N. and Randle, P. J. (1974). Immunoassay for insulin by insulin-antibody precipitate. *Biochem. J.*, **88**, 137

Ho, H. K., Ng. L. K., Thoa, N. B. and Colburn, R. W. (1975). *In vitro* interaction of synaptosomal uptake of morphine and biogenic amines. In D. Ford and D. Clouet (eds.), *Tissue Responses to Addictive Drugs*, pp. 209–218. (New York: Spectrum)

Ismail, A., Niswender, G. and Midgley. R. (1972). Radioimmunoassay or testosterone without chromatography. *J. Clin. Endocrinol.*, **34**, 177

Lal, H., Puri, S. and Volicer, L. (1975). A comparison between narcotics and neuroleptics: effects on striatal dopamine turnover, cyclic AMP, and adenylate cyclase. In D. Ford and D. Clouet (eds.), *Tissue Responses to Addictive Drugs*, pp. 187–207. (New York: Spectrum)

Midgley, A. R., Jr. (1967). Radioimmunoassay method for human follicle stimulating hormone. *J. Clin. Endocrinol.*, **27**, 295

Midgley, A. R., Jr. (1966). Radioimmunoassay method for human chorionic gonadotropin and human luteinizing hormone. *Endocrinology*, **79**, 10

Mitsuma, T., Colucci, J., Shenkman, L. and Hollander, C. S. (1972). Rapid simultaneous RIA for triodothyronine and thyroxine in unextracted serum. *Biochem. Biophys. Res. Commun.*, **46**, 2107

Müller, E. E., Nisticò, G. and Scapagnini, U. (1977). *Neurotransmitters and Anterior Pituitary Function.* (New York: Academic Press)

Müller, E. E., Panerai, A. E., Cocchi, D., Gil-Ad, I., Rossi, N. and Olgiati, V. (1977). Growth hormone-releasing activity of thyrotropin-releasing hormone in rats with hypothalamic lesions. *Endocrinology*, **100**, 1663

Odell, W. D., Wilberg, J. F. and Utiger, R. D. (1967). Studies of thyrotropin physiology by means of radioimmunoassay. *Recent Progr. Hormone Res.*, **23**, 47

Panerai, A. E., Cocchi, D., Gil-Ad, I., Locatelli, V., Rossi, G. L. and Müller, E. E. (1976). Stimulation of growth hormone release by luteinizing hormone-releasing hormone and melanocyte stimulating hormone-release inhibiting hormone in the hypophysectomized rat bearing an ectopic pituitary. *Clin. Endocrinol.*, **5**. 717

Prange, A. J., Lipton, M. A., Nemeroff, C. B. and Wilson, I. C. (1977). The role of hormones in depression. *Life Sci.*, **20**, 1305

Puri, S. K., Volicer, L. and Cochin, J. (1976). Changes in the striatal adenylate cyclase activity following acute and chronic morphine treatment and during withdrawal. *J. Neurochem.*, **27**, 1551

Sachar, E. J. (1976). *Hormones, Behaviour and Psychopathology.* (New York: Raven Press)

Schalch, S. and Parker, M. (1964). A sensitive double-antibody immunoassay for human growth hormone in plasma. *Nature (Lond.)*, **203**, 1141

Schildkraut, J. J. (1974). *Catecholamines and Affective Disorders: New Concepts in Brain Research.* (Bloomfield: Health Learning Systems)

Simon, M., George, R. and Garcia, J. (1975). Chronic morphine effects on regional brain amines. growth hormone and corticosterone. *Eur. J. Pharmacol.*, **34**. 27

Spector, S. and Parker, C. W. (1970). Morphine: radioimmunoassay. *Science.* **168**. 1347

Udeschini, G., Cocchi, D., Panerai, A. G., Gil-Ad, I.. Rossi, G. L., Chiodini, P. G., Liuzzi, A. and Müller, E. E. (1976). Stimulation of growth hormone-releasing hormone in the hypophysectomized rat bearing an ectopic pituitary. *Endocrinology*, **98**, 807

de Wied, D., van Ree, J. M. and de Jong, W. (1974). Narcotic analgesics and the neuroendocrine control of anterior pituitary function. In G. Zimmerman and R. George (eds.), *Narcotics and the Hypothalamus*, pp. 251–264. (New York: Raven Press)

Address for correspondence

Professor F. Brambilla, Ospedale Psichiatrico Paolo Pini, Via Ippocrate 45, Milano Affori, Italy

Index